1

The Land in Our Bones

"Feghali's evocative work grounds itself in the reclamation of land and plant sovereignty to at once refuse, defy, revitalize, and reclaim geographic and cultural concepts co-opted by fascist and nationalist movements in the SWANA region. Through an exceptionally attuned and affectively laden narrative texturing, Feghali enacts and animates for us what could be possible if we re-member ancestry alongside ever-emerging knowledge in service of liberated futures. In doing so, Feghali invites us into a world of *plantcestry*, one that distills with moving radiance how to move beyond familiar foreclosures insisted upon by borders, essentialism, sectarianism, and racism."

> —LARA SHEEHI, PsyD, assistant professor of clinical psychology at George Washington University and president of the Society for Psychoanalysis and Psychoanalytic Psychology

"As a clinical herbalist and member of the American Herbalist Guild, I have been waiting my entire life for an herbal book like this; a book in which the information shared about medicinal plants is firmly rooted in their historical, cultural, ecological, and mythological context. Feghali invites us to be in relationship with the plants, places, and stories which shape the culture of SWANA herbalism. . . . Feghali offers us all an embodied praxis to work with our plantcestors as a path of ancestral remembrance, reconnection, and healing. . . . This book is a masterpiece and an essential contribution to the canon of books on herbal medicine. It is a gift first and foremost to the people of the SWANA region, especially to those living in diaspora. Yet this book also is a tremendous gift to herbalists, gardeners, and plant lovers of all cultural backgrounds."

> —ATAVA GARCIA SWIECICKI, MA, RH (AHG), author of *The Curanderx Toolkit*

"*The Land in Our Bones* momentously affirms forgotten legacies of herbal and ancestral healing while potentiating urgent life-affirming visions for the future. By replacing dominant European approaches to Middle East/North African histories with restorative generational wisdoms, this book will transform our knowledge systems and the ways we reckon with land, life, and each other."

—DR. NADINE NABER, author and professor of gender and women's studies and global Asian studies at the University of Illinois Chicago

"As you read the pages of this book, allow yourself to hear the voices of OUR PLANTCESTORS. They are the ancient ones whose whispering wisdom is amplified by the clarity, the passion, and the poetry of Layla Feghali. This Daughter of the Diaspora has given us a passage away from the barren mindscape of colonial thinking, dehumanizing separation, and environmental devastation. In this work we are invited to heal from the wounds of war and the death of cultures. We may step carefully across the lines that divide us: race, class, religion, and traditions. If we walk softly, carefully, we may enter the Sacred Grove of the Plantcestors. This is the garden of Indigenous knowledge, where the herbs and flowers, the stories and prayers, the time-honored and reclaimed processes live and grow. . . .

Feghali walks with us. She takes us along on her personal journey in search of the Sacred Grove of the Plantcestors. As we walk, she picks sweet fruit from the trees, the juice moistens our lips. We listen carefully as she tells us the stories of our spirits' longing.

On this sojourn we pick up the pieces of our past, place the pain in the compost heap, and with knowledge and fresh soil we design a future scape. A vision of a new life that we have needed for so long. This is a monumental work."

—YEYE LUISAH TEISH, author of *Jambalaya*

"Although this book addresses the accumulation of knowledge by peoples of the Levant over several millennia, its strength is in demonstrating the depth of how these medicines were intertwined with our cultures and identities when our ancestors were more closely integrated into the ecosystems that generate and sustain life on our complex planet. The book also breaks the artificial barriers of history and politics that have been shaped by successive waves of colonization in West Asia and North Africa, that have artificially created divides between people deemed to be African or Arab, and demonstrates our deep connections through our shared cultivation of our plantcestors and ecologies. Drawing on this knowledge can be strategically employed in the healing work our generation must engage in, physically, culturally, and politically, in order to meet and overcome the threats of our age, particularly climate change."

—KALI AKUNO, author and cofounder of Cooperation Jackson

"The Land in Our Bones is so much more than an herbal reference book. It's a love letter to ancestors, a portrait of SWANA culture, and a symphony of forests and oceans. With it, Layla Feghali grapples with the tension of reconnecting to ancestral land while living in diaspora, away from a region disfigured by multiple layers of colonialism. The text blends deep herbal expertise with family anecdotes and vignettes of land wisdom. With her poetic prose, Feghali teaches us how to heal in our relationship with ancestral land. She does so with deep generosity, care, and complexity. This book is a gift, a path toward decolonized futures and one of those texts I will be returning to for many years to come."

—NOAM KEIM, Megaphone Publishing Prize winner 2022

"Layla is adding complexity and introducing plurality on identity and history that is purposefully erased and simplified in order to disempower the largest diaspora in the world in knowing where their roots belong."

—CÉLINE SEMAAN, cofounder of Slow Factory

THE
LAND
IN
OUR
BONES

Plantcestral Herbalism
and Healing Cultures
from Syria to the Sinai

LAYLA K. FEGHALI

North Atlantic Books
Huichin, unceded Ohlone land
Berkeley, California

Published by
North Atlantic Books
Huichin, unceded Ohlone land
Berkeley, California

Cover design by Jasmine Hromjak
Book design by Happenstance
Type-O-Rama

Printed in the United States of America

The Land in Our Bones: Plantcestral Herbalism and Healing Cultures from Syria to the Sinai is sponsored and published by North Atlantic Books, an educational nonprofit based in the unceded Ohlone land Huichin (Berkeley, CA) that collaborates with partners to develop cross-cultural perspectives; nurture holistic views of art, science, the humanities, and healing; and seed personal and global transformation by publishing work on the relationship of body, spirit, and nature.

North Atlantic Books's publications are distributed to the US trade and internationally by Penguin Random House Publisher Services. For further information, visit our website at www.northatlanticbooks.com.

MEDICAL DISCLAIMER: The following information is intended for general information purposes only. Individuals should always see their health care provider before administering any suggestions made in this book. Any application of the material set forth in the following pages is at the reader's discretion and is their sole responsibility.

Library of Congress Cataloging-in-Publication Data
Title: The land in our bones : plantcestral herbalism and healing cultures
   from Syria to the Sinai / Layla K. Feghali.
Description: Berkeley, California : North Atlantic Books, 2024. | Includes
   bibliographical references and index. | Summary: "A cultural history of
   the herbs, foodways, and land-based medicines of Lebanon and Canaan that
   explores how they connect family and kin in diaspora"-- Provided by
   publisher.
Identifiers: LCCN 2023031778 (print) | LCCN 2023031779 (ebook) | ISBN
   9781623179144 (trade paperback) | ISBN 9781623179151 (ebook)
Subjects: LCSH: Herbs--Therapeutic use--Middle East. | Medicinal
   plants--Middle East. | Materia medica, Vegetable--Middle East. |
   Flowers--Therapeutic use--Middle East. | Functional foods--Middle East.
   | Traditional medicine--Middle East. | Women healers--Middle East.
Classification: LCC RS180.M628 F44 2024 (print) | LCC RS180.M628 (ebook)
   | DDC 615.3/210956--dc23/eng/20230922
LC record available at https://lccn.loc.gov/2023031778
LC ebook record available at https://lccn.loc.gov/2023031779

1 2 3 4 5 6 7 8 9 KPC 28 27 26 25 24

Dedication, with Love.

To Cana'an and her descendants,
forward and back.

To kindred displaced and diasporic people,
looking for home in parallel.

To the Earth and her Indigenous and traditional
stewards globally.

Towards re-membrance, freedom, and deeper
care and belonging to life, land, and each other.

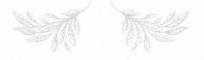

Contents

Acknowledgments

I am indebted, firstly, to Lebanon and my ancestors. Your seas and mountains, springs and valleys, cities, stories, and millennia of memory breathe inside my heart and bones—this book is in honor of you, and because of you.

Deepest gratitude to my parents and grandparents and these very places that raised them. Your generosity, resilience, and love has facilitated every grace in my life and inspired the very soul and possibility of this book. To my siblings, especially my beloved sister for your enthusiastic support and ever willingness to tend things each time I was away to write or for any reason at all. Thanks for existing.

To every single village, city, and elder of Cana'an and the Crossroads and their lineages who have shared with me the love and traditional knowledge in this book, and all the unseen moments of sheer generosity and grace in between their transmission and cultivation.

To the wondrous California lands that raised me, taught me, and nurtured this work into being.

To my lineages, to Ifa and Oshun, to the plantcestors and this miraculous earth, for illuminating and blessing this path.

I am indebted to every herbal teacher and traditional elder that has graced my path, influencing some aspect of the consciousness and personal development inside my re-membrance work and its underlying paradigms concerning the plantcestors and beyond. Be it learning in the classroom and herb garden, philosophizing in the ancient cedar groves of Lebanon's high mountains, praying amidst ocotillos or in traditional sweat lodges with Indigenous Aunties and Uncles who have welcomed me, harvesting songs for poppies in the native plant garden with beloved Olivia, interpreting coffee grinds and dreams with my Khaltos at the kitchen table, receiving limpias from Mexican grandmothers praying over my body with copal and roses, making dafa and learning Odu with Ifa priests, drinking water and sharing stories with Nubian elders on the Nile shores, learning Afro-Diasporic dances and their legacies of spirit and resistance passed down by brilliant Black women across Turtle Island (the US), collaborating on care with birthers and their tenders, or harvesting greens with my grandmother in her diasporic garden while we nurse a meal. I have re-learned and re-membered everything I know in relation to the lands I live on and come from alike, and the prayers, people, and plantcestors who have shared any expression of their own wisdom and love with me throughout the entire course of my life. My peers, kindred friends, family, comrades, cousins, and students—those who have received, entrusted, and helped shape, inspire, and re-shape my work over the past decade and more, making this work what it is, and me who I am—in the classroom, the throes of life, in ceremony, and the soil alike.

Amongst these people is an endless list of friends and peers who have supported me through various stages of this book, some revisiting text multiple times over, bearing witness to my every ebb and flow in bringing this book to life from beginning to end. To the friends unwavering in efforts to advise, affirm, hold space, and encourage me through even my most obsessive moments, I am eternally grateful to you—both named and unnamed here. Laureen Adams, mai c. doan, Noam Keim, sára abdullah, Shabina La-Fleur Gangi—this would not have been what it is without the container built by your sustained engagement, skillful feedback, enduring patience, and unflinching support and care. Infinite gratitude to the expert wisdom and guidance of Kali Akuno, Nadine Naber, Olivia Nigro, Raghda Butros, and Talitha Fanous. Thank you to every single beta reader and editor of any phase and portion of this book, to all who helped me think through any stage of its becoming, and to all who generously endorsed it. Special gratitude to extra efforts, resources, and willing support extended by Atava Garcia Sweicecki, Banah Ghadbian, Bothaina Qamar, Candice Valenzuela, Christina

Nesheiwat, Kati Greany, Liz Derias, Nico Acosta, Nirmala Nataraj, Nsomeka Gomes, Ramzy Farouki, and Tania Tabar. Thank you to Suheir Hammad, and to the RAWI team, especially Firas Hilal and Summer Farah. To my Aunt Mary, for entertaining my many phone calls for stories and ideas. Thank you to Yeye for first encouraging me to publish, moons ago. And to North Atlantic Books, especially my editor, Shayna Keyles, for all your efforts and this invitation to share.

May this book reach the hands and hearts of who needs it and will put it to use for our mutual liberation, healing, and re-membrance inshallah.

Introduction

HERBALISM IS A land-based therapy that emerges from generations of intimate relationship with place and practice. It is impossible to engage with its cultural legacies without confronting the ways our sovereign relationships with land and lineage have been interrupted. This work emerges as a reckoning with colonialism, nation building, and empire, and all that becomes lost and distorted in the land's desecration over eras. In the spirit of resurrecting from those impacts, I anchor this herbal sharing in lived experiences and the oral histories of my own lineages. Cultural wisdom is embodied and relational. I engage this sharing not for research's sake but rather as a practitioner and active participant committed to reviving land-based paradigms and nurturing ancestral practices that fundamentally aid the sovereignty, collective healing, and eco-cultural integrity of my own communities. The intention of this offering is towards deepening relationships, care, and engagement with the layers of ancestral medicine abundant still in our daily practices and places, and shifting worldviews towards a way of life that is more liberatory, embodied, and life affirming for all as we build new worlds anchored in the earth's most unwavering truths.

This book is about Cana'an (aka Canaan/the Levant—explained further on pages 23–31), about the long relationships between its people, land, and essence. It is about homeland, diaspora, and the constant cycles of departure and return, both physical and otherwise. Being a person of diaspora influences the way I relate to and extend the knowledge contained here. Just as the plants and earth itself encourage, I invite you to soften yourself to the sometimes nonlinear and often poetic nature in which I narrate and weave between my worlds to transmit something of these cultural legacies. The nature of diaspora—of me—is liminal, queer in its own right. Cyclical and migratory. I am constantly moving "in between" places, peoples, and ways of knowing. These processes are reflected in the writing and form of this book, shifting between storytelling and informational profiles as often as I do between eras of lineage and legacy. Scientific studies, family anecdotes, cosmological stories, political and historical context, and herbal folk knowledge all have their place and converse in some atypical ways through this text.

As much as this is a book about Cana'an at large, it is also a book about Lebanon and my own villages. I must name the incredible multiplicity of experiences and cultures in the makeup of our region—expansively diverse as it pertains to race, religion and spirituality, ethnicity, language, class, citizenship status, geography, and access to wealth and power in every way fathomable. Lebanon is made up of around 5.4 million Lebanese inside the country, with over 16 million living in diaspora. Likewise, approximately 50 percent of both Syrians and Palestinians currently live in forced dispersal. Lebanon contains the highest per capita number of refugees in the entire world, making up over 20 percent of the country's population.[1] Most of these refugees come from within the region's immediate borders, making Lebanon a complex microcosm of Cana'an's populations as a whole. Syrians, Palestinians, Armenians, Kurds, Iraqis, Assyrians, and onward, each transmit and continue aspects of traditional tending within shared borders, undoubtedly with varying layers of access and means in a country with devastating and rapidly multiplying factors of infrastructural and sociopolitical disruption. Alas, diaspora is arguably one of the most central aspects of the region's lived reality, with stark differences for those experiencing forced exile in a refugee camp of Lebanon versus migration to the suburbs of the United States or urban centers of Europe.

All this to say, my vantage point is particular, and this offering of story and knowledge is merely a sliver in the expansive puzzle of our web of relations. There are a few areas in which my positionality explicitly influences this text, which I would like to name directly:

DIASPORA | My positionality as a diasporic person raised in the Global North is different than those who grew up for a lifetime in the places I speak of, absorbing a different level of embodied experience and relationship to the land of Cana'an, as well as the challenges, understandings, and realities created by the wars, exiles, and occupations of my generation alone. Even within homeland, layers of cultural retention and traditional practice vary, especially on the basis of class, urbanization, education, generation, ethnicity, and the influences of neocolonialism; diaspora has distanced me in many ways from the integrated nature of culture, practice, and paradigms embedded in the continuity of place, identity, land, and language. Rather, these ways were transmitted to me in the time capsule of diaspora, its own vortex of loss and preservation severed from their original geographical terrains.

In other ways, diaspora offers me unexpected access and expanded intimacy with communities beyond my immediate familial/regional affiliation. On one hand, in diaspora, I live in cities cohabitated by people from all across the region's (and world's) sects, nationalities, ethnicities, and statuses; in a context where we are marginalized as a broader community, our similarities are emphasized, and intercommunity connection and friendship becomes a joyful and necessary aspect of understanding, cultural familiarity, and mutual care. This often looks different in the modern borders of Lebanon/Cana'an itself, where stratification based on identity results in a lack of interaction, or one laden with sectarian, racialized, and class-based divisions fed by recent wars and their imperial beneficiaries. On the other hand, dual citizenship to the US and Lebanon has allowed me an almost miraculous experience of (false) borderlessness throughout our increasingly militarized region; in homeland, I have the rare gift of mobility across borders inaccessible to most without a foreign passport, or in other cases ones which require a local passport. Even this basic privilege is not granted to many members of our region whose statehood is not recognized. The privilege of both enables me to experience a version of time, kinship, and mobility more reminiscent of my grandparents' era, where traveling between Lebanon, Syria, Palestine, Jordan, Egypt, and beyond was as easeful and common as the seeds and rivers that bind us, and fundamentally informed the formation of our cultural relationships, livelihoods, and bloodlines. My diasporic reality makes some altered version of this more seamlessly possible. Still, I experience it from the vantage point of a person with means to travel and who was raised biculturally in the US.

My specific diasporic experience is increasingly rare, with continuity of family in my own ancestral villages that I still have access to; many of my diasporic peers living in the US with roots from Syria, Palestine, and elsewhere are not able to return to their homelands even with privileged passports, due to exile, occupation, and war that has banned their families from return. They visit their families in refugee camps in neighboring countries, or the suburbs of Turkey, Jordan, or wherever it may be, often scattered across the globe as most of our families are.

Being from a family who has roots in two different villages from distinct parts of the country has also influenced my access to the place-based experiences that anchor this book. It is worth noting that until recent years, the cultures of Cana'an's villages have always had an integrated influence on the life of its cities. Today, Lebanon is one of the most quickly urbanizing countries in the world; in 1960, only 40 percent of its population lived in cities, and as of 2021, 89 percent live in cities.[2] Lebanon is also one of the most indebted countries in the world; due to a 291 percent inflation rate, income poverty went from 25 percent in 2019 to 74 percent in 2021.[3] Systemic failure, intense infrastructural collapse, and severe governmental neglect in the aftermath of the Beirut port explosion in 2020 have diminished access to many basic needs such as medicine, food, and electricity throughout the country. In the first four months of 2021 alone, 230,000 people left the country.[4] It has obliged others without this mobility to revive land-based ways like those shared in this book, just to survive. Inside the country, 5–7 percent of people have

migrated back to their villages, likely with more to follow.⁵ Even
those who live in refugee camps or cities can be found gathering
akoub عكوب and other wild food plants in the mountains in spring,
or growing tomatoes in pots on their urban balconies. This land-
based knowledge is in our collective bones, offering more than a
metaphor of kinship for the Western diaspora, but the actualized
sustenance that keeps our people alive when statehood and its cor-
ruption leave us to rot in their rubble. I hope this humble sharing
will be of service to those enduring these stark realities throughout
Cana'an and beyond it.

RELIGION, ETHNICITY, and SECT | There are numerous reli-
gious, ethnic, and ethno-religious communities in our region: Shia,
Sunni, Druze, Jewish, Bahá'í, Assyrian, Yezidi, Circassian, Orthodox,
Maronite, Bedouin, Kurdish, Nubian, Amazigh, and the list goes on
and on. I have more detailed context and personal relationship to
Eastern Christianity than to other religious lineages in our region.
References to Judaism in the cultural context of modern Cana'an are
particularly scarce; the Zionist project of Israel has physically and
ideologically alienated most of the Jewish communities native and
continuously inhabiting these lands—a wound still desperate for
repair. Despite their significant presence in Lebanon and Cana'an,
Druze practices and traditions are scarcely referred to, due to the
private nature of their tradition, even amongst their own initiates
and communities. Countless other religious and ethnic groups in
our region have maintained traditional practice, who I likewise do
not speak often of in this text, though I make every effort to acknowledge their traditions wherever I have the context to do so.

It is customary in Islam to offer blessings to the souls of the prophets, saints, and sanctified people after each mention of their names.
Please accept this note as an acknowledgment of the times they
are evoked throughout this text: عليهم الصلاة والسلام—may peace and
blessings be upon each of their souls. It is similarly customary across
religious sects to offer blessings to the spirits of ancestors whenever

mentioned; this is part of our living tradition of ancestral reverence. Please accept every word of this sharing as acknowledgment of my own ancestors woven into every single page: الله يرحمهم—may their souls rest in eternal peace. I invite readers to approach the entirety of this book with such care and sacred regard.

COLONIALISM | I am referring to all prior generations of conquest and empire in our region—not only European colonialism, though I acknowledge its particular impact on the current damage and accelerated loss of culture and land occurring regionally. All homogenization and erosion of localized cultures also erodes ecological integrity and the intelligence that emerges from autonomous intimacy with ancestral place. That being said, discussing what rests beneath colonial rupture is not meant to romanticize ancestral civilizations, which like all humans may develop their own systems of behavior that sometimes become oppressive. I am speaking to the essence and fundamental axis of the earth and our proximity to it as a compass for life-affirming habits, knowledge, and social systems, and the underlying protocols and lifeways which emerge from this center and generally become more distant the more conquest we experience. Still, it is not beyond our early lineages, or any human, to potentially corrupt and manipulate these things, as will be reflected in many of the cosmologies shared throughout this text.

LANGUAGE | Throughout this book, colloquial words from various Shami (Levantine) Arabic dialects are utilized to express the traditional knowledge native to this region. I often emphasize highly localized words, sometimes ones that vary even from one village to the next. I center these words because they embed the emotions and values within local worldviews and our specific relationships to the places, people, and events in our lives in incredibly poignant ways. For general Arabic names and language, I mostly rely on the Lebanese accent. For the romanization of Arabic, I use *a'a* to indicate the ع character except in some instances where it is the first letter in a word. *A'a* represents a voiced pharyngeal fricative. I use an apostrophe for the ﻋ character, which represents a glottal stop. *Eh* at the end of a word indicates ﻩ, pronounced with a silent *h*. *Kh* is for ﺥ, a voiceless velar fricative—similar to the sound of static on the television, and *gh* is for ﻍ, a voiced uvular fricative that sounds like a gently gargling or a rolling *g*. The remainder are loosely phonetic. I utilize the Arabic spelling/pronunciation of "Cana'an" throughout this book, typically spelled/pronounced "Canaan" in English.

REFERENCES | Written documentation of many oral history and ethnobotanical records are somewhat sparse as it pertains to plants in the traditions of Cana'an, particularly in the English language. Unfortunately, many of them are initiated by the occupying institutions and their settlers, which posed a painful contradiction and decision on my part as an author motivated by decolonization. The same forces which have intentionally and strategically eroded our rights and means of cultural practice are the ones examining and extracting land-based knowledge from us, often using it explicitly to strategize our further oppression. Where these sources are cited, I do so with an explicit will to reclaim what was ours to begin with, and with advisable discretion to readers and encouragement to my own community to take greater authority in the continuation and honoring of our own ways and stories, whatever form it may take.

I myself am in a constant process of re-membrance and deepening, my thoughts and understandings changing, expanding, and transforming. The work presented here attempts to articulate foundational wisdom and understandings towards land-based re-membrance from and for my own contexts; regardless, this is a profoundly personal and living dialogue, a lifelong stewardship that sharpens and shifts, revealing new layers constantly along the way. What you read here is the (partial) imprint of a particular moment within my lifetime of understanding and relationships fostered, anchored by personal stories I hold tenderly close and sacred. I have deliberated about whether to share these more intimate cultural layers in such a permanent and boundless form, knowing how often they get desecrated, misinterpreted, used against who it belongs to, and consumed without consideration, appropriate context, and attribution.

In the scattered reality of this era and its colonial imprints, cultural transmissions have necessarily expanded from their oral forms. This comes with risks. It is in the generosity and integrity of my own legacies, our fundamentally relational nature, and with a determination to keep these remnants alive that I ultimately chose to document personal cultural knowledge in this way. Before you read further, consider reviewing the "Meaningful Language" glossary (p. 299) to learn more about the way certain terms are presented in the book; I recommend doing so because language itself is a piece of cultural context, and it is used with great intention throughout the book.

This knowledge is in no way exhaustive. Still, I hope this reflection of Cana'an will honor some thread of the region's essence and some aspect of the unified lands that weave our kinships and experience as a collective. One of my wisest village elders of Lebanon's mountains tells me to "choose one thing in life or nature that calls you, and deepen in your study of that; to deeply know one thing is to deeply reveal the nature in everything." So, I share and study from where I am, acknowledging that "to know" is ongoing and not static in time like these pages. While I do not shed equal light on all of our parts at every moment, I believe the whole is reflected through the parts, and that is the foundational epistemology of re-remembrance as a living, evolving practice. The depth of my knowledge in some areas is greater than others, by the natural virtue of where and when I stand. I connect and illuminate through anchoring in the specific story which is mine to share today, with a steady consciousness and perspective towards the collective experience and future it is embedded within, and the ancient root it derives from. This re-membrance is moved by an effort towards what prevails beyond time between us: a study of the unwavering truths inside life itself—the love, the elements, the land and waters that ultimately unite, determine, and define us, and have since infinity.

Part I

TRACING ROOTS, TENDING FUTURES

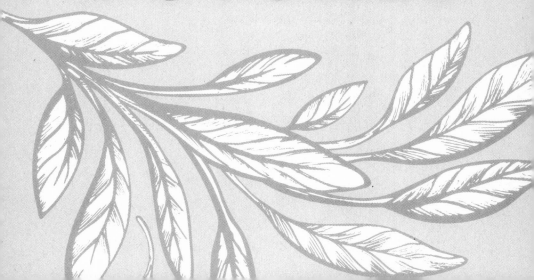

CANA'AN IS A crossroads of the earth. Be it birds or seeds, humans looking for life and refuge, or empires with a will to dominate for power and profit, this land has been frequented by many over the course of the past several thousand years. Our collective diasporas make one of the largest in the world, and our migrational lines are as complex with layers. Despite constant war, endless stories of exile, migration, language loss, and land degradation, there is palpable vitality and wholeness in the elements of place that still live through us. There is a lesson here—a medicine in this crossroads of rupture and immense resilience and revitalization at once, where loss insists on continuation, and life recreates itself constantly through the persistence of tending what remains, from wherever we are. No matter what has been lost or taken, a way persists as long as we do.

Plants of place and origin are an interwoven part of these understated worlds that mend and make belonging. They, like our ancestors, have adapted to the challenges of lifetimes, embedding wayfinding intelligence inside of us. When we are lost or have forgotten, they have the power to re-member us. They wake up the ancestral lifelines inside of us. Every time we eat our cultural foods, harvest and prepare our medicines, nurture the soil where we are, plant ancient seeds in new places, these legacies bless our bodies and guide our beings back into union with deeper sources of life's fundamental wisdoms and the earth's unfaltering guidance.

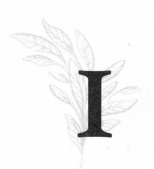

Re-Membering the Crossroads

I AM A CHILD of diaspora, born and raised to Lebanese immigrants in California in the 1980s. My mother comes from a tiny mountain village along the Awali River in South Lebanon, and my father from one on the northern shoreline neighboring the ancient city of Batroun. They both spent their childhoods raised between their villages and opposite sides of Beirut. They met in Detroit in the 1970s, a world apart from the ones they inhabited respectively in Lebanon, where it's quite likely they would never have crossed paths. My parents both embody traditional values rooted in the culture of Lebanese village life. They modeled strong communal sensibilities, traditional customs, and culinary palettes that built the foundational fibers of our diasporic home.

Like a majority of Cana'an's children, my parents left their country in an era of looming war. In Lebanon's case, a war that endured throughout most of my childhood, and in many ways, continues to linger with its imprints. The leadership of this same war is today still destroying lives in a collapsing Lebanon, creating a new wave of reluctant diaspora who feel no choice but to leave as I write this. I was protected from the visceral realities of such violence through a life in diaspora, which was not quite my father's plan but became both the privilege and sacrifice he and my mother ultimately chose for our young family as the war years did not seem to end.

My generation is characterized by many families just like ours, who often had much less choice in either direction. Some who left homelands in exile as refugees, and others who did not have the means to leave even the worst of conditions. My own family, like most from the region, was a bag of mixed experiences. My father's immediate family nearly all remained in Lebanon throughout the duration of the active war years, while my mother migrated to the US with her siblings and parents in the very early days of political tension that preceded the civil war. They lived in Florida, while we lived in California.

Our house was thick with other Arabic-speaking immigrants like us and their children, who became like siblings and cousins to me and my brothers and sister throughout our childhood. We shared similar stories of families scattered across continents and cities all over the earth. We navigated the tensions of negotiating cultures in our diasporic households, and homelands under the pressure of imperialism, occupation, and political collapse of many varieties. Many were from Lebanon, but also from Syria, Palestine, Armenia, Assyria, and Egypt. Even the neighborhood children my siblings and I played with daily after school were mirrors of the region's stories of continuation in diaspora and exile. On one side of our house, two girls near my age were raised by their family from Western Armenia (now occupied by Turkey), and on the other side, two Iranian Jewish boys near my brothers' ages who they played with as often. Our home was a gathering place for these strong social networks of survival and cultural familiarity sown by my parents to this day. It was also a revolving door for long- and short-term visitors who came directly from Lebanon to stay with us.

Family members and extended community would find reprieve under our roof to finish schooling, or simply exist for months or years at a time, where there was more promise for a stable livelihood. My paternal grandmother once came for a couple years' stay, filling my childhood with memories of kneading dough into small moon-shaped lamb pies that quickly became my favorite treat, and teaching me how to knit and play Basara and Tarnib with her playing cards. Though much was unspoken about the war they thawed from in our midst, the memory and energy each of these relatives brought with them became an intimate part of the underlying imprint in our home and in my own consciousness as I developed.

Immediately after the war ended and the Beirut airport reopened in 1992, I returned to Lebanon for the first time since I was six months old. It was a trip with only my father to visit a place that was intimately familiar somehow—already a part of me despite being foreign in so many ways. I was just eight years old, taking in a freshly postwar country that was still under military occupation by Syria in my dad's village in the north, and Israel in my mom's village in the south. It was a country with scars and open wounds on every limb of its body, many visible and many more internal. The Lebanon of that time was at once wounded and chaotic, yet hopeful for reprieve. The love I experienced there was immense and impactful. Every single painful and thriving thing I witnessed and felt there gifted me deeply, and nourished a seed I believe has anchored my path somehow since.

My dad often tells me about the day he took me to his village. He showed me around the church and communal areas, eager to tell me stories about his childhood adventures. Within moments of our being there, I looked at him and said, "Dad, when are you taking me to the grave of my Jiddo (grandfather)?" He was surprised that a child of such a young age insisted on paying homage to a grandfather I had never met or known beyond stories, in a place I had never grown up—embarrassed, even, that he had not thought to do this himself.

This memory reminds me that my gravity towards my ancestors and their places has been the primary relational thread compelling me since I was young. I still look to my ancestors as a compass in my call to re-member. Their reflection encourages me to listen towards the essence of older truths that are often convoluted and neglected within the splintering of modern wars and migrations. Where my living relatives have forgotten or have no guidance to offer, the memory of my ancestors and their love imprinted on me has lent me hope, purpose, and strength.

We are our ancestors. Their blood, their bones, their sacrifices and relationships to the earth are what have literally made us. It is not only their wounds that carry on inside of us, but their resilience, wisdom and power. Our ancestors and homelands weave a way inside of us that expands as we live and breathe. It is a legacy of love that continues through us, reinforced by habits of stewardship and care wherever we are. Deepening relationship with my ancestors has urged me closer to the land as our kindred source, most of all; immersion in the earth and waters of place has transformed and re-membered me in the most anchoring and ongoing ways, and brought me closer to the healing possibilities within and for my lineages, in the process.

Belonging to the bridging generation is complex, and perhaps by its nature compels a deeper seeking for clarity about one's purpose and place in the world. Unlike my parents, my own body was neither firmly rooted in one place, one identity, nor the other, though completely a product of both and the full spectrum of stories, generational memory, possibility and tension that lay between them. Diaspora is the land of "the in-between," of the everything and the nothing. Holy but shrouded, gestational and mysterious. This was not something my family could anticipate, nonetheless explain to me growing up, nor was it easy for any of us to verbalize or understand. It was a new terrain with no roadmap, no clear answers or linear guidelines, no apparent compass, and no real cohesion or generational social structures to support it. My life became a necessary reckoning within this tender terrain of liminality and the questions it beckons:

Who am I? What is "home"? What are the relationships that anchor and reflect me? What is this feeling? How do I heal? How do WE heal?

The more I matured, the thicker the layers inside these contemplations became. Identity was loosely footed from every direction of cultural influence surrounding me, compelling deeper interrogation and inspection for its own merit. Being Lebanese in an era notorious for its internal divisions only made the complications within this process more explicit. This challenge is one I have come to appreciate for the nuance it has necessarily instilled in me, shattering ideals of false nationalism, singular truths, and surface level concepts of culture and self. The contradictions and confusion surrounding these foundational questions of belonging and healing within my cultural context obliged me to reach towards deeper, more fundamental truths, if any were to be found at all. I have sought these sources of wisdom through every avenue I've had access to. Most of my efforts have been elucidated by the mirrors of an intimate network of intercultural kinships formed with chosen friends and communities in diaspora, wading through similar waters of reckoning and return, and lighting the way for me repeatedly through shared reflections. This has been one of the most illuminating and sustaining thresholds within the in-between life of diaspora; cross-cultural kinships with local Indigenous, Afro-Diasporic, and diverse immigrant communities have been the water that activates dormant ancestral seeds, potentiating their ancient stories that build towards rooted futures.

Once I became old enough to live independently, I moved for extended stretches of time to Lebanon, hoping to connect to these deeper sources in my own lineage lands. I have migrated alongside the birds in a steady cycle of departure and return between my homes across oceans, over and over again, living between my village, Beirut, and California for my whole adult life since, almost twenty years now. In diaspora and village alike, I have made a choice to follow the tiniest crumbs, listen with all the senses of my body, to collect what I could of these scattered bones.

Mostly, what tracing these roots has taught me is that the answers are usually closer than we think. It is the simplest rituals of everyday living that have built and sustained who we are. When I stopped looking for what was lost and started paying attention to what was still brimming with life around me, revelation was in the details of my parents in diaspora, of the kitchen table, my grandmother's bare feet, the daily routines of villagers seeking summer reprieve, the soil, the water, and the infinite web of communion that bustles in the body of the earth and our beings.

Diaspora is an ongoing and eternal reckoning, a continuous unveiling towards re-membrance, and the earth is my most unfaltering compass yet. The plants of address and origins have carried and guided me through all these passages, offering me profound wisdom, kinship and communion that anchors me tenderly in the land and healing of both my homes respectively, as it repairs my capacity to feel at home in my own holy body. These relationships have allowed and inspired me to steward the stories shared in this text.

Diaspora and the Colonial Wound

Diaspora is a fertile threshold of possibility, and a reckoning with severance at once. By its nature, displacement incurs losses. Once a place changes, customs naturally transform. So does the belonging and self-understanding that emerges from these rooted contexts. There is yet extra duress when a people are dispersed because of or during a time of genocide, war, or occupation. In these conditions, loss or rapid transformation of culture not only occurs for those who depart or are pushed into exile; culture also erodes more quickly in the original homelands left behind.

War and occupation alter culture by necessity, often obliging a people to lean on only bare basics as they manage to just survive. The need to survive reinforces certain cultural customs that can aid in sustaining life when access to infrastructural amenities are limited. Other rites, however, are interrupted, relationship to land is made less possible, and new patterns of relating and existing are born in the imprint of whatever survival means in that moment. Modern nation-building efforts infringe doubly on Indigenous communities; limiting their right to speak native languages, wear traditional clothing, and/or access ancestral lands are common tactics to erase, dominate, control, and secure power over Indigenous groups.[1]

Simultaneously, the pressures of modernization and capitalism in the past several decades have contributed to increased urbanization and the globalization of social cultures across the region, making traditional economies and their lifeways nearly impossible to maintain— and undesirable to many younger generations for whom Westernized expressions and professionalized careers offer more promise. This often pushes them towards migration to countries with economies that can adequately compensate their roles in the long run. For the people of Cana'an, this seems to increase more drastically every decade, economic and political collapse pushing anyone with the means to migrate to the Global North as local currencies decline and political instabilities constantly sharpen.

Cultural loss is a present and ongoing phenomenon. I cannot recount the number of times I have spoken to a traditional elder or village artisan whose skill of generations was approaching extinction due to lack of apprentices forward. Or the number of rural inhabitants who could recall a practice of their childhood that no longer had a living tender to refer to. All the while, natural areas that are not destroyed by war and the chemicals of its weapons and rupture left behind are increasingly privatized, settled by occupiers, and overdeveloped at an unsustainable rate for the sake of profit and domination, often with weak infrastructure to accommodate basic needs such as water, electricity, and trash maintenance, further diminishing local ecologies.

Colonialism and war not only erode culture and generational relationships to land, but they also degrade the ecologies themselves.[2] The intentional reconfiguration of landscapes includes the removal of local agriculture and the introduction of damaging invasive species by occupying forces, such as European pine trees in Palestine and eucalyptus in Lebanon;[3] both species spread aggressively and make the soil in their understory uninhabitable to most native ecosystems.

Ruling forces from within the region often leverage natural resources just as recklessly to consolidate political power; for example, Egypt's creation of the dams in Nubian Aswan dispossessed locals of generational wealth and land across some of the Nile's most fertile shores and ancient civilizations—and diminished the ecological integrity of the entire river.[4] This has impacted the culture and self-determination of peoples and nations across the eleven other African countries who depend on this waterway for livelihood.[5] There are numerous instances like this that demonstrate the fundamental axis between land, identity, and culture, and the ways they are extracted, exploited, and reconfigured by empires, occupying forces, and nation-building efforts, explicitly to serve its beneficiaries.

These extractive practices are eroding and actively degrading our native ecosystems and Indigenous relationships to them at quickening rates; as species and landscapes disappear, our traditions die with them. WE die with them. Traditional cultures are born directly from the land they are a part of. To damage land is to damage culture, and vice versa. We *are* (our) land, and (our) land is our culture, our livelihood, our self-determined possibility forward—whether we are conscious of it or not.

A Site of the Wound

The contemporary people of Cana'an make up a particularly large diaspora on this earth, and one that is constantly growing as our home cities continue to face violence and empire from every direction. When people are forced to leave or even when they choose to, these invaluable lifelines get interrupted quite literally.

It is like when an old-growth tree in the forest falls, and all the birds and fungi that made home in its branches cease with it. All the small plants growing in its understory lose their shade and moisture. The pollinators that rely on those small flowering plants lose a necessary source of nourishment. Everything and everyone has to reconfigure a new survival, re-acclimate to a new horizon. Some life manages to adapt and continue, other life flees to make a new home, some ends completely, and all life changes. In the dismemberment of our communities, pieces of us become scattered, changing who we are—whether we stayed, left, or ceased to be.

Diaspora is a visceral and bodily inventory of displacement's impacts, its losses and gains alike. Sometimes it is the place where old traditions linger on, stopping in time, evolving in new contexts, flourishing into something brilliant and new. In diaspora, survival often means remembrance, continuation of customs, stories, and memories that reinforce who we are and the last version we recall of the places we left. Most in diaspora either abandon it completely, or hold diligently to whatever crumbs of culture they can maintain. Sometimes things get kept in diaspora that have long transformed in the homelands that continue to change as life does. Still, diaspora is the site of a wound of profound dispersal and expansion, and the tender severance of connection to place and people—whose traumatic impact should not be undermined, even when departure is "chosen." Even when relocation provides relief and possibility, when it keeps some semblance of "home" alive, and cultivates new ones with their own richness to offer.

To be uprooted reminisces the visceral ways we are severed from the earth itself. Underworlds are exposed as we are removed from the womb of familiar soils that have nurtured us into who we are for generations. There is shock and often danger in transplantation. It is vulnerable, violent even. Our attention is necessarily called to the relationship between roots and soil, to its urgent need for tenderness and repair, and the damage caused by its disruption over lifetimes.

Diaspora becomes the echo of a more primordial wound of disconnection from our life-affirming kinship with the earth itself: colonialism. Colonialism degrades a primordial part of us, fracturing our most foundational sense of dignity, security, and connection, while damaging the land itself, and the fundamental power within our relationship to it.

Empire or colonialism has overtaken Cana'an repeatedly in different iterations over the course of the past 4,000-plus years, each time forcibly altering some aspect of local peoples' relationship with their place. Each time diminishing or reconfiguring culture, language, customs, and the land itself—so much so that even its native descendants do not always recognize what has been lost or taken along the way. Change is not bad. Change is a signal of life, resilient and healthy. Colonial interference, on the other hand, produces erasure of culture and of life. It is things taken and lost despite themselves, annihilated or disappearing inside the pressure of an outside force that intends to harm, eliminate, and dominate. It is a forcible attempt to homogenize and flatten us into identities that fortify nation over kinship with place. At the very root of its upheaval, colonialism severs us from the earth itself and our generational relationships with land and each other.

Cultures of Severance

My grandfather used to pick up local flint stones from off the ground, then strike them against one another to catch a spark bright enough to light his cigarette. Once the French mandate began, colonial authorities would give him a citation every time he was caught doing so. This criminalization was twofold: encourage the purchase of matches to support commercial interests, and dissuade the fundamental power embedded in the Indigenous act of making fire with only your hands and the intelligence born from generational intimacy with place. It is our relationship to the earth and its elements that ensures our self-determination.

The earth is our first and most foundational relationship of nurturance, anchorage, and agency that secures livelihood forward. Earth is our first mother—the generous lifeline every human and nonhuman on this planet shares in common without exception. Our relationship with the earth is a material, unwavering truth that determines our fundamental existence on this planet. In separating us from this relationship or reconfiguring and exploiting it on the occupiers' terms, colonialism interrupts our deeper contract as sacred living beings of a sacred living planet, and the practical ways we have evolved to navigate and mutually sustain life. It fractures our sovereignty in a multifaceted way.

We are the earth. An embodied relationship with the land imbues innate reverence for life, an embedded knowledge of its inherent dignity. We understand all beings have a consciousness, and we are a

20

fundamental part of the ecosystem. It teaches us how to steward life and land, through intimacy with its natural cycles. Our specific landscapes have sustained our bodies and provided for our societies generationally; they have also informed every aspect of our social structures, inspired our ancestral cosmologies, narrated our stories, animated our foods and agricultural practices, intonated our languages and the rhythms of our songs, revealed our gods, and inspired every aspect of our relationships, rituals, beliefs, and identities. These places have guided every aspect of our self-determined livelihoods and cultural formation, including our understanding of ourselves and each other in the universe.

For our ancestors, our village lands were the axis we organized our entire values and societies around, affecting the whole of our reality in not just practical but also spiritual, economic, political and social ways. Traditional cultures that emerge directly from intimacy with our ancestral places lend humility, responsibility, and intelligence to ensure sustainable continuation. They instill lifeways rooted in the balancing forces of nature itself and a respect for the deeper mysteries inside life's underlying creative force.

Colonialism intentionally disrupts this inherent relationship with the earth and replaces it with an ethos of domination and power that can be manipulated to sustain empires and generate wealth, rather than affirm life on its own natural terms. Severing humans from the wholeness of this relationship is the original rupture, the deepest trauma and most ravaging displacement, which has created space for every systemic and societal wound that has followed. It defiles our generational roadmap to good living rooted in agency and mutual care. The colonial wound creates a form of spiritual exile that dissociates us from the essence of life itself and displaces us from our cultural ways of affirming and stewarding it as a part of the living land that makes us. It shakes our sense of security and home in our own bodies and basics. These relationships are an objective truth that does not waiver despite these intentional disruptions, but we suffer to realize them as a result of them.

By displacing us from the inherent connection we have with the earth as a kindred creative and material source of life and nurturance, we lose leverage with reality itself as it becomes reconstructed around something contrary and rootless—something oppressive and damaging to the earth itself, desecrated as we suffer in unison. Colonialism not only displaces our bodies from the practices, ways, and places that have affirmed our connection to the earth and sustained our self-determined livelihood for millennia, but also displaces our soul from its connective source and fundamental nature as a compass. This is also why the reclamation of earth-based practices and ancestral traditions is such a deep re-membrance. It returns us to something essential, primordial in its truth, connective nurturance, and power, specific in its resonance; it repairs inherent roadmaps for respectful dignified life on this planet so that it may continue in integrity and reverence. Re-membrance is not to recreate or romanticize the past, but to build futures anchored in the foundational truths that still determine our lives today, and the generational wisdom that is already in our bones to nurture it with autonomy and sovereignty. These skills have been stripped from us on purpose. For the longevity of our species and the many who live alongside us, we must reclaim them. Our places are what make us, and what teach us who we are and how to live well across the spheres of time.

Original wounds require original medicine to heal. The earth is our origin. Recentering our relationship with the earth can begin to transform the traumatic wounding of colonial ruptures, and the "cultures of severance" that it has bred in so many expressions since. Mending a wound of origin returns us to the source of our basic existence in a way so profound it heals many other wounds in its path, transforming the very way we understand and relate forward, and slowly dismantling every system of violence and domination, of harm and disconnection, large and small. It returns us to ourselves and to life, which returns us to each other. The plantcestors (explained further on page 41) are a powerful and accessible way to rekindle the consciousness of earth's life-giving elements inside our own bodies, recalibrating the genetic map of our deepest source and nature from the inside out.

Remapping Cana'an and the Crossroads

Most of my recent lineage is from Lebanon, the primary place that has inspired the cultural sharing in this text. Lebanon is a small country on the eastern Mediterranean coast. It borders Syria to the north and east, and Palestine to the south. All these lands were once referred to as Cana'an كنعان (or Canaan, in English). Most Canaanite settlements emerged from around 3000 BC to 300 BC. The city of Jbeil in Lebanon, still named after its ancient patron goddess Baalat Gubal, has been continuously inhabited beginning as early as 6000 BC. In a certain era of time, the Greek name for Cana'an was Phoenicia, meaning "the Purple People," for the valuable purple dyes our ancestors extracted from the shells of murex that dwelled along the Mediterranean shore. Some scholars suggest that Cana'an also comes from the word for purple in the Canaanite language.[6] The Phoenicians, particularly those associated with modern-day Lebanon where boat building took place, were advanced sailors and traders of the ancient world, whose influence spanned across the whole Mediterranean coast and traveled far beyond.[7] They established cultural capitals along northern Africa's shoreline cities and southern European colonies, where there remain threads of interconnection. They are attributed with the creation of the first alphabet, upon which the Western world's modern languages are based.[8]

Cana'an is the ancestral civilization that originated in the areas between Syria and the Sinai region of Egypt everywhere west of the Jordan River, making up the physical borderlands between the African and Asian continents. Regional oral histories, historical records, and Abrahamic texts situate the Canaanites as a people with early roots between the Eastern Nile Valley and the Eastern Mediterranean, a mixed ethnic grouping of settled and nomadic-pastoral groups who intermingled on the eastern Mediterranean coasts where their civilizations emerged.[9] These lands and cultures are an Afro-Asiatic crossroads, a geographic extension of the African continent that is bridged by its legacies of medicine, story, language, culture, religion, and livelihood.

The Afro-Asiatic languages span across Cana'an and the Arabian Peninsula, the Horn of Africa, the Sahara, and northern Africa, including the Semitic, Cushitic, Tamazight, Omotic, Egyptian, and Chadic language branches. The origins of these language groups trace roots in the southeastern Sahara or the Horn of Africa, and speak to migrational relationships from this region for thousands of years.[10] Cana'an was also part of the Fertile Crescent, sharing significant relationships with ancient Sumeria (present-day Iraq and eastern parts of Syria). The cultures and migrational lineages of these diverse territories are born in relationship to Egypt, Mesopotamia, Anatolia, the Horn of Africa, the Nile, the Arabian Peninsula, and the Mediterranean Basin. Modern borders are insufficient at capturing these significant genetic, ecological, geographical, and cultural relationships, reducing them to geopolitical dynamics and modern cultural identities, many of which have been redefined and altered over time by colonial influences and empires.

In English, the term for this area is "the Levant," rooted in the word "rising" and the concept of the orient—an eastern place where the sun rises, which beckons the question Palestinian scholar Edward Said has posed, "East of where?"[11] It reflects a colonial hierarchy that situates Europe as center, much like the common terminology "Middle East," which activist scholars have more recently preferred to name geographically as Southwest Asia and North Africa (or SWANA). Whereas in Arabic, the Levant is typically referred to as "Bilad el-Sham بلاد الشام." "Bilad" means land or country, and "sham" has multiple meanings; it means Damascus, inferring a northern city, and mole or beauty mark, reflecting the ways our cities are scattered as freckles across the land. It refers to the children of Sham, the Semitic people of the biblical family tree, though Cana'an is actually a child of Ham in the Bible,* siblings

---

* The lineages of Ham became broadly associated with Blackness, the "curse of Ham" used to justify the enslavement of African people particularly in the advent of European colonialism/Christianity in the American South, but also at times in Islamic and Judaic traditions. It has simultaneously justified the subjugation of the Indigenous people of Cana'an by the Jews, and still supports Zionist mythologies of entitlement to "the Holy Land."

of Mizraim (origins of the Arabic word "Masr مصر," meaning Egypt), Phut (Libya), and Kush (northeastern Africa).[12] "Sham" also means left, translating as "the land towards the left hand," which positions it towards the west, whereas "Yemen" means right. Referencing a locality that centers the sacred Kaaba stone of Mecca in the Arabian Peninsula, this terminology emerged during a time when Arab caliphates had authority over these territories, starting in the seventh century AD. This influence still prevails over the regional identity in predominant ways today and has, over multiple eras of empire, slowly eroded the Indigenous pluralism embedded in our region's identities for thousands of years preceding.[13] This phenomenon is known as Arabization. Still, it was until the Ottoman empire that these lands existed as one unified entity, only partitioned into separate territories beginning in 1916 with the Sykes-Picot Agreement under the French and British, eventually becoming independent nation-states in the 1940s.

I find myself in an ongoing deconstruction of the colonial mappings used to name these lands and the neighborhood of relationships, ecologies, and cultures we are a part of beyond geopolitics and empire; current configurations have been intentionally constructed by colonists to leverage our geographical assets in their favor, and explicitly against the integrity of our own internal and intersecting relationships, and the dignity and wealth of our ancestral lineages and the African continental legacies in particular. Yet all across Lebanon, Palestine, and parts of Syria, you can still see 4,000-year-old Canaanite and pre-Canaanite archeological sites scattered across our villages. Our farmers still find their remains in our soil when they tend, and their blood still ripples inside our modern bones.[14] Our cities' names reminisce their stories, and our distinct dialects reference their legacies. Cana'an is the oldest and most local name known for the region we still inhabit today. Its influence is alive as far south as the Sinai, Egypt, where some Bedouin communities acknowledge Cana'an as their continuous genetic lineage. This is similarly true for the Qemant people (of modern Ethiopia), whose oral histories assert that their forefather was a man named Anayer who is a grandson of Cana'an (son of Ham and grandson of Noah), where they originally come from.[15] Their tribe faces serious threats today, under constant pressure to assimilate to Amharic and Tigray cultures, and subject to violence and dispossession from their lands due to the ethnic genocide committed by the Ethiopian state.[16] Both these tribal communities continue to heed remnants of the dying rituals born and evolved from Canaanite culture in their own respective ways, despite ongoing threats of erasure. Bedouin oral historian and traditional wisdom keeper Hajj Ahmad Mansour from the Gabeleya tribe of St. Katrine, Egypt, once shared this genealogy with me personally when I interviewed him in his traditional home in 2016.

Hajj Ahmad is one of the only in his generation to sit and learn at the feet of twelve traditional grandmothers and grandfathers of his tribe and continue to pass on and steward Indigenous ancestral knowledge to following generations. Modernizing trends and the increasing economic pressure imposed by global capitalism have slowly eroded cultural engagement amongst his peers and the youth of his tribe—a pattern prevalent increasingly across the practicing Indigenous communities of the Crossroads region (aka SWANA—explained in detail shortly). He is one of the few who still tends and lives as his elders did, in an earth brick home in the agricultural valleys of the high desert lands where we could only access him by foot. He instituted a school for learning about the ancestral plant medicine of their ecologically significant bioregion in the hopes of transmitting some of this generational knowledge forward. Unfortunately, it has since shut down due to the challenges of sustaining local engagement. Amongst the many wisdoms he shared in our short time together, Hajj Ahmad quizzed me on who my ancestors are. When I answered "we are the descendants of Cana'an," his demeanor softened instantly, eyes lit up with a deep smile, while he pointed his finger to one of the mud bricks in the wall behind him. It read "كنعان" (meaning Cana'an, in Arabic). He affirmed our relatedness, assuring me that this writing on his wall is a testament to the importance with which he asserts this lineage to his own children in homage of who they are daily, an identity shared with most of the

Bedouin in their local area despite the common misconception that all Bedouins come originally from the Arabian Peninsula.

Reclaiming Names and Pluralities

In the spirit of re-membrance and return towards an axis centered in the land itself and its original peoples and place, including the rare remaining practicing Indigenous communities and Elders like Hajj Ahmed himself, and in honor of the less-than-perfect process of deconstruction that I am still actively in contemplation of alongside peers, in this book, I will refer to these lands between Syria and the Sinai as "Cana'an." I do so within an understanding that the genetic and cultural makeup of modern people and customs have mixed and changed over time and always entailed some degree of migrational threads and mixed nativities, and that people with roots in this region currently identify in a variety of different ways ethnically, nationally, racially, and culturally. Cana'an was always the name of a place and people that encompassed mixed ethnic groups and sociocultural ways of practice, characterized by uniquely localized and diverse cultural expressions from city to city,[17] but unified by the overarching relationship to a shared land and waterways, and the similarities that yields naturally for earth-based cultures. I am choosing to use this original naming in recognition of the rooted and continuous relationship between this region's contemporary and ancient inhabitants. "Cana'an" is a place-based name that comes from the purple hue extracts of our shores, and acknowledges the intersecting lineages and heritage between the various African and Asiatic peoples of these Crossroad areas whose stories, ethnobotanical knowledge, cuisines, languages, cosmologies, migrational patterns, blood, and ecologies merged not just in recent history, but for thousands of years before colonialism.

I will refer to the broader SWANA region as "the Crossroads," or "ard el liqa' أرض اللقاء" in Arabic, meaning "the land of convergence." "Crossroads" is a descriptive word for this region that veers away from continental bordering that traditionally severs the African continent by delegating "North Africa" to the "Middle East" (or SWANA), an ambiguous collection of nations that seems to expand and transform every few years based on geopolitics, while subsuming more of Africa in a process of Arabization, and denoting colonial and racialized proximities to Europe versus the "Sub-Sahara." This has been a critique of African scholars and revolutionaries for a while now, who assert that the entirety of the continent belongs to an interconnected cultural legacy that cannot be dismembered to serve colonial interests and the racialized violence within.[18] Some even suggest a reconsideration of the continental borders all together, considering the ways in which reconceptualizing "Arabia" (Southwest Asia) as part of the African continent makes more sense given millennia of linguistic, cultural, genetic, and political relationships—"Afrabia," as Kenyan scholar Ali Mazrui names it.[19] Black historian and community organizer Sanyika Bryant speaks about this extensively in a 2017 interview I conducted with him called "Bilad il Asmar: Where Does Africa End?"; within our detailed conversation about these layers of relationship, he notes that "this region represents the homeland of the very first African diaspora," many of whom, he says, never left and continue living Indigenously in Black communities throughout the region to this day.[20]

Others resist this reclamation of territories on the basis of historical and persisting expressions of anti-Blackness and exploitation within this region, including legacies of enslavement, the modern Kafala system, general discrimination against local and migrant Black communities, and the ongoing ways that Afro-Indigenous communities such as the Amazigh, Nubians, and countless others are both socially discriminated against and politically dispossessed from cultural and territorial sovereignty due to the infringements of the Arab governments and societies they live within.[21] Others reject it on the basis of ethnic/geopolitical affinities and contemporary phenotypical associations. Arab nation-building projects have flourished on oppressive dynamics that persist for Indigenous, racialized, and marginalized communities regionally, including but not limited to relationships with the African continent and its peoples. A majority of the "Arabized" world exists on the current continent of Africa, and many of our ancestral lineages even beyond the continental borders are claimed by Africans themselves, including Cana'an.[22] This ancestral relationship is firmly attested within our own oral histories, languages, and the ecological territories that unite us. Both historically and contemporarily, Black people have always existed natively within Arab and Arabized identities and ethnicities all across the region, as have numerous Indigenous groups who fall into neither of these categories neatly. There have also been multiple invasions that have influenced the cultural, genetic, and racialized character of Cana'an over the past few thousand years, starting with the Assyrian and Persian empires in 900 BC, then the Greeks, Romans, and Byzantines before the Arab caliphates in the seventh century AD, followed by the Ottomans, the French, British, and Zionists. All these layers considered, neither Arab and Arabized populations nor Black communities are quick to claim each other as kin in the modern context.

After the rulership of the Ottomans and Europeans, Arab nationalism was reasserted as an attempt at regional reclamation against foreign imperialism; despite its liberatory aspirations, Arab nationalism reinforced racialized and ethnic hierarchies in the process. It built on a platform of national "unity" that relies on ethnic sameness and homogenous "belonging" to Arabness—which is often used to legitimize the extraction of resources from Indigenous and African communities that strategically fall within these territories, because "we are all one people"; it often does so while erasing the Indigenous pluralities and African character of national treasures, and subverting their sovereignties to reinforce Arab authority and cohesion.[23] This rides on a long legacy of European attempts to claim proximity to the ancestral legacies of Mesopotamia, Cana'an, and especially Egypt, racializing us within an insistence that Africans and those akin to them could not be capable of such genius—completely reconfiguring the Indigenous character of our region in the process of their renarration.[24]

Arabization is also a point of contention in modern Cana'an. While many see Arabness as a natural evolution of our native regional character, others have fiercely resisted it, understanding its dominance as a direct result of conquest and the forced flattening of our inherently plu-ralistic nativities.[25] This sentiment is more common amongst marginal-ized groups, some who did not even assimilate to Arabic language until the nineteenth century despite common rebuttals that "we have all been speaking Arabic for over a century now."[26] In truth, Cana'an and its people are diverse and multiple; we are both Arab and Arabized, Afri-can and Indigenous, with genetic and cultural roots that persist both beyond and between all these identity categories from family to family. Arab tribes and language have existed, originated, and intermingled in Cana'an since long before the Arab conquests, as have migrational and genetic relationships with the Arabian Peninsula in many of our lineages to varying degrees, but Arabic and Arabness were neither gen-eralized nor dominant as an identity in Cana'an until after conquest and its impositions. The relationship of linguistic and ethnic localities once inherent to our region should not be undermined for its role in the integrity of land and life; numerous global studies have proven the direct link between Indigenous languages and the maintained biodiver-sity and medicinal traditions of the specific ecologies they emerge in.[27] Pluralism is not only our nature, but a critical lifeline to our continua-tion as a species and must be respected for the life-tending relationships it reflects, encourages, and embodies. This said, resistance to Arabness becomes more complicated within the context of modern geopolitical dynamics and a white-supremacist world order; pan-Arabism as cen-tral to postcolonial liberation efforts creates a political binary around Arab identity and its rejection, and sometimes pushes those who resist it because of cultural erasure into more reactionary political alignments that are willing to acknowledge their mere existence as ethnically or culturally distinct peoples. This is often manipulated by political forces, driving even more polarizing dynamics that feed regional sectarianism that eats us from the inside, once again serving colonists ultimately while still neglecting the fundamental dignity sought by these Indig-enous groups.[28]

This region is constantly in a tug-of-war between empires and nations who try to claim its legacies for themselves, and more often than not in the modern context, explicitly do so by separating them from Blackness, while subsuming Indigenous pluralities in an effort to effectively do so.[29] By its inherently layered existence, the region elicits an interrogation of the fundamental constructs of race, identity, nationhood, and geography that we live within as a result of colonization, and the ways we ourselves allow our self-conception to be manipulated to serve its interests while dismembering our own indigeneities and kinships.

Ultimately still, the cultural and ecological continuity between these land bases and their people cannot be fully eclipsed by the racialized and political realities within. "Crossroads" evokes the positionality of this complex borderland area as a significant eco-cultural bridge between these multiple worlds—preceding colonial intervention and within its wreckage simultaneously. The term was offered by Sanyu Estelle Nagenda, a Ugandan Belizean claircognizant and soothsayer born and raised in California who has been involved in our ongoing conversations of communal remapping. This language resonates doubly for our still-in-process deconstruction, as we ourselves tend an ongoing intellectual "crossroads" to find more accurate language and remapping of this region and its multiplicities beyond the gravity of imperialism and anti-Blackness alike. It expresses an attempt to thoughtfully reclaim the dignity and truths within our layered ancestral legacies towards a liberatory praxis and self-determined realities for all involved respectively.

In returning to land-based practices and paradigms, unraveling these colonial reconfigurations of our region is an embedded process; the plants and their stories trace these roots and relationships in undeniable ways that support our re-membrance and integrity ultimately, recentering the earth's influence on our cultural formation and kinships. It is my hope that new mappings can emerge amongst our intersecting communities that follow the same suit: informed by the waterways and landforms that connect, intersect, and create us, rather than colonial objectives that redefine and border our worlds on the terms of profit and power.

Eco-Cultural Legacies and the Origins of Medicine

In the spirit of place-based remappings, it is worth acknowledging the ecological, medicinal, and cultural contributions of this crossroads on earth, and the critical impact of preserving and supporting its flourishment for planetary integrity across species. The Mediterranean Basin is an ecological hotspot of biodiversity, with over 13,000 endemic plant species (meaning they only exist in this part of the world), and over 200 endemic vertebrae.[30] Lebanon alone makes up only 0.0007 percent of the landmass of this earth, yet is home to 0.8 percent of the living species on this earth, and 12 percent of endemic land and marine species.[31] The Mediterranean Sea is the largest and deepest enclosed sea on the earth, with over 17,000 known marine species, one-fifth of which are endemic and face threat due to the habitat loss, pollution, overexploitation of marine resources, invasion of species, and climate change.[32] The Mediterranean Basin is considered one of the most significant areas for endemic plant life on the entire earth, with 10 percent of the world's plants found in around 1.6 percent of the earth's surface; it is also facing rapid degradation and species loss, with 5,785 of the endemic species assessed for the International Union for Conservation of Nature Red List, and 23 percent of them classified as globally threatened. Humans are merely one of the species that dwell and migrate through this fecund crossroad of lands and waterways to ensure and create life; in addition to 534 species of birds, including 63 that are endemic, the area makes up the second most significant bird migration route on the planet, providing habitat and sustenance on their journey between continents, just as it has for so many of our own as humans.[33]

There are endless layers of interconnection and particularity within the ecologies of this region, these aspects only scratching the surface. We have already overviewed the impact of colonization, empire, and capitalism on these numbers and the alteration of lifeways away from the consciousness of land. Protection and revitalization of this biodiversity hub cannot happen without restorative collaboration from the communities that have coevolved with it over millennia, political and cultural autonomy of our native communities, and reclamation of the traditional practices and intimacy with place that once allowed us to navigate these relationships in mutual vitality. For the people of Cana'an and the Mediterranean more broadly, our cultural re-investment in such stewardship and repair is also a responsibility—a meaningful life line towards the well-being of our interconnected planet, far beyond our borders.

Given its significant intersection, ecological lushness, and geography, it is no surprise that this region also makes up some of the oldest documented continuous civilizations in the world. Most of the Western world's modern sciences, medicine, languages, and major religions emerge from the Crossroads' ancient institutions and ancestral knowledge systems, born directly within relationship to those of the African continent we are a continuation of, and alongside those of China, India, and the various Indigenous communities globally whose lands Western colonists settled respectively;[34] in too many cases, these wisdoms have been appropriated by brutal imperial force. This is also true inside the realm of Western herbalism; Egypt and Sumeria have two of the most ancient written archives of herbal practice in the world.[35] Imhotep was a physician later deified in Khemetic Egypt. He recorded the treatments of over 200 human maladies in papyrus records over 4,000 years ago, from which the Greeks and Romans borrowed heavily to cultivate the "Western" standards of practice we still build on today.[36] When the Roman empire fell, these bodies of knowledge were further refined by the Arab, Persian, and African Sufi doctors, most famously perhaps Ibn Sinna (known in the West as Avicenna), whose canon of medicine and systems of practice laid the foundation for herbal and medicinal practices all across Europe; even modern allopathic systems in the West have evolved from it.[37]

This is not to discount or erase the many deeply localized practices of bioregional Indigenous and folk herbalisms all across this earth, and especially those tended in the private daily spheres of our matriarchs and midwives in villages worldwide, but simply to acknowledge that the lineages of lands represented in this text have contributed immensely to the Western world at large—and are a typically invisibilized, demonized, and exploited foundational influence to the Western herbal world in particular. While this book will emphasize relational, matriarchal, bioregional, and folkloric practices of story and healing over the more formal ones suggested earlier, this context is most certainly relevant to the reclamations at hand. This book hopes to dignify the relationships of colloquial care so profoundly embedded within our continuing cultural practice, recentering the soulful ancestral expressions of our lands and relationships to each other as the center of not just our own reality, but the foundations of the stripped and impoverished ones that were appropriated violently from our regions in the creation of colonial Europe and its pervading institutions across the Global North.

This offering of story, plantcestral anecdotes, and culturally anchored herbal wisdom is my own heartfelt contribution towards re-membrance of who we are when we are the center of our own stories, and the earth is the center of us. I dedicate it especially to my siblings of Cana'an and its diasporas who seek re-connection and healing homeward, earthward, soulward towards a liberated and dignified livelihood. To our elders who have built it for us over millennia. To every lineage and diaspora displaced and colonized yet persisting—our cousins from across the Global South who mirror and inspire, walk paths of re-membrance and reclamation in parallel, trace love in unison. The earth re-members everything, the primordial key and compass. The truest answer and unfaltering roadmap we need. May this sharing be a humble step towards it, towards stewardship, towards one another.

Plantcestral
Re-Membrance

"YOU HAVE TO lose something to remember something." It was 2016. I was in Armenia, sitting with my friend's mother in her living room. She was hosting me in the midst of a nine-month ancestral pilgrimage of re-membrance across the Crossroads. Every morning, we would drink thick bitter black coffee together out of tiny cups, then gaze into the grinds left behind to divine meanings from its shapes. Her message for me this day lingered more than most: "You have to lose something to remember something." This riddle somehow spoke into the theme of my life itself, and the call which brought me to her generous home in the first place.

My relationship to plants emerges within an ongoing stewardship of belonging, memory, and healing. An eternal affair of return compelled by my relationship to lineage, "home," and diaspora. Plants have been an intimate kinship and powerful compass in my reckoning with the fragmentation of migration and the vastness of colonial wounding in my own family and homes. There is incredible loss in these experiences affecting so much of our earth and communities. But the diasporic reality of being constantly "in between" has also anchored my call to re-member, and the steadfast longing to follow its deepest roots towards freedom, connectivity, and truth.

Re-Membrance: Collecting the Bones

The concept of "re-membrance" has been reclaimed by diasporic communities and culturally displaced peoples across the Western world. It is a movement centered around decolonizing identity and restoring relationships to one's Indigenous origins through reconnecting with land, traditional culture, ancestral spiritual practices, and pre-colonial identities. In the context of the Crossroads and the African continent, however, the notion of "remembrance" has older roots at the heart of the Sufi tradition for thousands of years.[1] For our Sufi siblings, the ritual of zikr ذکر, meaning "remembrance," is the invocation of sacred movements, the names and attributes of God, and sounds as a pivotal ritual of unity. Zikr is a prayer of return towards the ultimate Oneness of the Divine that exists in all life. It is a realignment of consciousness at the soul level, a trance-like portal towards embodied realization of the Divine Creative Source and the wholeness of its presence in everything. In the ritual of zikr, healing occurs through the felt memory of oneself as inseparable from the source of Life/God, which is also the umbilical of the earth. Since this Divine Oneness is our fundamental nature, the devotional practice of zikr simply reunifies us with it—with ourselves. It re-members us, so to speak.

In my own practice, re-membrance is an ongoing process of return and becoming "homeward," not only spiritually but in every way; "home" in the deepest sense is about belonging to our own nature, a reclamation of our truest essence that realigns us with our peace, place, and purpose in life and the universe. Re-membrance orients us back towards a profound root, potentiating the most radical manifestations of restoration, reclamation, and healing not only within ourselves, but within the land and collective we are a part of. Re-membrance is a source practice, which returns us to foundations of truth so deep and fundamental they can pierce multiple layers of the disruption in our

36

worlds: spiritually, emotionally, relationally, ecologically, culturally, and politically. When the axis our life rotates on is recalibrated, the essence restored penetrates everything.

To remember is to restore knowing. To recall and heed the essence of forgotten truths inscripted inside our bodies, the earth, and our lineages. To regain consciousness of innate parts of us that have been muted and eclipsed, lost and taken. It is to re-member. To collect and mend dismembered and scattered fragments back to unity. To renew membership and our place within our worlds. To re-member heals our capacity to connect. It is to reclaim ourselves as part of the land, and realize the foundations of our inherent interdependence and relatedness, even amid traumatic wounding. It is a choice to recenter our relationships of stewardship and care, as a pathway to belonging and freedom. Through regenerating the thriving ecosystems we inhabit and fostering the full spectrum of kinships within them, we begin to thaw from domination paradigms and their internalized harm, and recover pathways to sovereignty beyond their material grip.

Re-membrance unveils through intimacy with our specific places on earth, and the original cultures our ancestors created in reflection of them. It is to revive relationship with the most foundational intelligence inside our ancestors' legacies. It recalibrates us to the scripture of the creative force inside everything living, and our own particular place within it. To re-member is fundamentally, to align with the axis of prevailing truths that do not waver. The spine of life and its own laws as our systemic compass. It is to rematriate. To decolonize our ways of learning and living. Re-membrance repairs our severance from Earth, who is our first mother—our most tangible and intimate source of life and nurturance as humans, and the most immediate mirror and roadmap to the wisdoms that lie in the universe beyond. To center land and life itself, we are obliged to confront all the systems which operate in its violation, both inside, between, and around us. It is to find home in our bodies and each other again. To reaffirm our place in the life we inhabit, and all the relationships it contains. To re-sanctify life and the dignity it is inherently owed, as we lovingly invest in our responsibility for its tending.

It is to restore integrity to the structures of our world, and recommit to the life-affirming paradigms that can build a more dignified reality. To recenter and heed the Indigenous that still thrives amongst us, and humbly steward the wisdoms of where its memory still stirs inside our own bones. To reclaim what has been taken on purpose to deprive it.

It evokes for me the reflections of the goddess Isis in exile. Her sacred journey of re-membrance is yet older than the Sufis for the traditions of our ancestral region, and embeds profound lessons for the dispersed and exiled across this earth. Isis is our primordial Aunty, an embodiment of the Divine Feminine and a central goddess in the ancestral pantheon of Khemetic Egypt, whose story below was documented on stone walls over 4,000 years ago at the Temple of Abydos.

Isis was a respected and beloved leader, who reigned with her brother-husband Osiris and brought blessings to the people of Egypt. Her jealous brother Set became so thick with envy that one day, he devised a plan to trap and kill Osiris and take over the throne. His plan succeeded. He trapped his brother in a coffin and threw it into the Nile, where it tumbled, lost in the darkness of nighttime. Isis was pushed into exile, while the people of Egypt suffered under Set's leadership. For days, all she could do was cry and wail over the loss of her beloved. One day, when she was ready, she mustered the strength to pray over herself with medicine, completing this stage of her mourning ritual by cutting off a portion of her hair. She dressed in her mourning robes and went up the Nile in search of her beloved. Eventually, she found some children in the Delta area where the Nile meets the Mediterranean Sea who said they saw his coffin floating into the salty waters. She settled in the Delta region for a while, where she gave birth to her child Horus and prayed diligently for guidance until a path forward was revealed. After many unanswered pleas, the Divine Forces sent her a revelation. She was instructed to get on a boat and sail towards Byblos, the shores of Lebanon, where Osiris's coffin had floated onto shore, embedding itself in the trunk of a sacred cedar tree. The King of Byblos noticed this tree one day and sensed its power, crafting it into a sacred pillar in his temple where it now dwelled.

Isis left her child in the care of trusted Delta locals, dressed herself in commoners' clothing, and sailed to Byblos. On the shore, she used her enchantments to forge a friendship with the palace maids washing laundry. She found her way into the role of a night nurse for the royal family's baby. Every night, she performed fire rituals of eternal life on the child, revolving around this pillar where her beloved's coffin was contained. The queen eventually caught her, horrified at the sight of her child in the fire. This moment revealed Isis's true identity and purpose. The king took compassion on her situation, permitting her to retrieve her beloved's coffin from his sacred pillar, and supported her towards a safe return home to Egypt.

Impatient with grief, Isis opened her beloved's coffin and cried over his body in the middle of her boat in the sea. As she approached the Delta area, her envious brother Set was hunting nearby and caught sight of her. He immediately struck the boat with force, turning the coffin into the water, where Osiris's bones scattered and sank, lost to the watery realms yet again. Isis was steadfast in her pursuit, diligently following and collecting each bone until she had all of them except for his phallus, which was swallowed by a fish. Isis returned home where she assembled them back into form, re-membering the skeleton of his body into its wholesome shape. She prayed strong prayers and grieved deep wails over his skeleton with her sister Nephthys. Through the help of the other gods, she transformed into a bird, flapping her wings so quickly that the breath of life could re-enter him, and he resurrected back to consciousness. His journey, however, had changed him. Not even a god could return from the underworld unscathed. Instead, Osiris was given a divine seat as the God of Death and Rebirth, leaving the earthly realm to his son Horus, who would grow to restore justice forward in his legacy.

This cosmology gives meaning, sacred context, and possibility to the times we are in. Our ancients knew something of the future's trials and the many underworlds humans traverse on earth—underworlds not even the divinities are spared. Through these stories, our ancestors left us mirrors, roadmaps to make passage through the painful losses and conflicts within.

Isis's story reminds me that the violence of empire and patriarchal greed is not new, nor is the struggle against its reign. That even exile is as ancient as we are. So often, diaspora feels like this modern desert of despair, unredeemable fragmentation, and loss—a state of such profound displacement and banishment deemed by modern wars and the colonial culture of this uniquely unyielding era. Yet this sacred story was so significant to our ancestors that they etched it in massive stone temples to ensure it be remembered, learned from, and retold by us, their descendants, over and over again for infinity. Our cosmologies are inscribed with keys, arrows that offer hints and remedies for every version of personal and communal suffering in our lives. Mirrors and clues about the deeper values and holy codes in our tribulations, and the rituals of tending and coping that have supported us to evolve and ascend since the beginning of time.

Isis's story is mirrored by the Sacred Matriarchs of our lineages repeatedly across the Crossroad regions. Be it Inanna's solitary descent into the underworld, or Mother Mary's grief over the murder of her son before he resurrected, initiatory narratives of traversing underworlds of grief to rebirth new worlds are intimately woven into the Feminine Mysticisms of our ancestral legacies. They center heavily on stories of loss and re-membrance, death and rebirth, descent and transformation, self-reclamation and return. Our Divine Foremothers exemplify the possibilities of healing through even the deepest and most solitary pain. They mirror the regeneration of the earth and its persisting cycles.

Isis's story lends symbolic meaning to those of us who re-member in diaspora—that sometimes, leaving itself is what beckons re-membrance. "You have to lose something to remember something." Diaspora can feel a bit like a collective descent. We *are* the scattered bones that beckon retrieval. We are the exiled mother who tends loss and renews life at once, determined to repair what was ruptured. We often have no roadmap besides our love and the expanse of our longing, a nudging gravitation inside us that we know we must heed despite reason. Our reclamation is a slow mending in scattered crumbs and fragments, where each gain changes its shape a bit along the way. A delicate stewardship of pieces lost and taken to reconstruct a path homeward towards a place which has also changed and lost, grown with time, and been wounded equally by our absence. We trace the roots, follow the path of the water, submerge into its darkness to collect and reconnect the bones. To be reborn—reunited—in a necessarily transcended form. Our call and response homeward becomes a resurrection, a renewal. A re-creation of something old and novel at once. A transformational reckoning and return, to an unknowable but connected future. Isis's story reinforces that the road is a mysterious but holy one that reveals while we walk it. Even when we feel submerged in the waters of our own grief or the brutality of the world, we can indeed and must re-member parts of us that have been lost at sea, destroyed and buried on purpose, severed by traumatic violence, desecrated by force. Death has its own honor and wisdom, it requires its own devotion and regard. To mourn is a sacred doorway, fertilized by love's transformative possibility. Sometimes we have to descend, sacrifice, persist in order to be reborn.

That the retrieval in this ancient story happens on the shores of Lebanon, in a city just minutes away from my own village, offers personal significance and resonance. I am reminded that there is deeper sanctity to be had in this restoration work, and that my own lineage lands carry a particular memory in this imprint of healing and rebirth. That sometimes "you have to lose something to re-member something," you have to leave to return, and that the yearning to tend what was left by our lands and in our bones is not a path in vain, even when it feels vague and impossible. Our waters, this earth are a record of everything, and we are made of them. We are a continuation of our ancestors' stories—their power as much as their pain. Re-membrance is rooted in, anchored by, restored through these indestructible relationships. It is a call and response to who we have always been, and the earth is our ultimate compass.

Plantcestors: A Compass and a Mirror

The plants are our ancestors[†]—our Plantcestors, as I have come to call them. They are living organisms that surround and inform every single

41

aspect of our livelihood as humans. They are the air we breathe, the food we eat, the fibers in our clothing, the fodder of the fires our ancestors warmed and fed by, the wood that makes our houses, and the medicine we rely on for survival. Even allopathic pharmaceuticals come from the extracts of plants originally. Plants precede humans on this earth. They have adapted to life on this planet for millennia before we even got here, and as we relate to them, they show us how to do the same.

We evolved from them. They are our mothers' mothers' mothers, and have been in intimate relationship with our kind for thousands of years. They accompany us in our kitchens, native landscapes, and gardens, inspiring our cultural foods and recipes, absorbing all our colloquial chats and energies, and ritualizing our family celebrations and day-to-day lives with their nourishment. They color our traditional textiles and facilitate every ceremonial event of significance in our human cultures—weddings, funerals, births, and rites of passage of every kind. They help build the bodies of our traditional instruments and sacred tools, in creative intimacy with our hands and breath so we can express, sing, dance, pray, and emote in a fullest range of sentiments. They are our companions in every sense, blessing our lives with wisdom, healing, and profound beauty and affection as they fuel our existence.

Plants are sentient beings who not only nourish our bodies but witness, inspire, and respond to aid the experiences of our lives in infinite ways. They carry profound memory and consciousness, acting as bridges between the cosmic realms and the earthly ones, the human and nonhuman ones, weaving the wisdom of multidimensional worlds as they merge with each. They drink the minerals of the soil and water where we live, touched by every pollinator and organism in their midst, and absorb the sunlight, the moon and star patterns of constellations in the particular arrangement that frequents our specific place on earth. Then, we eat, breathe, and drink them, absorbing all this life and memory; all its mysteries, cycles, and medicines wake up in our

---

† Please read the entry about plantcestors in the Meaningful Language Glossary (p. 299) for significant context and acknowledgments.

own beings, attuning us to the life-affirming relationships of the lands we are a part of. Their bodies witness each mood of our private sphere, and record the grander wisdoms of the earth and cosmos we belong to, unifying these worlds inside of us so that we can heal and be more in sync with the creative forces inside and around us. It is no wonder they fill significant roles in the cosmologies, religions, and creation stories of traditional peoples all across the earth—in every ritual, symbolism, and the numerous amulets featured in the sacred lexicon of our traditional cultures.

The plantcestors make up the very foundation of who we are physically and genetically, but also culturally, spiritually, and vibrationally. They pulsate with the secrets of life in all its cycles, scriptures that exist mutually inside of us and are activated by these plantcestral encounters. When we work with plants as medicine, we call these relationships into conscious intention. Our attention activates the memory and transformation within their miraculous, life-giving secrets, harnessing and aligning us with their profound dimensions of healing, in re-membrance of who we are.

Plants of Lineage

The plants native and common to our ancestral lands have a particular affinity to our beings. They encode generation after generation of cellular memory, nourishment, and story embedded deep in the tissues of our own blood and bones. Our bodies, which have been informed and built by them for millennia, recall their flavors and chemistry, their essences and spirits. When we engage with our ancestral plants from wherever we live in the world, they light up these ancient parts of us, transporting us towards these first places inside of us. Our ancestral plants have the capacity to recalibrate us to the lands we mutually come from and its unique imprint of wisdom and resonance as aligned with our own soul's path. They remember us, activating roadmaps encoded in our DNA, and knowings blessed by the ages inside our flesh and bones and the specific ways our ancestors made meaning of life on this planet. They regenerate the soil of our internal universe, quenching the earth we are, reminding us and feeding us in a hue that is familiar and suited especially for us because it is part of our design. Our ancestral plants know us so intimately in fact that their mere presence in our lives can retrieve parts of us so deeply buried we do not even know they are amiss. They record the taken and untold memories of our ancestors and their embedded wisdoms too, because they are part of the source that created and inspired them since the beginning of time. Our plantcestors of lineage are such a foundational part of our cultures and legacies of knowledge, affection, and survival that we would not be who we are without them. To neglect them is to abandon a primordial part of ourselves. To steward them is to bless life forward and back, restoring something sacred and expansive in its healing and aid, especially for those of us who have been severed from our lands, lineages, or Indigenous cultures.

In my personal seeking to heal and make peace with myself through wisdoms of the land and my ancestors who lived closest to the earth, I have encountered many fractures and gaps of memory and insight regarding our rooted lifeways and understandings, sometimes broken from just one or two generations before. I have experienced a multiplicity of ways my own spirit feels lost, body untethered and stranded, looking for anchorage to guide me. But where my living elders have been unable or unwilling to remember or offer meaningful guidance, where the loss and ruptures of colonialism are simply too deep or long to reach beyond the splintered shards that remain preciously understated in our colloquial lifeways and kinships, the plantcestors and land itself have carried hidden keys towards restoration.

To rekindle relationships of listening and tenderness with ancestral plants has become a profound and pivotal part of my re-membrance and belonging on earth, and my humble homage of resistance to the persistent loss inside our land-based traditional cultures and their stewards to this day—not just in my own lineage lands, but across this earth plagued by colonial violence, ecological destruction, and imperial oppression. Likewise, to tend the plantcestors native to the places

I call home in diaspora and motherland alike has ushered meaningful care, beauty, and responsibility, a renewed sense of peace and place in my body and communities, and deep regeneration to the ecosystems I inhabit daily. Tending plantcestors and ecologies of place directly affirms Indigenous livelihoods in a simple but profound act that literally rematriates land and begins to heal colonial ruptures that have touched us all deeply. It is an ultimate act of love and reciprocity to our ancestors and future, the earth, and its stewards' life-affirming cultures globally. Tending our local habitats is an act of love and generous healing that returns us homeward and restores universal integrity in transformative ways.

Plantcestral Poetics:
Softening Our Senses, Tuning Our Bodies

Deepening relationship with the earth obliges us to soften the rigid colonial mindset and expand the rational intellect, embracing nonlinear cues and signals that attune us more deeply to internal, surrounding, and relational landscapes. It is a sensual realm that engages all our perceptive and bodily capacities to feel, receive insight, realize connections, and be responsive to life. I sometimes refer to this process as Plantcestral Poetics. Plantcestral Poetics immerses us in the minute details of the sensory body, nuanced observation, and the first language of symbols, patterns, and feeling between the lines, as a source of deeper communication, healing, and wisdom.

To attune to the plantcestral world, we must relearn to access and honor the multisensory ways we know and connect; first, we slow down, quiet down, and deepen presence with our body and spirit, familiarizing ourselves with the subtlest cues of somatic communication and letting these felt realms guide us. The plants reveal their nature through shapes, tastes, energies, and habitats that we engage with our embodied senses. Heeding the nonverbal details, synchronicities, and perceptive associations that emerge helps us unveil the dynamic story that lives between us and each plant, and honor its wisdom for healing.

45

The sensual nature of their kinship simultaneously weaves subtle containment from inside our bodies, recalibrating our nervous systems, and facilitating our capacity to return to ourselves; this repairs our foundation for healthier relationships with others. The plantcestors' mere presence begins to bring us back from fractured states, earthing us effortlessly. Through engaging our holistic body as a site of intelligence and connection, we naturally begin to deconstruct the fragmented paradigms that dominate so much of our contemporary world; the process unravels the ways we have internalized exploitive systems and dissociated to survive.

The plants by their nature instill reciprocity, healing the relational truth of our interdependence as species, as we care for them and they care for us and every other living thing in their midst. Through softening and rooting ourselves towards this stewardship, we relearn to feel, hear, and connect more authentically as we nourish and revel in life beyond just ourselves. The process repairs agency and security with our own body as "home," awakening the memory and medicine that dwells in the soil and soul of our tissues, where the deepest healing and reclamation lies. This is also where our ancestors live and continue through us.

The relationship beckons softness, revives intimacy as we regain the skills to arrive and interpret the unique dialect of our own body as an intuitive vessel and a compass and antennae forward. It is a reclamation of inherent guidance and generational wisdom, intentionally eclipsed by colonial conventions as a measure of control, and displaced by chronic states of traumatic stress so many modern humans endure. Deepening with the plantcestors recenters a mutual, embodied, and instinctual way of learning and being, reacquainting us with deeper faculties of our senses and spirits and rewiring not only the ways we "know" but the ways we exist. Through reconnecting to the earth's axis, we naturally realign to our own. In cultivating relationships with the plantcestors, we learn from the rhythms of every cycle in the living process of creation, immersing in life's seasonal transitions and the diverse personalities of our places on earth.

Building Plantcestral Relationships

I invite you towards this sensory way of relating and learning now. Take a moment to arrive to the experience of your own body in this moment. Begin by feeling the weight of this book in your hand. Feel the cadence of these words as they travel through your mind's ears. Notice your skin making contact with the air and your clothing. Are there temperatures? Textures you notice? Now feel the weight of your feet on the ground. Allow them to become heavier, softer, as you let the earth beneath you carry their entire weight. Give attention to the quality of this connection, feeling the security within the points where your body is in contact with the ground. Are there any sensations that reverberate inside you while you observe this? Use your senses to take inventory of the life that inhabits this moment inside and around you. Now take a breath and notice how it fills you. This oxygen is your first connection with the plantcestors. Feel into that relationship while the air moves through your being.

I invite you to engage in this detailed practice of sensory "listening" as you walk in the world day-to-day. Notice the conversation between the colors, feelings, and patterns of life as they unveil around you. Notice the places, people, and plants you pass by every day through this lens, and observe what changes. Lean into the subjective experiences and symbolic themes that appear, empowering the poetry of life's cues. Even as you read this book, the plantcestors may speak through your senses. This is an invitation to return to this sensory attunement periodically through your engagement, noting the way each layer of sharing reverberates through your body. You may choose to look up the plants' images while you read, or work with their remedies during each passage about them. Start to notice which ones soften, stir, or constrict you, and allow these threads to guide you towards deeper possibilities of relationship and learning. Take note of any specific plants that resonate with your senses as you read them, or other ones that show up in your daily life and conversations. Perhaps choose to cook, grow, or learn more about these plants in a more embodied way forward. Weave them into your existing practices: intentionally dance, paint, study, work and create alongside them, and see what emerges in the details of your living experience.

On a similar note, there are parts of this reading that may evoke tension or grief. As one of my teachers, a Mayan-Tzeltal curandera named Doña Lucia, always advises, consider the accompaniment of roses when tough junctures of ancestral longing, grief, or traumatic memory surface—in this book or otherwise. Roses are accessible in most parts of the world through rosewater, tea, oil, or plant cuttings. You can splash your face with their droplets, smell, eat, or drink them with sensory attunement and intention to initiate a relationship of healing. Notice how your feelings transform or deepen once they enter your being, and heed accordingly. Notice how your life interactions change while the roses work with you. This can initiate a simple experience of plantcestral relationship building in your life.

Original Medicines for Original Wounds: Plantcestral Re-Membrance Praxis

Like the land, our bodies harbor distinct memories. Dismembered and forgotten fragments of the earth's primordial and place-based wisdom leaves a unique residue, a lineage of knowing in each of us that sustains connection and transcends time and trauma. Each person carries their own wisdom and avenues of receptivity and connection, their own personal roadmaps and doorways to kinship with the plants and life in general. We, like our ancestors, and like every healthy ecosystem on this earth, each have a particular role to contribute towards the integrity of the whole. Our particular affinities and personalities, desires and expressions reveal layers of this perspective and the cues towards the deeper knowledge within. In reflection and exchange that honors one another's irreplicable place and purpose, we have the chance to realize and weave these threads into a tapestry of complex colors and shapes, to unveil and interpret a more cohesive story of meaning, memory, and wisdom that can only complete itself in living breathing unison. To do this work of re-membrance in a circle allows us to restore communally, learning not only through our individual practice but through the patterns and reflections of our ancestral relationships with one another and the lands that give us life. This becomes even more crucial in the scattered context of our displaced and colonized world. In a circle, our beings become an intimate mirror for each other's revelation and understanding. From the vessel of diaspora, we transcend imposed borders, reconnecting from across oceans, continents and lineages in a way that subverts lines drawn between us. We become a recollection of those lost bones, each retrieving a piece of what lies beneath the waters, breathing new life through our ancestral communion. We simply cannot re-member alone.

I call the practice of intentional partnership with our ancestral plants, stories, and earth-based legacies "Plantcestral Re-Membrance," a methodology truly inspired by the plants whispers in my own life as I sought a roadmap for reconnection, communal regeneration, and deeper healing culturally rooted in the earth and my lineages. Plantcestral Re-Membrance is an eco-feminist methodology that engages experiential (somatic), relational, and cultural practice as an avenue towards healing, collective reclamation, and the restoration of generational and place-based wisdom. Our philosophy of praxis incites the assertions of Black feminist Audre Lorde. In her poignant essay "Power of the Erotic," Lorde says:

> In order to perpetuate itself, every oppression must corrupt or distort those various sources of power within the culture of the oppressed that can provide energy for change. . . . We have come to distrust that power which rises from our deepest and nonrational knowledge. We have been warned against it all our lives by the male world . . . The bridge which connects [the false dichotomy between spiritual and the political] is formed by the erotic—the sensual—those physical, emotional, and psychic expressions of what is deepest and strongest and richest within each of us, being shared.[2]

In Plantcestral Re-Membrance, relationship building with land through embodied practice, communal exchange, and ancestral story encourages earthward paradigm shifts, as the central axis of knowledge revelation is returned to the lived and sensual realms of our miraculous bodies as a source of re-membrance and power. These realms inherently evoke the expanses of generational intelligence that made us, and they reattune us to the dialects of the earth we contain mutually.

In Plantcestral Re-Membrance Circles, intentional and closely held containers engage with cultural familiarities, anchored by but not limited to kinship with ancestral plants. Creative and emergent collaborations support the process of relationship formation and re-introduction to hands-on and multisensory ways of knowledge building. This technique re-engages and retrains us in deciphering our somatic compass, reviving internal sources of insight and elemental attunement through the implementation of Plantcestral Poetics. The overly cerebral training of lifetimes immersed in colonial schools and institutions often poses obstacles to embodiment and creative engagement. Through partnering with plants in an experiential and "listening" way first, these less linear senses are reawakened to initiate a deeper process forward inspired by the wisdoms of the land. Participants are provided with basic tools and techniques to recognize and reclaim the unique language and wayfinding mechanisms of their own being, supported and guided by the plantcestors directly. We study how this knowledge and memory is transmitted through communal reflection and reverential space holding; experiential revelation is supplemented by immersion in oral knowledge, medicinal records, regional cosmologies, and dream work to deepen and illuminate our learning. Intentional selections of ancestral plants and stories pair to help reveal original meaning through our bodies and the lineage lands we are a continuation of.

The container cultivated through this work supports the basic resourcing needed to gently reckon with what often dwells in the tender arena of our bodies and bloodlines. The plantcestors are masterful and personalized in the deep aid they provide, while the careful group container offers steady and intimate support for integration as layers of revelation take place. Through communal reflection and cultural study, the parts become woven into meaning that illuminates the whole, and a lexicon of patterns and symbols are realized through the collective body re-membered. Each aspect of the documented, folkloric, and experiential information contributes to the knowledge that emerges within. This work is an intentionally curated dialogue with the legacies inside our bodies and the stories inherited by our lineage lands.

This methodology is a framework capable of supporting numerous cultural re-membrance practices beyond work with plantcestors, though anchoring in their presence aids immensely. It was developed as a way to rekindle memory and deepen ancestral knowledge through embodying land-based cultural expressions such as dance, songs, basketry, textile work, culinary lineages, dream work, land stewardship, and traditional crafts of endless kinds. Our cosmologies and sacred sites have been pillaged and co-opted—repeatedly desecrated and appropriated by colonial entities that benefit and profit from generations of cultural theft at our expense; it is necessary for us to reclaim the generational axis of knowledge, re-anchoring in our personal and ancestral relationships to place as a primary site of re-membrance. This methodology allows us to do so, while also supporting us to wayfind within the many gaps in memories far and recent retold by our own families, that still find home inside these intersecting realms where our plants (earth), cultural arts, stories, sacred sites, and bodies meet. This intentional and full-bodied re-immersion is part of healing colonial wounding, repairing the earth severance of our communities, re-membering our ancestors, recollecting buried cultural wisdom, and healing personally and ecologically as we do so.

Some fundamental understandings that support this work are:

- **Our bodies are an archive, our bodies are the earth.** Our body, like the earth, is an agent and vessel of generational memory, healing, and primordial wisdom.

- **We must feel to heal.** The body's wisdom is realized through deepening sensory capacity and attunement. Restoring these capacities often requires, but also facilitates, healing on somatic, intellectual, and cultural levels.

- **The earth re-members everything.** Relating to land (and our traditional cultures as an expression of it) can help heal our sense of home and safety in our bodies. Through immersing our beings in elemental and embodied cultural practices and places, generational resilience can be realized and re-membered.

- **Stories and their places carry keys.** There are roadmaps and keys in the stories lived and shared by our immediate and distant ancestors, and the places where they dwelled. The plantcestors help unlock their memory in our own bodies, even when we cannot travel there ourselves.

- **Relationships determine life.** We heal and re-member in relationships—to each other, to place, to body/self, to land and lineage. Restoring these relationships is fundamental to healing from traumatic and colonial wounds, and supporting the rematriation and liberation of our world.

- **We are our ancestors.** Lost and fragmented cultural knowledge can be, in some form, revived and renewed through collective embodiment and reflection. As Lakota Elder Leola One Feather once insisted to me, each people across the earth have retained a piece of the larger cosmic puzzle that can mend our worlds back into integrity. We each must steward our piece, so we can share its valuable part to the re-membrance of the whole.

- **Re-membrance is return.** This work is sacred, holistic, feminist, and decolonial by its nature. It is transgenerational, eco-regenerative, and liberatory. It reconnects us to some of the oldest and most foundational ways our global Indigenous ancestors navigated life on this planet. To be in our bodies with the earth, is the greatest portal to restoration back and forward.

Regenerative Relationships
and Protocols for Practice

What is powerful about the plantcestors is that while each species carries its own steady signature of medicinal properties and vibrational patterns, they are also incredibly dynamic and relational, interplaying with the unique balance, spirit, and constitution of each person they relate to. This is why there are so many plants, for example, that have beneficial actions on the same organ of the body, but not the same one suits each person with that particular ailment. There is deep intimacy and complexity in the plantcestral world and the kinships they curate, which is why tending and working with them—and especially those administering them to others—requires great care, respect, and skill cultivated over a lifetime. Likewise, each plant has its place in the ecology of relationships it is a part of, which impacts the soil, water, animals, insects, fungi, plants, and humans who live there alike. It requires great respect and a sensitive relationship to know when, how, and in what context to harvest plants from "the wild" without damaging the balance of life it—and we—are a part of. To build slow relationships over many seasons in a certain place is what allows us to attune to these cycles with care, these relationships themselves facilitating the deepest medicine that the plantcestors have to offer—a detailed ancestral craft of its own.

When engaging relationships with cultural plants in their native habitats today, we must consider the delicate balance between participating in these hands-on practices and the important kinships they yield with our environment and ancestors, and counteracting the excessive burdens currently facing our ecologies. These relationships fostered are not merely transactional or one-directional; they require care in all directions to ensure the longevity of our collective livelihood. One of the most valuable teachings I learned in my training from Karyn Sanders at Blue Otter School of Herbal Medicine, was to spend time getting to know the places I collect from for multiple seasons before actually harvesting from them. This allows a person to observe the baseline distribution of a plot of plants in the wild and recognize how it fluctuates from one year to another, what needs might be present, and who else is harvesting from these same plots. For example, you may think that a stand of za'atar is incredibly abundant but do not realize that only two years earlier it populated more than 50 percent of that specific area. Before even considering harvest, asking permission from both the stewards of the land and the land itself is important. Besides this, one should never harvest more than what they need from a plant, and never take more than 10 percent of what is growing. We are not the only organisms who rely on these plants for sustenance. Being conscientious about the conditions we are gathering from is also crucial. With increasing toxicity in our environments, many plants flourish in degraded areas to support restoration of the land. Medicine is best avoided from major highways and other potentially toxic or polluted areas. Learning when and how to harvest is also important and changes with each plant. Some plants spread from roots and rhizomes, and even thrive when they are cut generously now and again, whereas others rely on going to flower and seed before harvest in order to reproduce at all, and can only be harvested from certain branches or windows of time in their reproductive cycle. Through taking the time and effort to learn these things, we honor the plantcestors who sustain us, and we ensure that they, and the interwoven web of species who depend on them for life, will continue to flourish in our midst.

Harvesting plants is not the only way to begin building meaningful relationships with their medicine. Just being in their presence provides profound healing sometimes, smelling them as your legs brush by them or intentionally making time to observe and sit with them to "listen" and learn from the ecosystem of organisms that surround them/us. Looking more closely to learn from what information their shapes, tastes, and colors evoke is an interesting way to warm back up to natural learning. Making flower essences is one of my favorite forms of plant medicine in this spirit of deeper listening, and requires very minimal harvesting at all. Watching which plants grow where and near whom, when they bloom or go dormant, and what climate and conditions help them thrive also allows us to know how to respect their cycles and support them.

Tending native plants is an incredible way to deepen relationship and healing as well. I highly advise anyone who has a garden, farm, or even a balcony to consider planting native species from your own bioregion—no matter where in the world you are. This helps both replenish the local habitat and foster an intimate connection with these plants, their medicine, and our own sense of place. In "the wild," helping spread some of their seeds around them when they have dried or removing invasive plants that are encroaching on their habitat is also a simple act of contribution towards their regeneration. Please ensure that you are identifying said plants accurately before participating in these ways, so you don't unintentionally contribute to more damage.

There is a strong impulse in the modern context to immediately begin harvesting and preparing plants to sell or consume. But these practices of reacquainting with place and giving back over time allow us to rewire the ways colonialism has trained many of us to relate (or lack relating) altogether. To connect is often more impactful than to produce, and how and why we produce and create are equally important. All this being said, hands-on practice is a central part of the ancestral relationship we are working to restore with our lineages and places, and has always been part of the traditional maintenance of our ecosystems and livelihood. My note is simply to consider the ways you reclaim these practices *within* a relational and cultural context, if you are approaching them after eras of severance. Reinvesting in your relationships with family members or local community who still live in these ways is a powerful chance for such integration, supporting and learning through shared practice.

Furthermore, to engage with intention in any and every aspect of work with plants and their preparations qualitatively changes the nature of the medicine we make. This is knowledge that has been reinforced consistently to me by traditionalists from every cultural lineage

I have been graced to learn from. Practicing presence, gratitude, and reciprocity restores a quality of balance and integrity to the food and medicine we cultivate and share. Speaking intentionally to the plants about the medicine we seek their aid for allows for more directed power likewise, as my dear Anishinaabe friend Sarah Headbird has taught me about immensely. To work with plants for sustenance and medicine is an exchange of life, so inherent and so profound at the same time. In my personal experience, the plantcestors I have gotten to know most intimately over time are the ones I first lean to for help with almost anything—even if it is beyond their typical range of biochemical action. These intimacies are expansive in their power and capacity to heal.

In this light, specific dosages and formulas are mostly not included here. This is in part to encourage a more careful and embodied way of deepening, redirecting people towards cultural recipes and research from their own immediate environments, and partially with respect to safety for those who are new to herbal practice. My sharing is not intended to diagnose, treat, or replace comprehensive treatment and consultation from a qualified health provider for any conditions that may be mentioned in this book. Particularly for plants whose stronger indications are mentioned such as in labor support or abortions, or for those of you who also are taking prescription medications for the conditions mentioned, wise precautions should always be taken with the use of the herbs and remedies of any kind. Please tread lightly and seek the expertise of an experienced practitioner for customized support, rather than endangering yourself with partial knowledge and protocols that can do more harm than good when lacking proper scope. Learning to identify the correct plants is a careful step of its own; many resemble others in their local habitats that may not be safe for consumption. Also note, in the Crossroads region, common names are often delegated to a number of different plants, fluctuating from village to village and country to country. Take extra care to identify the plantcestors properly before using them for the listed purposes, as their properties naturally vary. The Latin names can support your discernment when facing confusion, and give you a reference point to learn more about proper identification markers when learning about plants. It is best not to assume the colloquial name for a plant in one region refers to the same one with that name in another region before doing a bit of extra investigation. In addition to a plethora of books, there are some helpful online databases that may support plant identification in Cana'an, including documentation of some local names. These include www.mahmiyat.ps, www.barari.org, and the iNaturalist app.

The knowledge shared here is to inspire relationships and allow them to deepen with practical wisdom over time—just as our ancestors who pass this down from generation to the next. It is an invitation to begin with what you know, rekindle kinship with your families and the communities you inhabit to re-connect and re-member, and take time to listen and observe so that we may reintegrate a grounded practice of care for self and community slowly and safely.

Part II

FOOD IS OUR MEDICINE, LOVE IS OUR MEDICINE

MY MATERNAL TETA'S (grandmother's) house was a universe unto itself. Time and space would cease to exist there. Teta had been living in the US since the '70s but her house still smelled, felt, and tasted like the tiny southern village she came from, possibly even the same version of it she left before war and occupations, before the family moved to Ras Beirut, before they traveled oceans, before it all. We would come visit her often in the springtime when we were children. Easter was my Jiddo's favorite holiday, and I recall the festivities of that season and the rituals it entailed. All our maternal aunts, uncles, and cousins lived in Florida except for us, so our visits were special and brought complete-ness to the family for a moment. There was always lots of food.

Teta's house was a capsule of our memories. Every room contained its own secrets and stories from our childhoods. Etchings on the walls we got scolded for and height charts to archive our growth—our own lexicon of stories were left as testaments in every corner. Every drawer and closet had some old remnant from the family's life in Lebanon, or the handmade clothes our mothers crafted when they were our age. Every drape and couch, every item of Teta's clothing, all the adornments in the home were sewed by her hands. The whole place smelled like fresh grown za'atar, so much so that my clothing would always linger with this smell when I got back to California. At certain points in the day, all my aunts and uncles would arrive in a simultaneous cascade, the rakweh would boil and black bitter coffee would make its way to the living room where everyone collected to banter for a moment before going back to their daily work. There would always be a couple people playing tawleh (backgammon) on the other side of the living room while the rest of us sipped, and someone else in the kitchen rustling around for bizr (seeds) or fruit to snack on with the coffee. Undoubtedly, ahweh (coffee) was and remains the most steady and sacred ritual of all in my mother's family. The moment in the day when everything else would stop and we would all be together, in Teta's house, doing what families do, what village folk do, thousands of miles and decades of time away.

While the living room was the heart of the house where this ritual would take place, the soul of the house lived somewhere between the kitchen and Teta's prolific garden. For our people, and for my family, food is love, and culinary love is deeply and fundamentally communal. To share a meal or drink together is the most significant (and mundane) ritual of connective care, and it is also our primary vessel of botanical medicine. Our traditional foods are the first line of physical defense and fortification, as well as the initial method of treatment should an ailment arise. Furthermore, the seasonal nature of our traditional cuisine revolves around wild and baladi (homegrown, organic) crops whenever available, anchoring the traditional eating culture within the cycles of local land and its inherent intelligence and embedded medicinal properties and vitality. It is part of the unspoken way our communities calibrate to place and to one another.

This played out naturally in Teta's house. There was a tiny island in the middle of her kitchen, which always had a small container of za'atar next to one of zeitoon (olives), a bag of mar'oo' bread handmade by her, and a little jug of olive oil. At most points of the day, there would be at least a few of us sitting there, eating, snacking, or helping Teta roll grape leaves or prep a meal. In Teta's house, every ingredient and step of the food preparation process was approached with great respect. The kitchen led to a side room that stored additional cooking equipment, and a garage where her saj oven and distiller and an extra freezer dwelled, which led to the nursery of her garden where she grew parsley, za'atar, sage, and every other basic vegetable and herb of the Lebanese cuisine you could think of.

Teta's garden was her place of refuge and pride, and she was known in the family to have 'eed barakeh يد بركة ("a blessed hand," or what we call in English a green thumb) that could manage to help any plant live somehow. Okra, cucumbers, eggplants, tomatoes, figs, oranges, and of course, roses. All of these fresh greens would make their way into our meals prepared with undeniable love and packed with nutrients and protective medicine. The resourceful, seasonal, and natural qualities of the materials emphasized in Teta's house were always significant, and it was something my mother carried forward in our home too, she perhaps the most dedicated foodie of our whole family. Just as they insisted our clothing be made with cotton, silk, or other natural fibers, the grains, meats, and vegetables utilized in our meals were chosen with a grueling discernment and attention to flavor, freshness, and quality entrenched deeply in our land anchored culture. The love inside food prepared and shared was demonstrated by each detail of care and skill invested, the medicine ensured by insistence on cleanliness and homegrown ingredients wherever possible. In Teta's house and the lineage of her children, food is truly devotional.

The vibrancy of communal preparation, the songs, kinships, and comfort that naturally emerge in the process of making together is the unspoken niyyeh, the underlying intention and purpose inside Cana'an's traditional food customs. The colloquial and social nature of food in our culture is in and of itself medicine, reinforced by the potency of plants, reflecting a deep paradigm of health embedded in collectivism and mutual stewardship of season, kinship, and place. Companionship is the most consistent and primary ingredient in our traditional food remedies.

While my mother's family may be particularly invested in the ritual of traditional food preparation, its centrality in our home is not unique in our cultural context. Every aspect of culture across Cana'an centers around sharing meals—be it a regular summer day, a wedding, holiday, birth, or the death of an elder. It is somewhat offensive to refuse a meal or food item offered when visiting guests and family, and they will characteristically fill your plate with more than what you asked for. Food is an expression of love and generosity, which holds a high cultural value across our region. My father's family in Lebanon is just as food-centric; many of my favorite memories with my aunties and grandmother especially revolve around the conversations at the kitchen table while picking fresh mlokhiyeh off the stocks, or eating green garbanzos in the garden with them and my uncles—always with finjan ahweh (a cup of coffee).

The communal aspects of food in Cana'an's tradition exists in every stage and season of its preparation—from the growing, harvesting, and sharing of crops to the cooking and the consumption. My aunt reminisces about summer returns to the village during wheat season when she was a child. Wheat was usually purchased from villages in the Bekaa Valley, where it was known to grow well, and then brought to our own village in the south to be processed into burghul (cracked wheat used in many traditional recipes). A person would ride around the village with a loudspeaker announcing that today the wheat preparation would be happening at so-and-so's house. Everyone would then proceed to that family's house for a day of working together to prepare the grains that would nourish them collectively for the course of the whole year. In my own lifetime, I would most often arrive to my mom's village to find Great Aunt Lucy on the back patio with her husband and neighbors shelling pine nuts, drying sumac, or processing za'atar together, depending on whatever was in season. Locals would come and go to lend a hand as we bonded over a break to read the predictions in our coffee cups, delighting in whatever fresh fruit was currently growing. I barely know what the inside of her house looks like—most of our visits centered around the garden and its bounty.

In a similar spirit, I remember one beloved aunty in my father's village who spent her days walking around, with her umbrella for shade, arriving at the doors of extended-family homes with the special mission to help make ma'ajanat (dough pies) together. Her dough was famous for its delicious quality, extended family vying for her special touch and support in their kitchens. Food and its preparation has always been the central place of connection, nourishment, and day-to-day care across our region. Each person has a role, a hand to extend in the seasonal process, and the generosity to give of their abundance to one another regardless of how much or little they have. Even in my parents' home in diaspora, extended community arrives unexpectedly at the door with a huge bag of fresh tomatoes, pickled olives, or wild mallow from their garden as an offering of mutual care reminiscent of home with no return expected. It is at the very core of our culture to relate in this way. And it is also why there will always be enough to share when unexpected visitors appear.

Food itself is such a foundational and integrated part of our collective tradition that some people might miss just how meaningful it is as a form of herbal medicine. It is arguably the most tenacious, intact, aspect of our ancestral botanical wisdom alive today. Our traditional recipes themselves are balanced formulations we may not be conscious of, but we maintain in the continuation of our ancestors who first developed them, and are empowered by our union with one another in both their conjuring and consumption.

3

Tending "Weeds"

CROSS-COUNTRY TRIPS TO Teta Renee's house in Florida were characterized by food and garden exchanges between me, her, and my mom. I was merely the courier of these elaborate love notes packed in thermal bags to the utmost weight capacity permitted. There have been many TSA conversations about the frozen lamb sent back and forth, from my mom's end frozen whole, and back from Teta in the form of kibbeh prepared perfectly by her prolific hands. Anytime Teta or my aunt found an exceptional stock of perfectly tiny okra or fresh fava beans, they would mail a case to my mother and vice versa. At least half my own medicinal garden is made up of plants Teta Renee sent home with me—rue, aloe, rosemary, bay laurel, bitter orange, za'atar, and more. But Teta's most consistent request from our end was the California weeds that resembled those of her village ecosystems in the similar climate of South Lebanon.

Before my late-winter flights, my mother and I would go walking around the neighborhood, trowels in hand, to scout perfect patches of clean mallow and dock plants growing in sidewalks or abandoned hillsides. We would harvest them from the root, wrapping them with wet towels in a plastic bag so they could endure the journey across country. If the leaves were abundant, Teta and I would use them immediately in meals, while the roots would be planted in a special garden bed dedicated to these most beloved nostalgic foods that most North Americans discard as weeds. In fact, a great deal of my Teta's visits to California when I was young were characterized by her insisting we stop every time we saw a suburban fruit tree shamefully rotting its droppings on the ground, or a park lined with olive trees or prickly pears. Teta would embarrass us by knocking on the door and asking permission to harvest what was otherwise going to waste, in her fragmented English, or our mom and aunties harvesting olives during birthday parties at the public parks. Teta's resourcefulness and respect for the earth's abundance was undeniable, and she reveled in the chance to gather food from her environment.

There are many beloved "weeds" dense with medicinal values and integrated naturally into our seasonal and daily dishes across Cana'an. Many of them grow invasively throughout the Northern Hemisphere and make perfect complements to our apothecaries and kitchens in service of our bodies and the local ecologies at once, as their removal facilitates more space for native plants. While these recipes are quite likely the least elaborate or "sophisticated" of our culinary traditions traveling the world, they are some of my personal favorites. They are localized and economical food as medicine for and of the people who attune to the land they live on and its cycles. They were even more precious to me at Teta's diaspora house, where I got a glimpse into the deeply embedded relationship to the plants and seasons of her own childhood landscape that she learned to nurture and maintain connection to from an ocean away.

Energetics: Traditional Paradigms of Elemental and Bodily Intelligence

It is worth noting that the wild spring greens typically favored in our traditional cuisine often feature bitter taste palettes, as well as qualities that support the cleansing functions of the body, including the liver. In traditional concepts, bitter herbs known for their action on the liver are often characterized by a "cooling" and drying effect on the body. They support the secretion of bile, which helps us eliminate toxins in our digestive tract and beyond. Our ancestral systems of medicine classify the constitutional and energetic qualities of herbs as an important factor of effective formulation and understanding their medicinal actions. This is a common characteristic of traditional medicinal systems all across the Old World, first documented regionally by the Egyptians, and later integrated into Greek and Islamic medicine which make up the foundations of Western herbalism and allopathic medicine.[1] Simply put, our ancestors understood that our bodies are part of the earth, as are the plants, each containing their own unique makeup of the fundamental elements that make life flourish: water, earth, fire, and air.

Treating imbalances in the body involves not only identifying plants that address the direct action or organ needing attention, but a thoughtful matching of the elemental constitutions that make up our very fundamental life force. All life exists in an ecosystem of living relationships that must work to recalibrate one another based on their unique personal baseline. Successful herbal formulation requires a careful consideration of these elements in both the plants being paired and the specific nature of the body and ailment they are addressing. It is like matching personalities for compatibility, and constantly adjusting to the changing conditions to ensure their harmony and thriving. This is why qualities like "hot," "dry/astringent," "cool," "moistening" are often indicated in the medicinal profiles about these cultural plants shared in this book. These qualities lend information about the energetic and medicinal action these plants embody, allowing for more customized support when applying them for treatment. They allowed our ancestors to also learn something about a plant's medicine on the basis of their flavors, the ecology they grow in, and the sensations they evoke.

For a very simplified example of how this might be applied, many herbs "support the respiratory system" in a variety of ways. If I am suffering from a sore throat due to a dry cough caused by exposure to wildfires, I might choose a cooling demulcent respiratory herb such as violets, which means it has moistening and soothing properties to the tissues of the body, instead of a more hot and stimulating respiratory herb such as oregano. Violets' cool and moist qualities are an imprint of the ecology they typically grow in, often found on riverbanks or blooming after the cool snowmelt as the earth beckons spring. Whereas oregano's hot and dry nature is mimicked by the rugged arid terrain it is found in and its preference for minimal water and full sun to thrive. Both our own bodies and the plantcestors' bodies are influenced by the energy of the ecologies we have developed in, which inform the constitutional balance at play. Likewise, if I am treating a person who generally runs cold, I might choose to center warmer digestive herbs such as ginger into their formula, rather than a cold one like dandelion. Or if I determine that dandelion is necessarily indicated for them despite its cold quality, I might balance it with the addition of warming digestive spices such as cardamom or fennel to neutralize its energy.

The liver is a central organ in ensuring health of many bodily systems, including our hormonal cycles, digestive systems, blood, skin, and more. But the liver is also a spiritual organ in the older traditions of our region. There are multiple phrases in Arabic that demonstrate its importance in our ancestral culture. One of them is "awladna akbadna timshi ala el ard اولادنا اكبادنا تمشي على الأرض"—"our children are our livers walking on the earth." Other similar phrases across the Crossroads use the liver as a term of endearment, referencing the utmost value prescribed to loved ones. The liver is considered a seat of the emotions, much like the heart in Western paradigms. This concept has an ancient history in our region.

In general, our traditional healing concepts never separated the body from the spirit, as most physical illness correspond to spiritual disturbances. Ancient remedies reflect the integrated nature of addressing both to resolve an ailment. But the liver held a special role in our ancient practices that remains present in our language till this day. In Mesopotamia, the liver was considered the central organ of vitality in the body, and the seat of the soul, emotions, and intelligence alike. When ritual sacrifices were made, the liver of the animal was sometimes dissected to glean divinatory information about the state of spiritual well-being and how to resolve imbalances affecting the soul. Ancient Egyptians had a god dedicated to protection of the liver and regeneration of the corpse in the afterlife, removing it and placing it in ornate vessels to be cared for by the deity Imsety.[2] The liver in our traditional understandings held as much importance, even more so in some eras and places, as the heart and the brain. While adherence to many of these concepts has changed over time, it is worth noting that the liver is in fact an unusual organ with the unique ability to grow back and regenerate itself, and its health upholds the integrity of so many of our bodily systems needed to flourish and grow. In the pollution and toxicity of the modern world, extra care towards our livers is certainly indicated for most if not all people. Thankfully, the earth's abundance and our ancestors' herbal intelligence supports this possibility in prolific ways.

This chapter highlights merely a few of the common wild greens that are used as food and medicine in Cana'an. There are countless other greens which vary from village to village and season to season, embedding a specific imprint of the uniquely diverse ecologies across our lands and the infinite medicinal, craft, and culinary cultures born in our co-creative relationships with these beloved places over the generations. Plantains, parsley, wild lettuces, legumes, and edible grains and grasses of so many kinds are not included here—a gentle invitation to familiarize yourself with the expanses of these traditions as they manifest across families and subregions.

HAMAIDA | حميدة | DOCK | *RUMEX* SPP.

The Arabic name for this plant means "sour one" and is used to refer to various sour weeds growing around the region and world, including oxalis, a most popular one amongst the children, who like to suck on its sour stems in early spring. Hamaida root (yellow dock species, to be specific) is a well-known remedy in the Western herbal world for its healing properties to the digestive system, liver, and blood. It is a bitter herb that helps produce bile to support the digestive process and help the liver do its necessary cleansing work. It also fortifies and cleanses the blood. The combination of these factors make it an excellent one in the treatment of menstrual disorders, supporting the body to process hormones while also replenishing iron loss from monthly bleeding. Both aerial parts and roots are used as medicine. The plant is antibacterial, anti-inflammatory, antitumor, antioxidant, antidiabetic, and has cardiovascular supportive and anti-aging qualities.[3] The root can have slightly laxative effects so may be helpful in constipation but should be used in moderation and consideration of one's personal constitution.[4]

In Cana'an, its tender leaves are used in food, often mixed with mallow leaves, spinach, or other milder tasting greens and stuffed into savory pastries, vegetarian versions of kibbeh, sautés, or even raw in salads. This was one Teta and I would often harvest on our morning walks around the garden to tend and gather whatever was ripe. Teta would then bring them to the kitchen, wash them with a bit of salt, and talk to the plants while she chopped them for our meal. The thread of connection to these plants grown with care continued even as she consumed them, Teta modeling the relational ethos of our culture even when it was just her and her plants in the kitchen. As with many of the other spring "weeds," these mineral-rich leaves gently cleanse the body, preparing it for spring after the rich heavier foods and relative stagnancy of the winter season. In Cana'an, these greens conveniently become available around the time of Lent when it is customary to fast from eggs, dairy, sugar, and meat for those in the Eastern Christian traditions. A wide variety of traditional vegan dishes are cooked during this season, many of which feature these spring greens. These ritual observations mirror the cycles of the land and the needs of the human body in transitioning both spiritually and physically, replenishing itself in sync with the plantcestral world about to bloom. Hamaida is high in vitamin C, fortifying the immune system. It is also a diuretic, gently cleansing the kidneys and potentially supporting conditions such as UTIs and urinary stones. As a poultice, dock leaves have anti-inflammatory properties, applied directly to wounds, insect bites, rashes or burns to provide a cooling relief.

One year, I came at just the right time of year to bring plenty of mallow and dock leaves for Teta, and she prepared for me a special meal that I had never heard of or witnessed before or since. The dish is called ma'aeekeh and is likely specific to her tiny riverside village, located in the Jezzine district of South Lebanon. Not even my mother was familiar with it when I described it to her. Ma'aeekeh is a simple sauté of onions with tender mallow and sour dock leaves, cooked with a bit of hot pepper, plenty of olive oil, salt and lemon, and served on top of flour kibbeh. Kibbeh is a traditional staple in our region that combines burghul (cracked wheat), spices, and either meat or various vegetables to create a dough of sorts that is then roasted or fried—except in the case of kibbeh nayyeh, which is a raw lamb delicacy customary in Lebanon. Kibbeh is either served plain in hand-pressed patties, in the shape of oval balls stuffed with other veggies or meats, or in a flat tray layered with stuffings in between and decorated with geometric patterns on top. There are many varieties of kibbeh, including numerous vegan ones that feature commonly during Lent or as side dishes throughout the year based on what is locally available. My Teta Renee was famous for making kibbeh of multiple kinds, stocking our freezers full with lamb and pumpkin kibbeh especially, which nourished us for months even after she died. Pumpkin kibbeh, or kibbet l'ateen, is stuffed with chard or spinach, dock leaves, chickpeas, sumac and onions, and a delicious sweet pumpkin and burghul crust. But in ma'aeekeh I experienced for the first time a plain version of flour kibbeh, simply prepared with burghul and flour to make small dough balls that drink up all the juices of the wonderful wild greens sauté. This is a delicious, economical, village-savvy food that I have only ever known my Teta Renee to prepare.

KHEBAIZEH | خبيزة | COMMON MALLOW | MALVA SYLVESTRIS

Mallow is a well-beloved food and medicine across Cana'an, with its first records of human consumption found in Syrian archeological sites as old as 3000 BC.[5] It is one of my father's favorite herbs and amongst the first ones he learned about as a child. His father once advised him to put a leaf in his shoe as a remedy for stinky feet caused by fungal growth that embarrassed him as a school kid. My dad found it nearly miraculous how effectively it worked, and still has a voice of awe when he reminisces about this childhood learning. Antifungal activity is merely one of the medicinal actions touted by this abundant spring plant.[6] It is also anti-inflammatory, antioxidant, antimicrobial, and hepatoprotective and has been used to treat everything from colds and sore throats to wound healing, menstrual pain, eczema, liver and kidney diseases, and even cancer.[7] In the mountains of Lebanon, it is used as a first line of defense for infections of any kind, especially those that affect the respiratory or digestive system. The whole plant is boiled as tea and taken regularly at the first symptoms of illness, sometimes also bathed in to ease rheumatic and arthritic inflammation. It is also used to treat constipation, kidney stones, renal infections, and skin diseases.[8] It is a deep leafy green dense with essential fatty acids such as omega-3 and omega-6, calcium, potassium, and magnesium, vitamins C and E, protein, and general nutrition, commonly prepared as a food across the region.[9] The flowers are particularly high in flavonoids.

Mallow has a demulcent quality, soothing and easing dry irritations especially in the respiratory or digestive system. This makes it an excellent option when faced with a dry cough or recovering from exposure to smoke, chemicals, or fire that has caused inflammation. The mucilaginous slime produced by many forms of mallow is also a common quality in a variety of plants that balance blood sugar, and the deep green leaves provide abundant iron and nutrients to fortify and restore the body. Its cooling quality makes it well suited for the hot summer season when it grows. Regionally, we often use its flowers or those of its relative khetmiyeh (hollyhock) in tea for similar purposes. In California, a Raramuri teacher of mine named Olivia Chumacero taught me to boil the roots of common mallow for respiratory infections, and a Yaqui friend and mentor named Ericka Zamora taught me to collect the seeds for protein and use as a survival food for sustenance in times of need.

There are several native varieties of mallow in California and around the world whose flowers, leaves, and roots are used similarly for their soothing demulcent quality, often with affinities to the respiratory or digestive systems, though most are not edible nor as nutrient dense as common mallow. The most famous is perhaps marshmallow, its root and leaves used commonly in Western herbal practice for exactly these qualities. Another favorite edible of this plant family in our cultural cuisine is mlokhiyeh ملوخية (*Corchorus olitorius*), known as "jute" in English, "saluyot" in the Philippines, "ewedu" in Nigeria, or "murere" in Kenya. Like common mallow, it is a deeply nourishing supergreen powerhouse that grows as a weed in its native habitats, indigenous to lowland tropical areas of Africa and parts of Asia, and adopted into the domesticated gardens of Cana'an via Egypt. This vegetable is a well-regarded food all across West and East Africa, all of Asia, and the diasporic communities who have become accustomed to it as a food.

Mlokhiyeh is probably my personal favorite dish, usually harvested in mid summertime in Lebanon and prepared by my family fresh after my Teta Hind and aunt spend generous time removing the leaves from their stems around the kitchen table while we laugh and gossip over coffee. Others prepare it from dry or frozen forms, particularly when it is not in season. It's another plant that grew well in my Teta Renee's diaspora garden in tropical Florida, where she would harvest, clean, process, and freeze it for us to use in meals in our California home when my mother needed something quick to cook. The dish has an ancient history, said to be eaten by the royalty of the Pharaonic era in Egypt, and highly beloved by certain Arab caliphates in colonial eras following. It is so beloved in our region that each country has developed their own variation on its preparation. In Egypt and much of Palestine, it is served as more of a soup, finely chopped with plenty of broth and all its slimy mucilaginous qualities celebrated and enjoyed, whereas in Syria, it's cooked as a thick sauté served with chicken and rice with less detectable slime. In Lebanon, it's in between the two—a stew less finely chopped than Egypt but a bit more brothy than Syria, usually prepared with chicken, lamb, or both, then served over rice and topped with raw onions soaked in vinegar with crispy flat bread on top. It is an elaborate dish that inspires rituals of personal plating, each family member with their own preference and order of toppings. This made it a memorable food when we were children.

All standard versions of this dish are prepared with crushed garlic, cilantro, coriander, and lemon to flavor the greens, though I've seen Tunisian recipes that add tomato sauce as well. In my family, we roast the garlic and an onion to add to the broth, my mother's side preferring a combo of lamb shanks and chicken, while my father's side is partial to only chicken. I was joyfully surprised when I attended the wedding of a dear Liberian friend of mine and served a fluffy green rice onto my plate only to realize the familiar flavor of this beloved plant, which I have since learned is commonly eaten this way across West Africa.

HINDBEH | هندبة | DANDELION | *TARAXACUM* SPP.

With abundant medicine for the liver and digestive system and leaves that offer cleansing to the kidneys, dandelion is a common spring weed with profound medicinal applications. All parts of the plant are edible. It is cooling, anti-inflammatory, antimicrobial, antiviral, antihistamine, bitter, and diuretic.[10] It is dense with minerals and vitamins and packed with antioxidants. It has some blood-sugar-regulating properties, and the leaves have been studied for their cholesterol-lowering properties and blood pressure balancing, offering valuable contributions to heart health. Both roots and leaves can help alleviate constipation and slug-gish digestion. It is tonifying and cleansing to the blood and lymph. It has even been used in treatment of cancer.[11] Common folk usages also include decoctions and macerations of the leaf or root to treat kidney stones, fevers, jaundice, rheumatism, headaches, blood diseases, an enlarged liver, kidney disorders, and indigestion.[12] A decoction of the root in tea or extracted in wine or arak is prepared as a purgative, or dried and ground as a coffee substitute for those who drink excessively.[13] In Cana'an it is typically prepared in raw form as salads, in my family with raw onions, vinegar, salt, and olive oil. Or more commonly, as a sauté with fried onions, garlic, and a squeeze of lemon on top served with flatbread. Some regions serve it on flatbread as a man'ousheh or with other greens inside savory dough pastries that we call ftayer. The consumption of bitter greens is a welcome part of the taste palate in our traditional foods, naturally supporting the liver and bile production, aiding the cleansing mechanisms of the body, which supports hormonal health, digestive health, and so much more.

B'ALEH—FARFHEEN | بقلة—فرفحين | PURSLANE | *PORTULACA OLERACEA*

Purslane is an edible succulent-like round leaf that has a mild tang to it. It is packed with omega-3 fatty acids, making it a unique garden weed excellent for supplementing a vegan or vegetarian diet. It has a cooling and soothing energy, is diuretic, emollient, anti-inflammatory, antiparasitic, antioxidant, antidiabetic, hepatoprotective, neuroprotective, cardio tonic, antiseptic, and gastroprotective.[14] It is used to cleanse and cool the blood, making it great for fevers, as well as headaches, high blood pressure, and blood sugar balancing. But most of all, it is used across Cana'an as a delicious food. It lends its unique flavor to nearly any raw salad, and grows as a weed in gardens all over the Northern hemisphere. I once was studying with a teacher in central Mexico where she prepared a delicious soup of this green, with the stalks still attached almost becoming like noodles. An Anatolian friend has shared a recipe where purslane is prepared doused in garlic yogurt as a refreshing side dish. Purslane is found in many of the salads prepared in regional cuisines across Cana'an throughout the year, including fattoush—a favorite made up of mixed salad veggies such as cucumbers, tomatoes, lettuce, onions, and sweet peppers, depending on what is locally available, and sprinkled with sumac, pomegranate molasses or lemon, garlic, and olive oil as a dressing, and toasted or fried bread on top for a characteristic crunch. Fattoush is a regional staple in our culinary tradition.

AKOUB | عكوب | *GRUNDELIA SPP.*

The visual landscape of summer in coastal Lebanon is characterized by strange purple globe thistles called shawk il jamal شوك الجمل (*Echinops* spp.), growing abundantly along streetsides and undeveloped areas.

They range from periwinkle shades to deeper violets and blues, so compelling in their bright color when nearly everything surrounding them has already turned golden from the heat. They grow tall, making their flowers visible even from far away—the quintessential image of the Eastern Mediterranean warm season. One day, I returned to my Lebanese village home to find the neighbor kids in my driveway crushing these spiky flowers with rocks so that they could eat the heart meat within. I was endeared to see these young children originally from an urban area of Syria continuing this ancestral foraging practice with such joy. Once upon a time, across the villages of Cana'an, these plants were commonly collected and prepared into culinary delicacies, using both their inner meat and their young shoots and leaves. It has become less common as other foods are available and the labor-intensive process of shelling these thorny plants is not so necessary.

Medicinally, this gorgeous weed is a potent antibacterial that also improves memory, hearing, and vision. It restores the function of fine nerves and neural centers in the brain, used in conditions of paralysis, neuralgia, inflammation, and damage of the spinal cord, as well as a tonic for cardiovascular health. It's commonly used in Lebanon's villages for treatment of renal disorders. In Syria, its seeds are ground for use as an anti-inflammatory and galactagogue.[15] Its roots are anticancer, and like most thistles, it has healing properties for the liver, used in Chinese medicine to treat hepatitis amongst other things.[16] High in nectar, it provides important pollen to bees during the summer season when many of the spring flowers have already gone dormant.

Consumed similarly is the young thistle plant (*Grundelia* spp.) known as akoub عكوب in Arabic. This thistle has a unique flavor, making the labor-intensive process of searching the mountains and combing through thorns worthwhile to food lovers all around our region. The flowers and young stems are harvested, thorns carefully removed, and then cooked in a variety of preparations—in soup, grilled, cooked with garlic yogurt, or preserved in brine or olive oil to enjoy later in the year. In spring, mountain elders have even fed me the flower raw after removing the thorny exterior. Medicinally, it's helpful in the treatment of liver diseases, heart health, digestive issues, bronchitis, and blood sugar regulation. In our folk medicine, its stems, roots, and seeds are also a treatment for colds and fevers, kidney pain, and constipation. Its latex is a treatment for swelling, toothache, skin discoloration, and inflammation.[17] It is antioxidant, anti-inflammatory, antiseptic, hepato-protective, and anti-parasitic. An elder from the village Bsharri in Lebanon insists to me that akoub is supreme for healing the bones, especially supportive to those who are unable to move or get up easily due to pain in their bones.

In Palestine, the harvesting of this early spring plant has become criminalized by the Israeli settler state, who claim that its presence in the wild has been diminished due to overharvesting hence the imposition of this law. But the plant has been traditionally consumed by Palestinians and all across Cana'an for hundreds of years. Surely, the development of settlement after settlement and the introduction of invasive plant species by the colonizing culture has been more of a threat to Indigenous plants and ecosystems—humans included—in recent decades.

Sadly, the Israeli settler state has used claims of sustainability and preservation to control the traditional harvesting practices of native Palestinian communities, in attempts to strangle local micro economies, further sever land-based access and relationships, and eliminate the continuation of culture—all hallmark attributes of settler colonial strategy. It is in fact the relationship between Indigenous peoples and their native lands that have allowed many of these plants to remain present and regarded in the culinary and medicinal traditions of our region for thousands of years. We have developed alongside each other, and the people of the villages where plants like akoub dwell have developed their own intelligence about the cycles of regeneration and proliferation by the species of native plants, adhered by traditional harvesting protocols. The real focus of sustainability should be to recenter these Indigenous technologies rooted in multigenerational relationships to place, and teach younger generations how to harvest in ways that ensure the life of these plants will not only continue but spread per this ancestral knowledge. This is our responsibility to our own traditions, ecosystems, and cultural legacy as we ensure their continuation. The Israeli law banning the harvesting of this plant as well as other staple cultural herbs including za'atar and maramiyeh (sage) claims that it is only banning the commercial harvesting of these crops, not the personal collection and use of them. However, a fourteen-year-old boy named Yusef al Shawamreh was killed by Israeli soldiers in 2014 for doing exactly this.[18] These traditions are our own—the people of Cana'an, and not for the jurisdiction of any outside government—no less the settler state economically and politically strangling the Palestinian population, who never needed to commercially collect and sell such crops before the colonists' presence. The settlements have severed access to lands we harvested and stewarded for years, and created unimaginable economic pressure to ensure the most basic needs for families living across Palestine. The self-determination and return of Palestinian lands to its people would be a more appropriate solution to the protection of precious wild plants and the cultures from which their culinary usage emerged and belongs.

TAYYOUN | طيّون | STICKY FLEA BANE | *INULA VISCOSA*

The resinous smell of tayyoun is the summer hallmark of coastal Lebanon, including my own village. For me, it is the fragrance of home and connects me to the deep memory and emotion that lives in my father's town where I dwell whenever I return to Lebanon. Even Fairuz, one of the most famous and nostalgic singers of the region, sings of "reehit il tayyoun" (the smell of tayyoun) in her sentimental song of longing for her grandmother's tenderness from the ghorbeh, the "foreign" state of living in diaspora.

Tayyoun is probably the first local plant medicine I ever learned about in my father's village, popular for its miraculous ability to heal wounds and stop bleeding quickly when applied directly as a fresh poultice, a tincture, or a powder of its dried leaves. My father and his cousins reminisce that as children, they felt safe knowing this plant was around, confident that as they climbed on rocks and ran around the coastal and mountain trails, any injury could be mended by this accessible plantcestor. Tayyoun is an incredibly resilient plant that grows abundantly and remains green year-round. In the height of summer when nearly every other shrub has gone dormant, tayyoun is at its prime, blessing our vision with remnants of green. It has bright, sticky resinous leaves that make it easy to recognize and lend its antimicrobial, antifungal, anti-inflammatory, and antiviral qualities to the wound-healing process. It is likewise laid out on baskets before drying fruit, helping ward off unwelcome critters and organisms and repel mold. Someone from a mountain village named Aa'oura in the north of Lebanon told me his village adds a couple leaves to jam when they are boiling it, adding a slightly aromatic taste and likely supporting its preservation as well as thickening.

Tayyoun is excellent for the treatment of everything from respiratory disorders to rheumatic and musculoskeletal pain, teeth and gum infections, fungal infections of all kinds, diabetes, high blood pressure, intestinal worms, fractured bones, and cancer. Taunt Violette from my village shared its usage for treating bedsores as well as athlete's foot. Imm Elias from the Bsharre area of Lebanon shared uses collected from all over North Lebanon, with elaborate stories about the plant's effectiveness at easing general digestive distress when taken in small consistent doses as a tonic tea, treating cancer, and healing bruises and hematomas when used as a soak. Infused in oil, it is used to relax muscles as well as remedy infertility.[19] I infuse the plant in olive oil to make a salve for treating muscular and joint pain, excellent for arthritis and rheumatism. Its infused honey or tea is supportive in treating respiratory disorders and easing inflammation in the body. It has helped me soothe an itchy throat and allergic cough attack. It makes an excellent steam or foot bath for pain relief, respiratory irritation, and treatment of fungal skin infections. In Palestine, one of the names for this plant is Rara, or Rara Ayyoub, referring to the Prophet Job (Ayyoub) who relied on this plantcestor to help him endure pain when he was being tortured. In the Book of Proverbs, the Bible notes this plant's aid in healing wounds, bruises, and abdominal ailments.[20] One aunty in my father's village shared a story about her neighbor using it as a hot compress for her daughter who had a horrible and painful ulceration on her hand. Her mother infused the plant in boiled water, then added sea salt. She soaked it in a towel and used it as a compress to dress her daughter's wound every day. It relieved her pain and inflammation better than the allopathic medicines were, helping her heal within a few days.

This potent plantcestor grows in the most degraded areas, thriving in compacted and eroded soil. It is extremely hardy, popping right back up even between the hardest rocks or after being chopped down to its root year after year. It blooms with generous flowers through the fall, making it valuable food for pollinators when few other flowers are available or nearly as abundant. Last but not least, I have used this plant to make an incredibly rich dye for natural fibers. Its flowers and leaves yield an incredible gold color with a slightly green undertone.

HASHEESHIT IL BAHAR | حشيشة البحر | ROCK SAMPHIRE/"WEED OF THE SEA" | *CRITHMUM MARITIMUM*

The Arabic name for this plant translates as "weed/grass of the sea." It is an almost succulent type of plant that grows directly on the coast, often in the crevices of the rocks that line the eastern Mediterranean shores. It has small yellow flowers that typically bloom in fall. In my father's village, one of my dearest elder friends named Jiddo Hanna Chahine used to share with me about the local plant medicines often, including this one. We would admire the ful فل (Arabian jasmine) plants in his garden, and he would share with me old remedies from the Arab medicinal traditions and local folk practices. He was one of the few traditional elders left in my father's village who still lived his day-to-day life nearly completely in interdependence with the local ecology. Every day, he would walk to the shore to catch local fish for food, and annually, he would collect his own salt and harvest this plant to supplement his family's diet. He would collect in the spring, when the shoots were still tender, and then pickle them. Eating at his house was a soulful immersion into the flavors and feelings of every element our village contained.

This plant is believed to benefit the thyroid with its exceptionally high levels of iodine, and the roots have been used by coastal communities as a general tonic as well as a remedy for constipation and liver support.[21] It is enjoyed as a humble village delicacy with a wonderful subtle flavor of the sea, alongside the small round fish native to the local coast. The American University of Beirut has validated its high levels of protein and nutrients, and suggest that its capacity to grow near salt water make it a promising source of accessible nourishment for poor coastal communities.

4

Man'oushet Za'atar: Street Food Staples

FRESHLY MADE MAN'OUSHEH on paper-thin warm mar'oo' مرقوق bread (known as shraq شراق in Jordan and Palestine) is another hallmark of my childhood food memory made by Teta Renee's diaspora universe. My mother and her family spent three months upon arrival in the US testing every brand of local wheat to find exactly the right combination that would ensure its perfection. Even in Cana'an, this bread requires particular skill and special varieties of flour that could withstand being flipped from arm to arm to stretch until thin as a sheet of paper. The women who prepare it practically dance with the dough like an appendage of their body, swaying in rhythmic motion to stretch without breaking, before they rest it on a big round pillow used to flip it evenly onto the round oven.

My family lugged the traditional dome-shaped saj oven across oceans and seas so Teta could continue this traditional culinary art, selling this bread to many in the diaspora who were finding their way to the US in the midst of wars and occupations at home. Their bakery became a meeting place and arrival hub for recent migrants and refugees from across the region, a place where many would find and support one another, and simply replenish in the comfort and nourishment of flavors, sounds, and welcome that reminisced home. My grandparents' house became a first pitstop for many newcomers via the connections made at the bakery, a natural extension of resources and hospitality considered standard in our cultural way. After my grandfather got mugged and lost his vision, Teta sustained a livelihood in Florida by making and selling this village bread for years out of her house. For us children, it was the hallmark of arrival to my grandparents' home. The first morning always began with her flipping dough at the saj in her garage while the smell of za'atar and fresh village olive oil wafted into the hungry kitchen. We would sit at the counter eating them warm, perfectly soft and crispy, and unlike anything you could buy in a market. It is no wonder I always left Florida smelling like za'atar. It will forever evoke the emotion of Teta's house, our sense of smell known to be the most ancient in our body, connecting us to primal body memories and epochs long past.

Za'atar wa zeit (za'atar and olive oil) is a staple in every household across Cana'an, with various versions and unique blends customized across villages and country lines. Za'atar is the name of both individual herbs (*Thymus capitus* and *Origanum syriacum*), as well as a spice blend eaten commonly at breakfast or prepared on flatbread as street food called man'ousheh, enjoyed at any time of day. The za'atar blend is a perfect example of brilliantly balanced medicinal herbal formulation with profound tonic capacities in our day-to-day diets. There are many versions of the blend, with multiple varieties in Jordan, Syria, Lebanon, and Palestine, and every household with their own variations on top of that. In some regions the blend includes cumin, marjoram, crushed biscuits called ka'ik, mistica, or other things. In Lebanon the standard ingredients include za'atar herb (regional thyme and/or oregano), sesame seeds, sumac, and sea salt. It is typically doused in olive oil or occasionally sprinkled on top of other foods as a spice.

In my family, while a large portion of my Teta Renee's Florida garden was dedicated to growing za'atar despite the unideal tropical weather, it was my paternal Teta Hind whose blend took precedence in our house. Teta Hind, or Tetitna ("our Teta") as I affectionately called her, made za'atar with generous proportions of sesame, toasted perfectly for an extra crunch that my mother loves. Every visit to Lebanon was completed with her praying hands getting busy in the kitchen to make huge batches of her special recipe especially for my mother to travel home with. For the medicinal aromatics of the thyme to come out, the sesame should be toasted in a pan first, then the fire turned off and za'atar mixed over it immediately while still warm to bring out all the volatile oils, and the sumac and salt mixed in just after. In Los Angeles, we have a perfect climate for growing potent za'atar, which my mother now dries and prepares herself in an attempt at Teta Hind's recipe. Like many mothers in our region, she would insistently prescribe this food before any important school exams or while studying, insisting that both the sesame and the za'atar encourage memory and stimulate the brain.

Za'atar as a blend is potently antiviral, antimicrobial, and tonic to nearly every organ in the body. It balances both flavor profiles and energetic qualities, curbing the dry and hot nature of the thyme with the fatty oils of sesame and olive oil, and offsetting the spicy sharpness of oregano with the sourness of sumac and the salt of the sea—its own sacred medicine in our cultural repertoire. It is delicious, healing, and fortifying to the body as a whole—a perfectly integrated medicinal tonic always in arm's reach at the kitchen counter, or when walking the streets of Beirut, or a day trip in the mountains nearly anywhere across Cana'an.

ZA'ATAR | زعتر | *ORIGANUM SYRIACUM* + *THYMUS CAPITUS*

As mentioned earlier, za'atar is a name used interchangeably for a number of native herbs from the *Origanum*, *Thymus*, *Thymbra*, and *Satureja* genuses that have very similar medicinal profiles. There are two

85

particularly common species that are used for their medicine and food regionally, *Origanum syriacum* (which is technically called zoubea'a زوبع but commonly referred to as za'atar) and *Thymus capitus* (which is often referred to as za'atar barri زعتر بري or "wild" za'atar). Both are native to the temperate areas of Mediterranean and West Asia, and they have a hot and dry energetic quality, lending a stimulating and circulatory action to the body. Za'atar is typically harvested in the summer season when it reaches its peak and flowers.

Origanum syriacum is antioxidant, antimicrobial, antifungal, antispasmodic, antiseptic, anti-inflammatory, analgesic, anti-parasitic, and carminative.[1] This plantcestor is useful in the treatment of all respiratory ailments, infections, and pulmonary diseases, including allergies thanks to its antihistamine properties (an infused honey would be wonderful for this). Its antispasmodic and expectorant qualities make it particularly helpful for coughs that have excess phlegm, and equally in boggy gastrointestinal infections as it simultaneously fights bugs while easing intestinal spasms and alleviating diarrhea. It has been useful in treatment of ulcers and helps to clear "wind" in the gut, including for infants which is amongst its many folk usages. It is also a diuretic, and used to treat headaches.[2] Due to the presence of thymol, it is an excellent candidate for oral health, supporting healthy gums with its antiseptic powers. Za'atar is an excellent menstrual tonic, balancing hormones, encouraging uterine stimulation and easing cramps especially when taken regularly. I met one farmer in South Lebanon named Abou Kasem who swore that his daughter and wife taking one capful of distilled za'atar water per day blessed them with perfectly regulated pain-free cycles. It also supports the liver and has been studied with some promising anticancer and tumor-fighting potential.

Za'atar supports the cardiovascular system and healthy blood circulation throughout the whole body and nervous system, increasing memory and stimulating the brain, hence its common attribution to students across Cana'an and its diaspora. It is a powerful nervous system tonic with studied antidepressant and neuroprotective qualities,[3] and also relieves muscle pain and stiffness in the joints and is used as a remedy for rheumatism. It is highly antimicrobial and antiviral, appropriate for cleansing the environment or body from potential infections. Along with internal uses, it makes an excellent steam, smoke, essential oil, or bath for this purpose. It has been helpful in the treatment of headaches, bug bites, and wound healing, and is a good herb for treating candida overgrowth and other fungal conditions. My Teta Renee swore it was a primary benefactor in her infused herbal oil for the treatment of lingering skin itching that no allopathic remedy would heal. In the folklore of the region, za'atar has a strong association with ritual cleansing. It is a likely theory that this was the "hyssop" of the Bible used by Jesus to perform his healing miracles of both body and spirit. It was also used in the Old World to repel against the poisonous venom of snakes. In our Re-membrance Circles, za'atar revealed its consistent power to support creative practice and break energetic stagnation, inspiring clarity and self-trust.

The plant is very important for pollinators and especially depends on them for effective pollination. A study performed in Jordan documented that wind plays almost no role in the pollination process of the *Origanum syriacum* flowers, but that twenty-one different species of bees were recorded visiting it, including eight that were never before seen in Jordan.[4] There is some inherent wisdom in the fact that my own and most families traditionally harvest za'atar after it has flowered, ensuring that both we and the pollinators can benefit from its generous gifts and continue its reproduction forward. This is unfortunately becoming an increasing problem for this plant regionally.

Za'atar is the most heavily harvested and traded plant in Lebanon and has recently been put on the "near threatened" list by the UN Development Programme.[5] Increasing competition in the market has led to earlier and less sustainable harvesting practices, including repeated collection of early shoots that prevents long-term reproduction ability as the plant is unable to drop seeds. Poverty has driven an increase of unskilled harvesters from surrounding areas making pilgrimages into mountain villages of Lebanon, where they pull such wild plants from the roots in order to sell as much and collect as quickly as possible. Increasing incidents like this are cited in my conversations with friends from numerous towns surrounding my own, sadly. Farmer Abou Kasem has established a farm in the Nabatieh region of South Lebanon especially dedicated to the sustainable propagation and harvesting of this beloved cultural plant. Developing methods of agricultural tending for this wild plant has supported the economic sustenance of his family while ultimately contributing to the plant's longevity in our wild for more years to come.

His is a model that could show promise across the region as demand for za'atar continues to grow. While maintaining a relationship to the wild growth of this plant is important culturally and ecologically, relearning how to care for these plants in our own gardens may encourage greater respect for their reproductive cycles and temporarily alleviate the burden on our wild landscapes as they endure increasing stress from urban development, climate change, and commercial overharvesting alike.[6] It is righteous for us to tend rather than take from the wild stands we have cherished harvesting from. In some years, for example, we can protect and support their replenishment for a while by supplementing with food from our home and community gardens. Particularly because of those exploiting this plant for commercial purposes, a balance of both relationships may be necessary as we face the changing conditions of this time. To allow at least a portion of the plant to go to seed and then help spread them nearby in the fall is one simple way to facilitate rather than tax the longevity of this precious cultural plant, while deepening a different kind of relationship and reciprocity of care.

In addition to the dry za'atar spice blend, this plantcestor is commonly prepared as a tea, a distilled water extract, pickled (the wild variety in particular), infused in oil, utilized as a steam or bath, and eaten fresh in the form of salad. Throughout my childhood, my mother's village was difficult to visit due to the fact that it was occupied by Israel along with the rest of South Lebanon until the year 2000. Since nationality in Lebanon is passed down paternally, me and my siblings had ID cards locating us in my father's northern village, which required special measures to permit visitation to these occupied areas. We did not have much immediate family living there any longer, so this wasn't something my parents bothered to do often. I have very few early memories of my mom's village as a result. What I remembered most vividly was the uneven terrain of the roads en route to her village, the vibrant garden of my great-aunt's house, always with fresh fruits and coffee on the porch, and the chilling remnants of a shot-up hospital left over from the civil war with warnings to tread lightly due to the presence of mines.

I starkly remember eating a fresh za'atar salad one of my first times there as an older child. I was with my aunt and her husband on a rare visit to my great-uncle Kamel's house before he died. He lived in a humble village home with one of the old-style toilets that required squatting over a hole, an experience that was new to me. He hosted us outside, a customary preference across Lebanon's village in warmer seasons. I vaguely recall him wrestling around the back garden as we waited for him, rinsing off veggies. Not long after, he brought out a small bowl of delicious salad made with fresh za'atar leaves topped with sliced raw onions and dressed with village-pressed olive oil, vinegar, and salt. The pungent kick of the wild leaves was perfectly offset by the sourness of the vinegar and the sweetness of the onion, and everything felt like it had just come out of the earth. I have had the same salad many times since, but never with such a lingering impression as the one prepared by his hands, grown in the generous terrain of my mother's riverside mountain village.

Za'atar was the first of the edible cultural plants whose traditional harvest has been criminalized by the Zionist government in Occupied Palestine as well as the Golan Heights (Occupied Syria).[7] Since 1977, anyone found in possession or trading the plant in any amount can be imprisoned for three years or fined, or in Yusef al Shawamreh's case with the akoub plant, even killed. There is no village or city in Palestine, Syria, Lebanon, and Jordan that does not lean on this medicinal blend in our daily livelihood year-round. Arous za'atar, a simple flatbread wrap of this spice spread with generous olive oil, constitutes an economical meal on the go for people all across our region. A school lunch, a breakfast before work, a late night snack. To criminalize our generational relationship with this plant is so explicitly an attempt at Indigenous erasure and control. It is part of the ongoing colonial effort to sever and absorb Cana'an's ancestral legacies of sustenance, and legally punish the kinship with place and its continuation amongst our Palestinian and Syrian siblings under settler occupation.

5

Floral Foods

FLOWERS ARE A SENSUAL delight of this earth that have rightfully earned our reverence as human people. Each shape and color, each fragrance, the whole spectrum of expression they embody and evoke have endowed healing and holy symbolism for the rituals of our lives. They have a way of animating the creative force present in alive beings, nudging that God part of us in this enchanted way. The flower world is one of true sensual immersion, effortlessly drawing us into the experience of our sensory body, while awakening the transcendent nature of our deeper spirits. They expand us, softening that line between worlds by imbuing our physical vessels. Whether they crown our heads or adorn our graves, flowers' energy comes with meaningful healing in human rites of passage since the beginning.

Flowers prepared in the life-giving element of water have their own significance. In a modern practice, one version of this preparation is called a flower essence—a vibrational remedy made with the delicate collection of blooming flowers in spring water then exposed with intention to the sun's light for a number of hours and preserved with 35–60 percent brandy. This solution is put in small dropper bottles and a few drops are consumed orally for treatment in the tradition of Dr. Edward Bach, a British doctor and homeopath who developed a system of flower essence therapy.[1] He believed this new model was the true "medicine of the people," and it has become renowned across the globe since it first developed in the early 1900s. Whereas tinctures are macerated extracts of plants that optimize their biochemical components, flower essences are lightly infused waters that heal through an imprint of their energetic essence. They are indicated for treating the emotional and vibrational roots of imbalance, distress, and illness. They require very low dosages, minimal plant material, are easily reproducible, affordable, and typically have no contraindications.

While Bach was the main person involved in the systematization of this technique in its modern application, the use of flowers and the elements for healing are as ancient as time itself. Traditional iterations of this wisdom manifest in flower baths and similar infusions of water and other sacred elements, such as the sun or moon, to bless or cleanse the spirit in a variety of ways. One Afro-Brazilian grandmother named Maria Alice Campos offered in a workshop I attended with her that flower essences are specifically indicated for supporting the transformation and healing of consciousness, noting them as a most appropriate medicine for our times. I could not personally agree more with her assessment.

In the traditions of the Crossroads regions, flower waters are prepared most commonly through distillation and incorporated into our daily practice and cuisine in a variety of ways. Distillation is an ancient practice whose origins may come from Sumeria or Egypt thousands of years ago, and whose modern tools and practices were refined by Arab alchemists in the eighth century AD.[2] In particular, Abu Musa Jabir ibn Hayyan designed the alembique pot, also known as a still. The origins of this practice were fundamentally spiritual in their nature, the process of separating the vapor of a substance seen as a purification and concentration of its deepest essence. Hence why alcohol is sometimes referred to as "spirits." This process applies in a metaphor of spiritual rebirth and elevation as human souls as well, and it utilizes all the sacred elements of creation to assist the process towards this transformative means.

Distillation can produce alcohol as well as herbal hydrosols, such as orange blossom water and rosewater, and is also where "essential" oils come from. The plantcestors are immersed in water in the copper pot, which is heated by fire that releases all their volatile oils into the steam, which is cooled as it collects and drips out completely transformed, its spirit concentrated into an elevated material form which is deeply aromatic but with no plant matter to detect. On the very top of this soulful water, the essential oils rise in a layer to the top and can be collected with a syringe and used in perfumes or otherwise, a tradition which also has deep roots in our regional medicine practices. In the Western herbal tradition, these distilled waters are typically used for topical purposes as sprays or in lotions. But at the attar عطار, the Arabic word and concept for apothecary, this form is the primary internal extract employed as medicine, similar to how tinctures are utilized in the west. Many aromatic herbs, flowers, and alcohols are produced through this ancient technique, which originally was bound as deeply to the planetary transits as it was to the earthly elements leveraged.

While the alchemical philosophy of practice has lost quite a bit of traction in current-day Cana'an, the karakeh كركة, or alembic still, is a common tool present in many households to this day. Arguably, the best quality aromatic waters and alcohols in our region can be found in unlabeled and recycled jars filled by village aunties and grandfathers who still integrate this craft into the preservation of annual harvests. These sacred waters are used in mundane ways in our cultural cuisine and home apothecaries daily, the floral ones being amongst the most precious and celebratory.

ZAHER EL LAYMOON—BOUSFEIR | بوصفير—زهر الليمون | ORANGE BLOSSOMS—BITTER ORANGE | CITRUS AURANTIUM

When my mother's family first migrated, their livelihood was tending a citrus farm on land owned by another Lebanese family. This terrain was familiar to them, because they came from a part of South Lebanon known for its citrus production. There are a variety of regional culinary preparations involving every part of the orange. Most of them come from the bitter orange tree (*Citrus aurantium*), known as bousfeir in Lebanon and khishkhash خشخاش or zefer زفر in Palestine (whereas khishkhash is the name for opium poppies in Lebanon—note these are not the same plants). Orange blossom water or mazaher was one of the primary goods my mother would prefer to purchase from her village, where the quality and authenticity could be ensured due to the crop's local presence and traditional customs. This old-world species of orange is the one specifically sought for the production of mazaher and other medicines, still a bit feral in its nature, preserving aromatic potency and medicinal chemistry. Its flavor is a bit like the combination of grapefruit, lemon, and a tangerine at once. The tree is native to South and East Asia, common throughout Cana'an, and by a stroke of luck also present in Florida where my mother's family arrived. Every spring, Teta Renee and my family would collect the petals of the zaher (flowers) in their grove to distill them in her copper karakeh she managed to haul somehow from Lebanon. They would do so carefully, removing only the outer petals and leaving the inner stamen so that it could continue to be pollinated by the bees and mature into fruit. Citrus is one of the symbols I associate with my mother, born of these contexts.

My mother's family eventually relocated to another part of Florida, where they established a small bakery dedicated to Arab sweets, where these oranges and their floral waters make a particularly prominent appearance. My mother apprenticed under a professional Lebanese baker there, mastering the preparation of everything from ba'lawa to halawet il jibneh (a sweet cheesy dough infused with syrup or stuffed with cream) to ma'amoul (crumbly buttery cookies stuffed with dates, pistachios, and walnuts) and beyond. Orange blossom water is central to each of these desserts, continuing the thread of relationship between this tree's essence and my own family's labors of cultural love in the form of food. The flavor and aroma of orange blossom water is so quintessential in our cultural context that the name mazaher alone carries it; it translates literally to "the water of flowers," defining somehow what "flower" itself even means. In the cuisine of Cana'an specifically, I would say that it is even more prominent than rosewater, which makes similar appearances but is used more sparingly for most dishes.

There is no part of the orange that goes unused in our kitchens; the inner peels are cooked in syrup and wrapped to make a marmalade that my mother and aunt especially love. Some areas use the fruit's juice in the common breakfast ful mudammas, a hearty fava bean dish with origins in Egypt, usually prepared in Cana'an with fresh tomatoes and herbs dressed with olive oil, garlic, and lemon or, when available, bousfeir juice. The juice is prepared in another regional dish specific to my mom's southern family. It involves a stew of il'as قلقاس (malanga root) and chickpeas sautéed in onions and tomato sauce with the juice of bousfeir to add a uniquely tangy flavor not quite comparable to any other citrus fruit alone. It becomes thick with the flesh of the root vegetable, and turns a compelling orange hue due to the tomato and bousfeir base. This is another dish I've only ever seen in my mother's kitchen but presume may be common in other southern villages due to the prevalence of these particular crops.

Mazaher also features prominently in a hospitality custom across Cana'an where guests are offered the option of regular black coffee or ahweh baydah, which translates to "white coffee," an infusion of orange blossom water with sugar served hot like tea in a small demitasse cup. Mazaher is an aromatic remedy used to ease anxiety and depression, calm digestive distress, and fight insomnia, making it a wonderful alternative to black coffee when served at night.

Alternatively, a cool drink variation is the sensuous inclusion of orange blossom water into the regional preparation of lemonade, particularly famous in the Batroun district of my paternal lineage. This floral addition is one of the cooling comforts my mother used to prepare for me when I was feverish or ill as a child, and one I delight in for refreshment on any regular summer day. My Teta Renee added drops of mazaher to a bottle of water or rubbed directly on the gums of colicky or restless babies. It is also a common ingredient in skincare, spritzed on the face as a toner or incorporated into creams, its essential oil known as Neroli regarded amongst the most valued alongside its sister plant rose, across the cosmetic and perfumery industry worldwide. Its aromatic oils have also been used as an effective aid for relief of pain and anxiety during labor.[3] The peels are likewise helpful in the treatment of digestive disorders such as indigestion, constipation, ulcers, and heartburn, as well as a calming effect on the nervous system and the muscles of our body. All parts of the bitter orange have been used for their antimicrobial, antioxidant, carminative, anticancer, antianxiety, antiinflammatory, and antidiabetic qualities. Its fruit and peels have been studied with promising effect in the treatment of cancer, supporting the immune system, helping the body's mechanism to break down tumors, and preventing metastasis. Its juice helps fight infections including salmonella and staph. Its floral aromas are used as a sedative with relief for depression and anxiety.[4]

WARD | ورد | ROSE | *ROSA DAMASCENA*

Maward is the sister of mazaher. "Ma' ماء" for "water," and "ward" for "rose," meaning rosewater. This is one of the first and most important herbal distillations from the ancestral traditions of our region, used similarly in the contexts of desserts as well as a common facial toner, an eye wash, and a potent medicine for nearly every organ in the body. Of all the beloved plants in my apothecary, rose is amongst the ones I reach for most often, incorporating it into numerous formulas and leaning on it often as a singular remedy of its own. Rose is an underrated panacea of medicine for the body and soul, with several wild species growing across the region and world, as well as important heirloom species cultivated by our ancestors specifically for medicinal use. Amongst them is *Rosa damascena*, known to us as ward jouri. In the mountains of Lebanon and beyond, old grandmothers and grandfathers can be found lovingly growing this treasured rose and distilling it in their homes for use throughout the year. It is even made into a delicious floral jam and a sharab (syrup) colored with beet juice for a bright pink coloration.

Sharab is diluted in water to make a refreshing summer drink, which I personally like to mix with a splash of pomegranate juice for extra tanginess and refreshment. The hips are also prepared as teas or jams in parts of the region, as they're packed with vitamins C, A, B1, B2, B3, K and E, niacin, bioflavonoids, iron, calcium, magnesium, and phosphorus.[5] All parts of the plant can be used as medicine.

Rose's association with the heart is not merely symbolic. This plant has tonic usages for the cardiovascular system, as well as treating colds and flus, supporting the brain, nerves, immune, and menstrual system. It is anti-inflammatory, antiviral, antimicrobial, refrigerant, emmenagogue, aphrodisiac, astringent, tonic, nervine, diuretic, hepatoprotective, analgesic, and diaphoretic.[6] Its astringent petals and leaves have been used in healing of the ears, mouth and gums, headaches, the digestive system, and beyond, and its fragrance has been used to clear the mind and strengthen mental faculties. It cools the liver, has been employed as a salve to heal burns, ulcers, and hemorrhoids and cool fevers. Its extract in water or as an alcohol tincture has even been studied with effectiveness in the treatment of HIV, preventing and slowing down viral replication.[7] Ibn Sinna noted that the rose "addresses the soul," with a calming effect on the heart, mind, and spirit alike, strengthening the brain and capacity for comprehension and sharpening the senses. It may be helpful in the treatment of anxiety that causes heart palpitations as well as other mood disorders such as depression and nervous stress.[8] The smell of rose was understood as a primary vessel of its medicine in the Old World, where it has been regarded as a spiritual medicine with purifying qualities to the heart and associated with the Prophet Muhammad as well as the Virgin Mary, who now and again performs miracles of apparition by crying rosewater tears out of her statues tended as altars all across places like Lebanon. This grandmotherly plant has endless medicinal uses for essentially every system in the body, and has been utilized by our ancestors for over 5,000 years across the region, with precious species such as the jouri co-created specifically for medicinal applications for generations by our stewardship and care.

BANAFSAJ | بنفسج | VIOLETS | *VIOLA ODORATA,* SPP.

Violets beckon the start of spring in the hills and mountains of Cana'an. They carry an association with renewal and rebirth, amongst the first flowers to bloom after winter's snowfall. My mother reminisces about their common use as a dyeing agent for easter eggs when she was a child, the violet's flesh gently wrapped around the eggs and covered with tight stockings to leave an imprint when dipped in onion water. Violets are small unsuspecting plants, with deep green heart-shaped leaves that sprawl in low-to-the-ground stands scattered with purple flowers. They can thrive in the most neglected conditions, though they tend to prefer some coolness and moisture. Violets are so humble they are often bypassed for their power. I am convinced their purple hue has something to do with their regenerative secrets.

The first time I worked with this plant, I was on the verge of a downward emotional spiral in a town where I felt isolated and out of place. A few minutes of meditation with merely a couple drops of violet extract swept through my body like a pristine river, clearing stagnations and debris of physical and feeling kinds, and completely transforming my state of mind in no more than an instant. Their association with grief is common in folklore—"violets are blue"; they support the release and expression of repressed and difficult emotions, helping us "feel to heal." Violet was one of the first plantcestors to "show" me just how profoundly flowers can heal us, and how potent the vibrational impact of their spirit can be on our own. The violets effectively interrupted a spiraling emotional descent, helping me move effortlessly through the densest places inside of me while filling me with a sense of embrace and love in its trail. I could feel this full somatic *knowing* that I was supported—an "I've got you," imbued with the rare intimacy and loyalty of a lifelong friend.

I have since affectionately incorporated violet leaves and flowers often into remedies for emotional restoration, or instances characterized by stagnated or sinking states. Violets epitomize the intelligence of water, softening us within a knowing of the life-giving element's sheer strength. Just as their energy encourages "flow" on the emotional level, they are reputable for their gentle support in the lymphatic system— the cleansing waterways of our own body, which help keep us healthy. Violets are expectorant, antitussive, diuretic, and antiseptic. The leaves and flowers are cooling and soothing, used traditionally for treating respiratory illness and colds, inflammation of the intestines and stomach, as a diuretic, an antiseptic mouthwash, and to treat skin irritations.[9] They have been used to eliminate cysts, tumors, and as a poultice for cancer in the breast.[10] In Lebanon, they are also used to treat sprains, for sore eyes, hemorrhoids, heart disease, rheumatism, jaundice, and as a laxative (their roots are emetic). Their leaves and flowers are pleasantly sweet, edible as an addition in salads, candied and sugared in some parts of the world. On occasion in Lebanon, you can find their flowers prepared into a jam.[11] Medicinally, they are used as teas and topically in oils and poultices for their emollient and soothing effect. In Lebanon, they are used as a tea for lowering hypertension.[12] They make an excellent child-friendly syrup for instances of sore throat. I often infuse them in honey likewise. In Syria, they are used as foot baths for insomnia.[13] There are numerous viola species that grow generously all over the globe, aiding some of the most painful discomforts of our inner lives as humans as they signal hope, spring, and rebirth.

KABAR | كبار | SPINY CAPER | CAPPARIS SPINOSA

In early summer, the golden wheat stalks and grasses are interspersed with these thorny ground-sprawling plants with deep green leaves and almost whimsical white flowers with tall stamens that poke out of the center in a deep shade of fuchsia. You can see the flowers nearly melt away as the day gets hotter, lasting for just a moment to lend its color to the landscape. This plantcestor has always captivated me visually and energetically, embodying sharp resilience and ethereal and fluidly feminine qualities all at once. It is basically a "weed," growing between tiles and sidewalk cracks nearly as persistent as tayyoun and in the same ecosystems usually, and an underutilized weed at that. I cannot tell you how many times I have found a plumber or technician removing these plants from my garden offering me unsolicited "help," as they see this plant as a thorny nuisance to "real crops."

It may not be conscious to many, but pickled capers featured in bourgeois restaurants across the Western world are in fact the flower buds of this unsuspecting plant growing abundantly across the Mediterranean. They are one of our most ancient sources of food, gathered lovingly by the god Enkidu as an offering of food in the Sumerian Epic of Gilgamesh nearly 5,000 years ago, alongside jasmine, figs, and fragrant flowers. The caper plant was so significant to our ancients that its creation story is cited in the Sumerian cosmology known today as Enki and Ninhursaga. The story takes place in the sacred paradisiacal land of Dilmun, where Ninhursaga, the Mother Goddess of fertility, pregnancy, creation, transformation, and nurturance of living things, creates the caper plant alongside seven others. They sprout from the semen of Enki, god of wisdom and freshwater, when Ninhursaga wipes and buries his semen in the ground from between the weaving goddess Uttu's thighs. This act is Ninhursaga's response to Uttu's lamentations about Enki disrespecting her, as he had seduced and discarded several other women in her lineage before her. The eight plants born from this act are so precious to Ninhursaga that when she returns to Dilmun to find that her lover Enki ate them all, she casts the "eye of death" upon him, cursing him before she leaves the world again to a place where nobody can find her; eight organs of his body become afflicted for each of the plants he devoured. Worried for Enki as he begins to die, the other gods send a fox to find Ninhursaga and reason with her, leading her to a change of heart eventually; Ninhursaga is the only one with the power to heal Enki. She takes him into her vulva where she inquires attentively about each pain, transforming them one by one through the birth of eight new healing gods. He repents for his indiscretions against the women and the land upon his healing.

In this story, the creation and consumption of the caper plant leads to the creation of more gods, more healing, and more life on earth. The power, duality, and necessary respect of the mother as an embodiment of the earth, and the earth/mother's creative and sexual capacities as ultimate healers and transformers, are highlighted in the themes of the story and the various iterations of life and desecration that take place. This matriarchal myth is considered by some scholars to be the origins of the Garden of Eden stories and the biblical inception of life on this planet as recorded in Genesis.[14]

All parts of the sacred caper plant are medicinal. Caper is antioxidant, anti-inflammatory, antidiabetic, anticancer, analgesic, antispasmodic, antiviral, antifungal, carminative, aphrodisiac, emmenagogue, expectorant, stimulant, diuretic, neuroprotective, and an all-around tonic. It is classified as warm and dry energetically. Different parts of the caper plant have been used to support everything from blood pressure regulation to intestinal worm removal, thyroid function to cancer treatment, malaria to liver disorders, skin issues, toothaches, kidney and spleen disorders, digestive issues, infertility, headaches, and more. They are a panacea of medicine and nurturance for nearly every organ in the body. Capers are also high in fatty acids, proteins, and fiber.

While their consumption as food is not nearly as common in modern-day Cana'an as one might suspect considering their prominent presence, soil deposits and archeological excavations in Syria and Palestine have proven their usage as food in Cana'an for over 10,000 years.[15] The plant's use as medicine has been documented amongst Greek, Egyptian, Iranian, and Chinese traditional medicines for thousands of years, as well as in Ayurveda and traditional Arab medicine. Most parts of the plant are edible. Its ability to tolerate salinity makes it a useful nutritive food and remedy in coastal areas where access to fresh water is an issue. The plant is high in fibers and B and E vitamins, the buds also high in vitamin A, C and K. It is rich in iron, calcium, potassium, phosphorus, magnesium, zinc, and manganese.[16] It is used regionally as a blood purifier and diuretic, to relieve digestive discomfort, treat kidney stones, support the liver and spleen, and treat eczema.[17] In Lebanon, it has also been used for treatment of malaria. Bedouins in Palestine use it to treat infertility and erectile dysfunction. A common folk remedy shared with me in my paternal village and across a number of villages in North Lebanon is use of the root in alleviating pain and inflammation from spinal discs or in the joints.

The root has a very hot energy, so it must be treated with care. It is mashed then wrapped with a towel or thin cloth applied as a poultice to the area where pain is present, making an herbal heat pad of sorts. Bedouins boil the leaves and use it similarly for the same purpose. They are highly anti-inflammatory hence indicated in a variety of remedies for arthritic and musculoskeletal pains as well as sciatica. In other parts of the region, the seeds are crushed to treat painful periods as well as infertility.[18] Their remedies are countless, expansive across all systems of the body, many different types of herbal and culinary preparations, and various parts of the plant. I recently met a microbiologist in Lebanon named Hanan Bou Najm who has dedicated herself to reviving local knowledge and practical use of this plant and others. She emphasized the probiotic support offered by pickled fermentations of the flower buds, leaves, and berries respectively. She emphasized that the berries carry similar medicinal qualities to the flowers but are much higher in calcium. When I asked her about the medicine of the leaves, she said, "They are our local moringa," meaning a deeply nutritive, mineral- and vitamin-dense "superfood," growing generously across our land.[19] This incredible medicine grows abundantly alongside the people of Cana'an, the earth providing answers and remedies much closer than we often seek.

TEEN—JEMMAYZE | تين—جميز | FIG— SYCAMORE FIG | *FICUS* SPP.

One of the stars of our summers are the plump fig trees yielding colorful fruit across the region for thousands of years. An ancient archeological site dating back to 4000 BC was found in my village near Batroun several years back. It was believed to be a village itself, in which amongst other things many seeds were found in clay pots, documenting seed saving or farming endeavors and giving us a glimpse into the crops most common since that time. There were four primary kinds found there that are still staples in our culinary traditions today: wheat, olives, grapes, and figs.

Figs are in the floral food section because their fruit is in fact an inverted flower, pollinated singularly by a specific wasp who binds their destinies together. Besides only the varieties of common fig (*Ficus carica*) we are used to enjoying as fruit across the globe today, our region used to be full of sycamore figs (*Ficus sycomorus*), or what we call in Cana'an jemmayze trees. My Palestinian friend Muhammad Abu Jayyab shares a colloquial name for the jemmayze tree, "shajar sabeel شجر سبيل," meaning "tree for those on a journey." He shares the way these trees offer reprieve and nurturance to those who are far from home in our cultural references—an appropriate symbol for the migrational crossroads and expansive diasporas that embody our region, and the ways we tend home and those who are far from it as a sacred task wherever we may find ourselves. Jemmayze trees were once so prominent in Lebanon that a whole section of Beirut is named after them, though most have been chopped down over the years due to urban development unfortunately. One huge one still stands at the very entrance of the city from the highway, greeting me each time I arrive from my village to the city center.

The jemmayze trees are African in origin and considered sacred in Khemetic Egypt, where they carry an association to the maternal sky goddesses Nut, Isis, and Hathor, who mutually carry a role in the provision of nourishment to the soul of the dead. The fruit is connected with the resting place of the soul, as well as a place where lovers meet. It was often grown next to pools or offering basins in the temples as well as in people's homes, and it appeared in various remedies in the Ebers Papyrus, an ancient record of Egyptian medicine.[20] Interestingly, in a document dating 2575–2565 BC from Snefu, the first king of the Fourth Dynasty in Egypt mentions these figs as "the tree on whose fruit the people of the Land of Cana'an grow and flourish." Another famous record from the Sinuhe Papyrus dating 1800 BC makes reference to the figs that grow in Cana'an, which they called "the fertile land of Yaa."[21] Cuneiform tablets from Mesopotamia in the Akkadian period also feature the importance of figs as an offering to the deities and to one another, as well as a medicine made from both the fruits and leaves to treat headaches and respiratory distress respectively. There are countless references to figs in Greek and biblical stories, and all across the Mediterranean, India, and beyond. Many of them are associated with life's drunken pleasures, the goddesses, and the bounty of the earth. Some suspect that this was the original forbidden fruit of the Garden of Eden.

Figs' leaves, fruit, latex (milky white sap that oozes from its branches), and bark have been referenced in traditional medicine systems all across the Eastern traditions for their use as anti-inflammatory and anticancer agents, since researched with proven potential by modern science.[22] They are also antibacterial, antispasmodic, and laxative, and have been used in the treatment of digestive issues, cardiovascular health (to lower cholesterol), support the regulation of blood sugar, and their latex to heal warts and other skin ailments.[23]

All around Cana'an these trees are found growing both wild and domesticated. I have cited the jemmayze tree at the temple of Karnak in Egypt, and seen the common fig growing wild at Astarte's throne in the temple of Eshmun (Phoenician deity of healing) in Saida, Lebanon, in the Byblos temple dedicated to the local goddess Baalat Gubal (known to the Greeks as Atargatis, the mermaid goddess of fertility) as well as Isis, and countless other sacred sites of our ancestors across Cana'an today—including the archeological village recently found in my own town. They are abundant in association with our regional goddesses and grandparents alike, who are known to share these homegrown floral fruit with pride all across our cities throughout the summer season, as they have been for thousands of years. In addition to enjoying them fresh, we often prepare them into a jam with sesame seeds, dry them for consumption in winter, and make them into molasses (though this tradition is less common today).

ZA'AFARAN | زعفران | SAFFRON | CROCUS SATIVUS, SPP.

Saffron is a native of Iran and Southeast Asia known worldwide as one of the most expensive spices in the world, made from the carefully collected stamens of the crocus flowers. Saffron imbues everything it touches with a sunny yellow tint and has been used ethnobotanically as a dye as well as a medicine. This plantcestor is a powerful aid for the treatment of depression and anxiety of severe and mild kinds. With species native all across the Mediterranean and the Crossroads regions, crocus are a fall-blooming flower whose harvest typically takes place around November. Saffron features as a common ingredient in most Iranian dishes as well as several Mediterranean ones, particularly in rice dishes and sometimes desserts. It has an earthy, sensual quality to it, but also a soulful flare, energetically endowing a lively quality to all it touches.

It is considered hot and moist energetically. It is highly antioxidant, an expectorant and sedative, emmenagogue and adaptogen.[24] It is used in pain relief and the treatment of asthma, supporting the heart and brain, balancing blood sugar, aiding neurological health, and antican-cer activity. Some villages in Lebanon regard it highly for its antiseptic, antispasmodic, and tonic uses, making its flowers or leaves into a tea to treat children at the onset of infections such as mumps, chicken pox, or the measles.[25] It has a number of other healing actions on the body per regional traditions, including lowering blood pressure, cholesterol, supporting digestion, and easing insomnia, mood disorders, and hor-monal imbalances.

SAHLAB | سحلب | ORCHIS MASCULA, ORCHIS MILITARIS

There are over fifty gorgeous orchid species that grow natively across Cana'an, including the sahlab flower whose tuber is used as a flavoring and thickening agent in desserts, rice puddings, winter milk prepara-tions, and sometimes in the making of Arabic ice cream, which has a stretchiness a bit like gelato. The sahlab orchid is considered generally fortifying to the health and body, providing sustenance with mineral-rich components while also being an aphrodisiac, calming the nervous system, soothing digestive distress, and soothing inflammation with its mucilaginous properties.[26]

Unfortunately, this plant has been overharvested over the years, and its common cultural use has been replaced with artificial reproductions for the most part, due to its lack of availability in the market. I do however still see it while walking along the village trails in rural parts of Cana'an, lending its gorgeous towering fuchsia flowers to the spring landscapes. Since its tuber is the part used, harvesting of this plant does not allow for natural reproduction, and so its presence in the wild needs a great amount of extra care and protection.

LOOF | لوف | BLACK CALLA LILY | *ARUM PALAESTINUM*

The stunning black calla lily would captivate the eye of any viewer, deep hues of midnight enshrouding the tall stamen as though the whole universe lives inside its black velvet core. It is rare to see such deep dark colors in the flower world. This plant is native across Cana'an and other parts of the Mediterranean, and is beloved as a medicine and a food alike, especially in Palestine where villagers eat the leaves cooked in lemon and olive oil. Take caution, as the raw form of this plant is toxic. This plant and others of the loof (calla lily) family are employed regionally in the treatment of cancer, constipation, as an abortifacient, vermifuge, bone strengthener, wound healer and cleanser, and in the treatment of kidney stones. In traditional Arabic medicine, it is also used to heal disorders of the circulatory system, poisoning, and beyond.[27] Interestingly, this rather phallic-looking plant is specifically studied in support of prostate cancer treatment, synching up with the "doctrine of signatures," an ancient method of gleaning insight about the medicinal qualities of plants based on the way their shapes mimic particular organs of the human body. This plant demands such attention that it is engraved on the ancient walls of Thutmose III's temple at Karnak, brought to Egypt from Cana'an over 3,000 years ago in an era when he asserted rulership over Canaanite territories. The plantcestor maintains this tribute till today, with whatever mystical secrets and symbols are within contained.

6

Fruit of the Tree

SUMMER AND FALL in the Mediterranean are a chain event of one delicious fruit after the other, including both domestic and wild varieties and several highly medicinal ones. Amongst my personal favorite are mulberries, myrtle, prickly pears, cherries, green almonds, and pomegranates. The list is endless, and in many cases the extra harvest gets turned into dibis دبس (molasses), sun-dried snacks, sharab شراب (syrups), or mraba مربى (jam) to extend shelf life and availability for supplementation in winter months, when most fresh crops have gone dormant. All of them are dense with vitamins and minerals, but it is perhaps less recognized how many medicinal actions our wild fruits in particular have. The folk use of these accessible foods as medicine has become less common over the years, though these are exactly the medicines that have sustained our lineages for generations and that can continue to hold us steadfast in difficult times.

Many of these wild trees have been stewarded with care by our ancestors because of their nourishing capacity and healing, demonstrating our relationship not just with our domestic gardens but with the whole of the lands we live on. We have had rituals over time of stewarding wild trails just as well as our own gardens, our hands making up parts of the landscape just as the animals that "prune" them in their seasonal consumption and the crafting of their nests and dens. My grandparents' stories are full of long walks between one village and the next, from one small town to the city capital, all traversed by foot until relatively recently. Along these slow journeys, these trees have provided shade, replenished nutrients in transit, and acted as familial landmarks. So while we have many domesticated fruits beloved in our cultural cuisine and home gardens, I dedicate some special attention here to merely a few of the "wild" varieties that make up our local ecologies without the need for additional water, fertilizers, or any manipulations of the natural territory. These trees are the ones that mark the paths our recent ancestors walked in their own day-to-day lives, our endearment towards them cultivated by these intimate and generous relationships to place. Fruits are incredible in that they culminate every season's minerals, drink sun and moonlight for months, and are visited by nearly every pollinator you could imagine before they arrive to our bodies with their nectar. Their rich nutrient content is the cumulative life force of so much elemental abundance and relationship, feeding all our cells and organs with irreplaceable sweetness, sunshine, and sustenance.

SUMA' | سماق | SUMAC | RHUS CORIARIA

Just down the road from my great-uncle's house is the original village of my mother's family, resting alongside the river Awali in South Lebanon. A big earthquake in the 1950s destroyed many of the homes, obliging my own family and others to move to the neighboring town. Every time I go there, I drive down to the original village, where the ridge overlooks a gorgeous river that many of my mother's childhood stories in the village center around. Her family has a tiny piece of land along that ridge, left to them by my grandparents, where the foundation still stands for a house, unconstructed. This tiny plot of land is surrounded by sumac trees and the sound of running water below. If I go at the right time of year, I can see the heads of the sumac berries drying in trays on village balconies. Truth be told, these balconies are always covered in some of earth's bounty, each season its own plantcestor featured. My mother's trips to her village always include visits to local neighbors for the purest, freshest harvests of wild plants tended by hand and heart year-round, with no cutting corners around the traditional processes of ideal preparation.

Sumac is a shrub-like tree found in subtropical and temperate regions of Africa, the Mediterranean, and West Asia. There are native species that also grow across the Americas. It has a cooling and astringent quality and sour-tasting berries that yield a deep red hue after which it's named in Arabic. Its berries are typically ready for harvest in late summer. It is a generally fortifying herb, endowing a quality of strength and vitality resembled by its blood-red color.

Sumac is a powerful herb, practically a panacea. It is rich with all kinds of minerals, vitamins, and antioxidants, especially potassium and calcium, as well as vitamin C. It is also dense with fatty acids and a multiplicity of medicinal actions for nearly every organ in the body. It is an excellent blood builder and can help prevent blood clots. Its potent astringency indicates it in any conditions that are characterized by excess liquid. Swelling, boggy infections, excessive urination, sweating, or bleeding. In my family, it is most notoriously reached for when someone has diarrhea. We sprinkle some on eggs or boiled potatoes to help settle the stomach and fight infection in the gut. It is a common spice in many of our daily dishes, serving tonic health upkeep. Sumac is a potent anti-inflammatory and immune-supportive herb, excellent for flus, colds, viruses, fungal and bacterial infections of every kind. It is used to treat headaches, muscle aches, and general body pain, and has healing properties for the heart, kidneys, liver, blood, and lungs.[1] It is hypoglycemic, helping stabilize blood sugar as well as lower blood pressure and cholesterol, and its astringency can help stop excessive bleeding (including after birth, during menopause, or otherwise). The astringency and diuretic qualities support the treatment of kidney infections and UTIs. It has liver-protective qualities, and has been used to yield breastmilk (though it is contraindicated beyond moderate food doses during pregnancy).

Sumac has been studied recently with some promising possibilities in treating covid, thanks to its neuro-protective, cardiovascular, immune-modulating, and anti-inflammatory qualities.[2] It improves circulation and reduces inflammation in the blood vessels and is considered a mild cardiovascular tonic. It's been used for treatment of hemorrhoids and varicose veins and is antimalarial. While we don't think about a lot of these medicinal attributes in our daily consumption of sumac, the cultural cuisine of Cana'an most certainly integrates this powerful tonic as a daily fortifier and defense for our whole system. While its most common form of usage is the berries dry, ground, and separated from the seed, its leaves can also be used as a tea for medicinal application. Because of its high tannins, sumac has also traditionally been used as a dye for leather and fabric.

Za'atar is only one of the many recipes that features sumac in our cultural cuisine. Sumac is used as a garnish on all kinds of foods, including eggs (my favorite), as well as a primary spice featured in several other meals. Salads such as fattoush are one common example. Msakhan مسخن is a Palestinian dish prepared with sautéed onions, chicken, and sumac wrapped in olive oil–slathered bread. Sumakieh سماقية is a name in this spice's honor, used to refer to various dishes across the region that feature it as a primary flavor. One version is kibbeh sumakieh كبة سماقية, known in the Beqaa region and other villages of Lebanon, where flour kibbeh is served with a sour sumac sauce on the side, prepared with lentils and potatoes, or the flour kibbeh is served with sumac mixed into the dough. Another is the Gaza sumakieh, a dish of lamb, chard, and chickpeas made with sumac, and I do not doubt that there are other versions of sumakieh prepared across the region. A common sumac dish my own family makes is a'adass bi hamod عدس بالحامض (lentils in lemon), a lentil and chard soup spiced with generous sumac to give a sour flavor. But probably my favorite sumac dish of all is il'as قلقاس, which is fried, boiled, or roasted malanga root served with a side dip of sumac and garlic infused in water to give a delicious sour-savory flavor. Sumac berries infused in water with sweetener added make a wonderful pink lemonade, a recipe I learned from Indigenous communities in my diasporic California home, whose colloquial name for their native sumac tree is "lemonade berry."

A'ANAB | عنب | GRAPES | *VITIS SPP.*

It would not be complete to talk about the medicinal food repertoire of Cana'an without discussing grape and its derivatives. Grapes have been cultivated regionally for thousands of years, originating from the wild grape ancestor *Vitis vinifera*, native to the Mediterranean. The fruits themselves are vast in their medicine, all parts of the plantcestor utilized in the cuisine of Cana'an. They are eaten fresh, dried as raisins, or prepared into molasses. Wild grapes are prepared into a sour liquid called husrum حصرم, which was the predecessor to lemon in many of our traditional foods. The leaves are eaten raw when they are tender, used as a bread-like vessel for tabbouleh in my family, deliciously tangy and soft. They are also used fresh, pickled, or frozen to make warak a'arish ورق عريش or warak dawali ورق دوالي, a stuffed grape leaf dish with vegetarian and meat variations regionally. One of my personal favorite foods is the lamb version, with lamb chops lining the bottom of the pot, a stuffing of spiced ground lamb with rice, plenty of olive oil and even butter, and lots of lemon juice. The flavor of the grape leaves and lemon saturate the lamb, which melt with tenderness by the time the cooking is over. It is delicious! It can be served with yogurt on the side, and some variations use a tomato-based sauce instead of lemon as well.

Grapes, especially wild grapes, are nearly miraculous in their potency as medicine. They are antiseptic, anti-inflammatory, analgesic, cardio tonic, circulatory, hemostatic, diuretic, and full of minerals and vitamins. They treat everything from colds and flus to menstrual disorders, digestive distress, pain, heart and blood deficiencies, skin irritations, and even cancer. Juliette De Baïracli-Levy was a Turkish and Egyptian herbalist whose life was spent in the company of traditional peoples all over the world exchanging cultural herbal knowledge. In her book *Common Herbs for Natural Health*, she asserts that wild grapes are so powerful in their restorative capacities that if a person found themselves with an illness lacking further remedies, their salvation may be found fasting exclusively on the fruit, leaves, and tendrils of these plantcestors for a period of time.[3] It is no wonder that grapes have featured meaningfully in the sacred and medicinal repertoire of Mediterranean peoples and beyond for thousands of years.

The earliest evidence of wine production is from clay vats with sediment aged around 8000 BC in the Caucuses. The earliest record of wine as used for medicine specifically is from a Sumerian box from 2500 BC, and again in 2200 BC, where it features in a cuneiform tablet documenting the oldest remedy in the world.[4] Wine as medicine has been documented in ancient Egyptian medicinal records likewise, both territories where grapes did not grow easily but were imported with regard to its profound value medicinally. Records suggest that the Canaanites were central in the spreading and exporting of wine across the Old World and to Europe, whose wine-making grapes are thought to have roots in Cana'an to this day. Wine itself was a medicine, used both internally and as a poultice for a wide array of remedies. But it was also a menstruum within which other herbs were extracted and formulated for potency.[5]

While the practice of alcohol tinctures is not as common across much of Cana'an today, and the contemporary culture of Islam further discourages the presence of alcohol in many parts of the region, alcohol tinctures through herbal wines, beer, and hard liquor in fact all have origins in our region, where they have been produced and utilized for remedy making for thousands of years. Furthermore, their origins are embedded within the sacred codices regionally, be they alchemical, Pharaonic, or Abrahamic. Jesus himself is associated with the grape vine and with wine in particular. His first miracle was turning water into wine in the city of Qana in modern-day South Lebanon. Jesus's blood is ritualized with wine in the church to this day, and in fact, a passage in the Bible says the Good Samaritan heals the wounds of a beaten traveler with no other than olive oil and wine, our two steadfast plantcestors till this day. Wine has become more of a social drink in the modern context, and its production remains a notable craft in Lebanon and parts of Palestine especially.

Furthermore, our local grapes are highly sought for the production of our beloved arak عرق. Arak is a distilled grape alcohol infused with anise seed and produced traditionally across the villages of Cana'an. It is made by fermenting grapes, distilling them three times with yansoon يانسون (anise seed), and allowing them to age in a clay vessel for a year or more before being ready to drink. Yansoon is a trademark flavor of the region, lingering with a licorice-like sweetness and countless medicinal actions from respiratory to menstrual to digestive support and immune fortification. "Arak" refers to "sweat" in Arabic—araq عرق, a name referencing the distillation process in which the "sweat," or steam, of the plantcestors distilled is collected. The commercial industry of arak production is centered almost exclusively in Lebanon, but one of the pleasures of visiting the mountains and local towns is tasting the exceptional homemade brews. The drink is served in a tall shot glass with ice, then topped with water that magically transforms the clear liquid into a milky white due to the anethole component in the yansoon seeds. When I was a child, my Jiddo used to drink one small kess (glass) every day with his lunch, a tonic that every child in my maternal family was familiar with from a very young age due to this ritual. There were certainly some tricks played between children, convincing one another to "drink some milk" only to be met with the sharp flavor of this strong beverage.

My Teta Renee would likewise lean on this cultural drink as a remedy for a sore throat, rubbed on the gums of a teething baby, and an antibacterial digestive agent amongst other things. Regionally, it is necessarily served with any mezzeh, but especially with our raw meat dish kibbeh nayyeh alongside raw onions and mint; the arak ensures any bacteria in the raw meat be thwarted before affecting your organs, and the flavors complement it divinely—another natural medicinal food formulation executed with communality and the artistry of complementary flavors. Arak, like wine, maintains the healing cardiovascular elements of the grapes as well, with antioxidant, antiseptic, and anti-inflammatory properties intact. Celebratory and medicinal at once, this drink is a cornerstone of Cana'an's food legacy.

HEMBLAS—RIHAN | ريحان—حمبلاس |
MYRTLE | *MYRTUS COMMUNIS*

There's a story in my paternal village about Taunt Violette, whose house was right on the coast where a myrtle bush grew near the rocks, and she loved it very much. The myrtle became a large shrub providing shade for fisherman and others, until one day, somebody cut it down. She was so angry that she cursed the man who cut it with the rage of her words, damning the hand who desecrated her tree. The next day, he got into an accident of some kind that permanently injured that same hand. Taunt Violette's hands, on a contrary note, blessed nearly every new baby in the village with her postpartum massages, bathing them with the leaves of this exact hemblas plant to heal their skin whenever infection arose. She is the one who eagerly awaited the opportunity to perform zalghoota in our village, a chant of blessings to the bride and groom traditionally offered at weddings by elder women. They start with the rhythmic phrase "*aweeeehhha*" followed by riddling prayers of good wishes and familiar village anecdotes about the dynamics of new marriage, and completed with the collective vocalization of our ululating celebration call "*lililililili.*" How the joyful utterances and righteous rage of village aunties travel alike. How words are prayers, potentized and reflected by the energy of this mystical plantcestor she partnered with so intimately, and whose stories over the ages reminisce this living legend somehow. The mother's love that devotes itself to life's stewardship protects it just as fiercely.

Hemblas, known in English as myrtle, is a fragrant shrub native to the Mediterranean, with gorgeous white flowers that bloom at the height of summer and berries that grow ripe in fall. The leaves have an aromatic quality to them and can be used as an alternative for bay leaves. There are a couple different varieties of this tree that grow natively around the Mediterranean—one that produces yellow berries, another bush with black berries, and one with no berries that is traditionally planted at gravesites in Syria, where it's known by the name rihan (note that this is the same name for basil in many parts of Cana'an yet this is a completely different plant). Syria is not the only part of the region that subscribes a spiritual position to this common plant; its leaves are used as protective medicine across Iran's diverse ethnic communities, from the Kurds to the Afro-Iranian communities of the southern gulf coast where I commonly observed it in incense blends for spiritual protection and cleansing. I spotted the plant at important shrine areas within multiple Zoroastrian temples when I visited there in 2016, in whose tradition it's associated with Ahura Mazda, their Creator deity.

Myrtle is dense with folklore all across the Mediterranean, where the Black Madonna is said to live under its boughs in Italy, and it helped the Greek goddess Daphne shapeshift into its form so she could escape the rape attempts of Apollo.[6] In the Abrahamic traditions, Adam took a myrtle tree with him when he left the Garden of Eden, and Jewish tradition recites another story in which a woman accused of being a witch was transformed into a myrtle tree after being murdered by her town. There is yet another tale from Arabic folklore that involves captive French men who were transformed into a myrtle bush until the protagonist of the story could defeat the spell cast by the witch who placed them there. The through line of stories about myrtle seems to involve the mystical realms, protection, shapeshifting, and a particular association with feminine power. It also carries an association to the Venusian deities across the Mediterranean pantheons, with a particular association to love and (re)birth. In rural Lebanon, there are still reports of using this plant in religious rituals associated with the Eastern churches. Some churches use it to endow divine blessings and expel evil spirits, as well as in funerary rites as symbols of eternal life.[7]

In contemporary Cana'an, myrtle is often enjoyed as a fruit. It has a peculiar flavor with a strong astringency, but they are one of my mother's favorites and I have grown to quite regard them in my own medicinal practice as a result. This beautiful plant is antibacterial, antirheumatic, antiviral, astringent, carminative, analgesic, antifungal, tonic, and so much more. It is an excellent tonic for the cardiovascular, reproductive, and respiratory systems, lowering cholesterol, healing bronchial infections and coughs, and aiding fertility for all sexes. It can support healing from diarrhea and general indigestion, help heal gum infections, hemorrhoids, and acne, and heal conjunctivitis. Decoctions can support treatment of urinary and bladder infections, while baths and internal applications may ease rheumatic pains. It is an excellent tonic for the nerves—both flowers and berries alike—and in India has been used to treat epilepsy. It is generally a healing plant with restorative qualities for nearly every organ in the body. In Italy, it is turned into a delicious liquor called mirto, and in ancient Egyptian texts the leaves were crushed to treat fever and infection.

KHAROOB | خروب | CAROB | *CERATONIA SILIQUA*

Interspersed between the native ecosystem of oak, pistachio, and strawberry trees across the coastal scrublands of Cana'an are the generous kharoob trees whose bean pods have provided sweet sustenance for animals and humans alike across the ages. In September, the pods mature and are collected from the trees typically to be prepared into thick molasses that supplies minerals, protein, and medicine year-round. The part of my paternal village my family's house is built in contains some of the oldest kharoob trees, including one in our back yard which me and my parents can be caught snacking underneath in hot summer months. There are not many large native trees that grow across the coastal landscapes, making kharoob's large canopy a grace on multiple fronts.

Carob has become well known around the world as a "chocolate substitute," though their tastes are quite different. Kharoob is naturally sweet with an earthy flavor. It is typically eaten as dibis bi tahini دبس بالطحينة in our cultural cuisine—a swirl of carob molasses and sesame tahini dipped with bread for a simple dessert with layers of rich flavor. I recall this dish from a young age as it was my father's favorite treat, transporting him perhaps to his childhood home every time a relative managed to bring us a jar from his village. Molasses is prepared of many fruits in our region, which can all be used interchangeably in dibis bi tahini depending on what is available locally. Some common alternatives are grape molasses or date molasses. Other preparations for dibis il kharoob (carob molasses) include sfouf, a cake-like cookie prepared in some regions with carob molasses, olive oil, anise, and flour, deeply localized flavors dense with nourishment and accessible to make.

Most molasses concentrate the minerals and vitamins in these crops, making them excellent supplements of iron and vitamins. Kharoob in particular is also high in protein, phosphorus, and calcium, and has antimicrobial, anti-inflammatory, and antioxidant actions. One of its folk uses is as a remedy to constipation, though its pulp is also used in treatment of diarrhea. It is also excellent for respiratory health, having been studied with some promise in the treatment of chronic obstructive pulmonary disorder and lung cancer. It promotes healthy cholesterol and general heart health, and even the treatment of diabetes. Kharoob has a low hypoglycemic index, making it an appropriate alternative to processed cane sugar for diabetic patients as it does not create spikes in blood sugar. It is a good supplement for those with blood-deficient anemia, providing iron in a more digestible form than most pills—a wonderful supplement for prenatal fortification—and it has been used to treat heartburn, coughs, digestive complaints, infections, intestinal worms, pain relief, and more. A decoction of the leaves is used for lip sores and herpes.[8]

Carob bean gum has been extracted for use in food preservation and was also used in the mummification process in ancient Egypt. The wood has been used traditionally for fuel and carpentry. Its seeds were traditionally used as a measuring unit for gold, after which the measuring units are named after kharoob to this day—"carat" (*Ceratonia* is this tree's Latin name). It has been a good source of food for both livestock and humans, and it is economically significant to the rural economies across the coastal region.[9] I can only presume that this native food played a significant role in the sustenance and survival of Lebanese communities during the grave famine of the early 1900s when nearly 40 percent of the population was killed due to the lack of wheat and the political blockades and rationing of the Ottoman empire at the time.

One of its names is St. John's Bread, since the Bible mentions it as the food he ate when traversing the desert. I wonder if this name carries a double meaning, hinting at its use for nourishment when bread was not in fact available. Kharoob is a staple food and distinctly regional flavor with unique significance to our native lands, where they are endemic and abundant.

ZA'AROUR | زعرور | HAWTHORN | *CRATAEGUS* SPP.

Famous worldwide as a supreme heart medicine, in Cana'an za'arour is most beloved as an edible wild fruit, sold commonly in local markets and harvested across villages when they mature starting in August. My mother reminisces about long walks to the village spring with her uncle, how tired they would be until they saw the za'arour tree. If they were lucky enough, it would be fruiting with some berries close enough to reach and replenish them to complete their walk. She says they were not that common, making their appearance feel special and celebratory. In addition to being eaten fresh, the fruits are sometimes prepared as jams locally, and in Lebanon, some families have made them into a wine for use as a heart tonic.[10] There are several species that grow regionally and natively all across the Northern Hemisphere where they are thick with folklore across the board. In the Mediterranean, the white flowers have symbolized purity and have been used in spring celebrations, fertility rites, and marriages for thousands of years. In ancient Anatolia, the Hittites noted the tree for its protective qualities and spiritual cleansing from "evil" and the "wrath of the gods." They were used as a threshold plant, growing around the edge of sanctuaries.[11]

Medicinally, all parts of the tree are used, including the fruits and seeds, the bark, and the flowers and leaves, which are amongst the most common teas found in bulk in the apothecaries of Cana'an. They are most famous as a powerful heart tonic with a very effective hypotensive action, and hence it is advisable to take caution if one is on prescription heart medications. They are also sedative, antimicrobial, anti-inflammatory, hypolipidemic, antispasmodic, diuretic, and antioxidant.

They support healthy blood circulation, and have been used regionally to support kidney health, eliminate gallbladder and kidney stones,
reduce fever, stop coughs and ease menopausal symptoms including
curbing instances of hemorrhage, treat anxiety and headaches, insomnia, diarrhea, and diabetes.[12] The hard wood has been used to make
tools.[13]

GHAR | غار | BAY LAUREL | *LAURUS NOBILIS*

Bay laurel is associated with everything good in our region. My grandmother used the common phrase "nefaa mitil zeit il ghar نافع مثل زيت
الغار"—"as beneficial as the oil of bay"—to describe the essential value
in any exceptional person or thing. Bay leaves are an ancient plantcestor
used traditionally across Cana'an to cleanse—the body, the spirit, and
our foods. It is one of the first medicines introduced after birth, massaged into the skin of newborns to bless them, and between their toes
and armpits to prevent fungus and odors as they grow.

The trees grow abundantly across the Mediterranean, leaves boiled
into nearly every stew or broth prepared in our region to remove the
zankha of meat and add an aromatic flavor to the base. "Zankha" is a
culturally specific word describing a particular stench of meat, fish, and
eggs when they are prepared in particular ways or the plates they were
served on are not cleaned properly. Bay has been used in the preparation of saboon baladi صابون بلدي (traditional soap) for thousands of
years, with potent antimicrobial, antiviral properties, as well as analgesic, antifungal, and anti-inflammatory qualities that support healing of the skin, relief of pain, and relieving all swelling, burns, bruises,
and other topical conditions, as well as a hair tonic. Internally, they aid
digestion, support the kidneys, and help regulate diabetes. In ancient
Greece, their boughs were used as crowns to adorn heroes and victors.
They were also associated with the delivery of oracles, as they were
chewed upon and waved by the priestess Pythia while she delivered
sacred prophecies. Romans associated them with immortality and utilized them in ritual purification.

BUTUM | بطم | MASTIC TREE | *PISTACIA PALESTINA*, SPP.

The butum tree has a mystical energy across Cana'an, storied with the sites of saints and local folklore in the places where its oldest trees grow. Varieties of this tree have been found in excavations over 7,000 years old, demonstrating the lengthy relationship our regional ancestors have maintained with this plantcestor.[14] This tree is part of the Pistacia family, with a number of species in our region that all contain medicine. Some such as *Pistacia palestina* grow abundantly across the lowland scrublands of the Eastern Mediterranean, and others such as *Pistacia lentiscus* that mastic gum, or mistica مستكة, comes from or the *Pistacia terebinthus* have become more endangered over the ages. This species also contains the tree that produces fisto' فستق, the pistachio nuts which are enjoyed both fresh and dried in regional dishes and desserts across the region. All these species contain medicine, mostly associated with the fruits and the musky resin that grows from their immature fruits and bark. I delight in rubbing their sticky beads between my fingers to smell their resins, and making infused oils for use in healing salves, particularly the common and pervasive *Pistacia palestina* species.

They can also be eaten as a crunchy snack, raw or roasted, lending a mildly sour flavor. One aunty from the northern Lebanese mountains tells me they are eaten or brewed into a tea in her village to treat kidney stones. They are antibacterial, anti-inflammatory, antioxidant, anti-ulcer, antidiabetic, cardio-protective and anticancer, and have been used for over 5,000 years as medicine for healing the skin, digestive system, blood sugar balancing, oral care, as an incense, and in culinary uses.[15] They add a distinctive flavor to delicious Arabic ice cream, are sometimes ground and added to za'atar mixes, and are commonly used to preserve and thicken jams and other desserts. They also are the base of traditional chewing gum regionally, elastic while also supporting gum health. In spring, tender shoots of the *Pistacia palestina* species are collected and consumed steamed or in other food preparations.[16] This is known by the name of shabshoob شبشوب.

Species of this tree have also maintained a ritualistic quality and spiritual importance across the ancient Mediterranean, particularly the *Pistacia terebinthus*. My friends in Jordan involved me in a group of artists pilgrimaging around the sites of the oldest remaining trees around the country, thick with local stories involving the honoring of saintly figures and revered ancestors where each tree dwelled. In Cana'an, the tree was associated with fertility and the cultic worship of Asherah. The Egyptians imported the resins for use as an incense, in purification rituals, and mummification.[17] The plantcestor carries a symbolic relationship to the life-death-rebirth cycle across our ancestral traditions.

MAHLAB | محلب | SOUR CHERRY | *PRUNUS MAHALEB*

Similarly to sahlab, the pits of cherries from the mahlab tree lend a distinctive flavor to regional desserts, prepared into a milk pudding known as mahalabieh مهلبيه seasoned with rosewater, and playing an important role in the dough of our ancient ritual dessert ma'amool معمول, alongside mistica مستكة. Mahlab has anti-inflammatory, antioxidant, antifungal, antibacterial, and sedative properties.[18] Like sahlab, it is considered generally fortifying, with high protein and plenty of carbohydrates, and a generally tonic effect on the body. It is easing to the digestive system and used in folk medicine to treat kidney stones and urinary issues. It is consumed boiled with sugar as an intestinal tonic, for treatment of dysentery, as well as to ease the nerves.[19]

Zeitoon, Tree of Life

FEW ANCESTRAL FOODS impact me with the power that zeitoon does. The bitterness of fresh olives softened in sea salt rewires me cellularly. When I taste them, I can feel my spirit vibrate, as though my body is expanding and condensing at once. It's like a part of me swirls into timeless universes I cannot see, and in doing so ushers the rest of me back to myself. My body arrives, returns to itself almost abruptly. In an instant, I regain a sense of place in the moment I occupy, its visceral physicality and whatever is beyond it, restored completely to fullness for some time. Zeitoon is holy food for me, doused in the sea's residue —sacred doubly. It is a food that re-members and recalibrates me at a soul level.

I cannot even recall the first time I ate zeitoon; it is synonymous with us, so embedded in our home that I cannot separate it from my life's beginning. I do however remember the first time I had the fortune of being in Lebanon near the fall when harvests occur. My mother taught me a simple preparation to cure the fresh harvest, allowing me to eat them before being pickled in jars of brine for longevity. We aim to collect them while they are still green, but not too small. In her recipe, we simply pound each olive with a rock or mortar and set them in a dish with coarse salt for a few days until they sweat and sweeten a bit. They transform into a darker, deeper hue of green when they are ready to eat. In this form, their true flavor is fully experienced, their natural bitterness and thick texture preserved while drawing out buttery rich oils from inside their flesh yet undiluted by salted water. My mother simply adds some fresh lemon and we eat them with village flatbreads of any kind for a divinely medicinal treat. This preparation does not preserve very long, so it is only prepared in the beginning of the crop in a very small batch, making it a seasonal delicacy of sorts and my personal sacrament.

I recall moments of my mother pounding olives rhythmically on the back patio while I sat with her in our California home, the fruits collected from local trees in our diaspora neighborhood or brought to her by friends from their gardens. We have one tree of our own which my mother cures from annually, often sharing jars with her friends in return. While many of our cultural foods maintained some level of consistency in taste and feeling through my mother's hands, likely due to the fact that we lived in a place with a similar geography, weather, and landscape to Lebanon, I will admit that olives are one exception. These fruits appear to be more impacted than others by the flavor yielded through the soil, sun, and elements of place, or perhaps it is the generational relationships of endearment that enshroud these village harvests with a particular touch of potency and love. Whatever it is, they simply taste and feel different when they come from their native Cana'an. My family would savor whatever jars managed to make their way to us from either of my parent's villages, and it is always obvious to me when the oil used in a meal comes from the blad (homeland). Plant-based foods record the literal flavors of place, each mineral in the soil, each cycle of sun and rain feeding them particularly, zeitoon seemingly more than most. This is part of why cultivating relationships with the crops native to where we live is so crucial—even more so than exclusively replicating our ancestral cuisines from ingredients foreign to place. Perhaps this is also why eating the fresh harvests of zeitoon in Lebanon had such a visceral impact on me, the quality and feeling of the fruit quite different than those we maintained regular access to, and more resonant to the memory in my generational body in its unique way.

In Cana'an, zeitoon harvest arrives in the season of thinning veils. Come autumn, we transition into darker days when even the plantcestors settle more deeply into the underground world of roots, evoking the spirit of our own roots and the honoring of our ancestors. The earth communicates a natural continuity across life's cycle, this time of dormancy and darkness simultaneous with that of falling seeds that gestate future lives. In the fall, the roots of most native shrubs become fortified, ideal for harvest as the vitality inside leaves and flowers "dies" back completely, in fact regenerating themselves while initiating a whole new life cycle. The mirror offers: to nourish our origins is synonymous with renewal and securing future generations. The darker seasons are where new ones get created. Olive trees convey as much, regionally stewarded by one generation as a barakeh بركة, a blessing of livelihood and wealth to the next and the one after and onward.

ZEITOON | زيتون | OLIVE TREE | *OLEA EUROPAEA*

Zeitoon is our quintessential Tree of Life. Our most precious heirloom and steadfast plantcestral kinship. A mutual stewardship whose steady care ensures generous sustenance of oil and preserves that nourish the people of Cana'an year-round. There are olive trees over 3,000 years old in our region who still produce fruit. My own Jiddo Salloum's spirit is close to me through these trees, he himself once a loving tender of his village garden and our family trees. His grove is interspersed by a whole ecology of local plants I enjoy each time I visit them. There are honeysuckles and wildflowers, sages and hyssops, carobs, oaks, and even a hawthorn tree that surround their periphery and crawl on the stone terrace walls. Though I never met him in person, the village home my parents eventually built is proximal to the groves he tended and passed down to my father as an ultimate grace, and perhaps an intentional lifeline of sustaining connection and responsibility to this ancestral land that my father had to leave. Besides the practical blessing of these divine fruits and their oils each year shared with my aunt and her family, my closeness to this land itself lends me a tender thread of connection to Jiddo's spirit, and the care of his hands embedded inside the memory of this family grove. I come to know Jiddo through time on this soil and stories sown steadfast inside the tales of the people who never left this part of Lebanon's coast.

Olives are traditionally harvested after the first strong autumn rain, naturally cleaning them from dust and debris while also plumping them up a bit for harvest. This is typically between late September and early November. These resilient native trees do not typically get additional water during the year, not even in the hot summers. The potency of their flavor and medicine is in part due to the arid nature of the terrain they thrive in, a quality shared with the largely aromatic repertoire of plants growing natively across Cana'an. In my family, my mother's southern village tends to produce the most delicious oil, while my father's northern village excels in the olives themselves, typically preferring the green variety though we also have preparations for black olives regionally. My mother's family used to tend the traditional oil press of her village when she was young, a large stone disk that would be turned repeatedly on top of the fruit to extract the oils. Pits and bits left behind were used in the production of saboon baladi, a traditional olive oil–based soap, or for coals. Now it is more common to find mechanical presses, each village or town with their own. The system in our village works through an option of either bartering part of the oil pressed as payment to the family who runs it, or exchanging cash. It is similar for those who now hire people to complete their annual harvests as families have become more urbanized over time. The harvesting family can be paid in money or in a portion of the olives or oil to feed their own families. This model allows the abundance of the land to be shared and the stewardship mutually tended, even for those who may not have trees of their own.

There is not a single table, home, or apothecary across Cana'an that is absent of zeitoon and its golden zeit (oil). It is by far the most foundational food ingredient alongside salt. Every part of this tree is blessed with nourishment and medicine, the leaves, fruit, and oil named in the Bible for as much and equally sacred in the Quran. Interestingly, while olives are harvested in the time of darkening seasons, the Abrahamic traditions associate the olive tree as primarily a bearer of light, utilized for medicine, spiritual blessings, and food alike. The tree itself is a co-creative testament between our ancestors and the land, with this particular association starting long before the Abrahamic inceptions. It is believed that the olive tree in its native form was a fruitless evergreen shrub growing across the Mediterranean until, over 4,000 years ago, one ancestor grafted it with a fruit-bearing branch to create olives. These trees reflect not just the land itself but our proactive stewardship and intimate relationship with it, co-created by us, and each year beckoning ritualistic harvest, preparation, and tending by local families. This is undoubtedly why it has become such a significant symbol of Indigenous livelihood in the context of Occupied Palestine, where images of settlers uprooting the ancient trees is synonymous with their attempts to erase the original people who tended them, and testaments of our continuity in that land. In the Canaanite cosmologies emerging in this same territory over 3,000 years ago, the olive tree as a bearer of light is central to the creation story of Sour صور (pronounced "soor"), the southernmost Lebanese city, known in English as Tyre, and one of the most important city centers for the Canaanite civilization, where its temples remain visible still today.

> There were once two floating rocks off the shore of the sea that wandered aimlessly across the waters. The people of the shore were the First Humans of that place, holy and eternal as the earth itself from where they themselves one day emerged. On a particular day, the god Melqart evoked himself in a form familiar to deliver an oracle to these Earthborn people. With conviction, he instructed them how to make a "chariot of the sea," a vessel to traverse the salty waters where they could reach these wandering Ambrosial Rocks. Melqart described the vessel in detail, that they may build one to navigate the waters with success. He

prophesied that once they arrived, they would find an olive tree on one of the rocks which is as old as the rock itself, with an eagle perched on its top, and a snake wrapped around its trunk. They would find a self-generating fire that makes sparks from the center of the tree, its glow enshrouding the tree completely but not consuming it. Neither the snake attempts to make the eagle its prey, nor does the eagle attempt to consume the serpent. Melqart insisted that these People of the Earth must journey to this rock, catch the wise eagle and sacrifice him to Yam, Lord of the Sea. They must pour the eagle's sacred blood onto the wandering cliffs as an offering to the god Baal and all the Blessed, so that these rocks would no longer wander over the waters, but rather join to make a city where their people could dwell.

These First People embarked to heed this calling, guided first by the sight of a nautilus fish jumping from the sea. His body mirrored exactly the intelligence of the boat they were meant to build. They constructed it effortlessly through mimicking the creature, what being more masterful at navigating oceans than the fish himself. Once they began the voyage, the crane flew over them, a new compass; the balance in her wings catching wind as should their sail, reflecting how they may glide gracefully along the living waters.

When they arrived at the island, the eagle immediately flew down to meet them, willingly joining his fate. The Earthborn took his life with reverence. Stretching his neck, they sacrificed him with a knife and fed his blood to Baal and the Lord of the Waters. As each drop of the divine blood sank, they turned into roots, fixing the rocks to the place that they would no longer wander. This is how the city of Sour was born, and how Melqart became its patron and god.

This Phoenician creation story is retold from the original records of the old-world Greek poet Nonnos, who documented a version of it thousands of years ago.[1] While it is not often recited anymore in contemporary Cana'an, the name "Sour" itself means "rock" in Arabic and presumably our earlier languages. The story demonstrates the sacred beginnings of olive as a part of us as much as our lands themselves, both of us mutually born of this soil since inception and nurtured by it since. The olive tree is the eternally burning heart, the light-bearing energy that harbors all the creatures dwelling upon it, a center point of life on our land, surrounded by the divinity of the sea. The story expresses a balance of relationships between the various creatures and elements of place, a reverence and humility with which our first ancestors heeded each living entity as a teacher and counterpart in collaborative stewardship of life's calling. The whole story centers the water and earth as a mother and compass from which our livelihoods and civilizations were built, the gods themselves embodied within these sacred elements from which we and our purpose both directly emerge. It also builds the origins of Canaanite sailorship as a Divine Calling and Craft. The regional trade as sailors was a unique aspect of Phoenician civilization's identity that allowed our ancestors to expand, transport, and exchange all across the ancient world.

It is also worth noting that the people of Sour had their own names for the gods and their own unique stories corresponding to the local landscape and culture, showing the ways that Cana'an was both a unified territory expanding across continents and one that maintained space for specificity across its various centers. The old-world culture of this region naturally celebrated and curated itself around unique expressions yielded by highly localized places and its people. This element of unity within diversity is one of the many things that colonialism erodes—and has especially degraded in our contemporary region. Empire harps on separation from localized and self-determined relationships to land, imposing the homogeneity of more nationalistic identities that turn the land into an idea and a resource, while absorbing the power of Indigenous relationships to it for their benefit. These ancient stories offer testament to our place-born relationships beyond flattened colonial inflections, harboring keys of re-membrance, and deepening insights rooted in the Indigenous consciousness of the Earthborn in our blood. They require us to thaw linear paradigms to even grasp the layers within, like all sacred stories and the codes they harbor—like our plantcestors and the stories they re-member when we commune with them.

Despite these losses, in this anchorage, this place of shared beginnings, olive continues to provide in deep and expansive ways to address almost every human need. It is a nutritious, abundant food, whose oil features in countless remedies of our region, every part of the tree a supreme tonic for the heart, skin, hair, liver, immune system, blood sugar, and on. It has a cool and dry energy with diuretic, anti-inflammatory, astringent, hypotensive, antibacterial, antiviral, hepatoprotective, and tonic qualities.[2] Leaves and branches are prepared as a decoction in Syria for treating diabetes, hyperacidity, skin diseases, hypertension, and as a laxative.[3] Extracts of the leaves have been studied in the treatment of countless cancers, infections, and viruses of common and complex kinds, treating nearly every malady and illness the body could conjure.[4] They are practically miraculous, extremely accessible, and with no known contraindications.

Olives have an almost adaptogenic quality, meaning they generally fortify our bodies against the multiplicity of stresses humans endure, serving as a foundational support for both prevention, fortification against, and treatment of a variety of disorders. I find myself leaning on this tree's medicine even for support through layered conditions such as interfacing with trauma, calling upon them to anchor and nourish my body while I re-call and gently rewire my spirit and mind. The top of our spine where it meets the brainstem is called the "olive," forming a pivotal place of communication between the spine and the brain—a neurological borderland for integration between the body and mind. A dear Turkish friend of mine named Emel Orhun shared with me once her powerful experiences making olive flower essences with ancient trees in the Mediterranean, where the remedy revealed an ability to help create new neural pathways, perhaps an affirmation of its vibrational support in the recalibration from traumatized states. More typically, its flower essence is utilized in cases of emotional and physical exhaustion, supporting a quality of deep rest where it may be resisted or inaccessible.

All parts of this tree have an affinity to the heart, reminiscing the image of the sacred fire that emanates in Sour's creation story. The oil of this sacred plant has been used as a menstruum for anointing oils for this quality of luminescence, as well as the fuel of the actual lamps of our Old World. A mystical elder friend of mine from up in the ancient cedar groves of Lebanon's mountains asserts that, second only to the cedars, olive trees carry the highest vibrational frequency of all the trees in our region, endowing healing and mysticism in their presence alone.

Zeitoon trees typically have a larger fruit harvest every other year, in which we lay sheets on the ground beneath the trees as every member of the family or community gently rakes the fruit off the branches where the sheets can catch them. Fruits are immediately taken to the press where a portion of them are made into oil, while the rest are rinsed and soaked in new water for three consecutive days to sweeten the bitterness a bit, then pounded, and pickled in salted water for a few weeks before consumption. Oftentimes lemon, hot peppers, rue, olive leaves, or other herbs are added to the brine to lend additional flavor. I like the way this fruit itself mimics the landscape, immersed in sea-like water to become ready. Each part of this communal harvesting process comes with its own rituals of connection, expressed in regional folk songs called dala'aouna دلعونا, popularly sung in Palestine during the olive harvests but popular across Cana'an in the expression of various local traditions. The phrase itself comes from the Arabic word "a'awn عون," which means "to help." It speaks to the spirit of mutual aid, a collaborative spirit of helping neighbors; this quality is required in the annual olive harvest and labor intensive land-tending village customs across the seasons more generally. These songs ritualize communal work but also express the foundational place for communality within our food and land culture, full with metaphors and affections about the crops themselves as well as the anecdotes of village life that are born alongside them. The songs birth one of the rhythms of the regional folk dance dabkeh دبكة, in which we circle together performing a pattern of stomping motions.

My father used to take me to cultural events as a child to learn and practice this dance in diaspora. He explained to me that the movements emerged as an expressive way for village folk to join forces in building the clay roofs of traditional houses, in which earth and straw needed to be compacted well into even flat surfaces to provide protection needed from the elements. These roofs required maintenance every now and again, each home and its family needing the village's support to maintain adequate shelter. What I love about this aspect of our culture is the way coming together out of need lends to expansive opportunities for soulful expression, and the intimacy and relationship building within communion—even beyond the practical intent.

The contents of the songs lend yet deeper emotion and meaning, evoking a sense of vulnerability and a container for longing as the people gathered with the land soften towards what dwells within. The rhythm of the song is established as a template of sorts, the words changing with each singer, sometimes with a call and response for the chorus—just as the dance follows the patterns of the leader in the line, who has the authority to customize per their liking as the others follow in the basic pattern established. The response aspect lends to a feeling of witness and affirmation, an unintrusive container of acknowledgment for whatever emotion emerges by the leader in that moment. Sometimes the lyrics speak to the love of land and endearing acknowledgement of its endless abundance, for example in this popular Palestinian version for the olive harvesting that starts:

a'ala dala'aouna a'ala dala'aouna, zeitoon bladi ajmal may koona, zeitoon bladi wil looz il akhdar, wil meramiyeh wla tinsa il za'atar

على دلعونا على دلعونا زيتون بلادي أجمل ما يكونا زيتون بلادي واللوز ا لأخضرو المرامية و لا تنسى الزعتر

It hails the abundance of the land in its various expressions: "the olives of my land and all their beauty, the olives of my land and its green almonds, and its sage and don't forget the za'atar." Or another that begins:

a'ala dalouna a'ala dala'aouna, wil blad il helweh zahrat il koona, wil blad il janeh wili ma ahlaha

على دلعونا على دلعونا و البلاد الحلوة زهرة الكونا و البلد الجنة و إلي ما أحلاها

This means "a'ala dala'aouna and this beautiful land and its world of flowers, this land of heaven how beautiful it is," and continues in a prayer of safekeeping for the land and an acknowledgment of its lineage passed down by generation and into the future. A Lebanese version by Tony Kiwan recites:

a'ala dala'aouna a'ala dala'aouna, raho el habayab ma wada'aouna, a'ala dala'aouna a'ala dala'aouna, Allah ysamih-hon shu a'azabouna . . . ya tayr el tayer sawb el habayeb, salemli a'ali kano yhebouna

على دلعونا على دلعونا راحوا الحبايب ما ودعونا على دلعونا على دلعوناالله يسامحهن شو عزبونا . . . يا طاير الطاير صوب الحبايب سلم علي كان يحبونا

This means "a'ala dala'aouna, our beloveds left us without saying goodbye, may God forgive them for the torture it caused us . . . oh, bird flying close to the loved ones, say hello to those who used to care for us." The song becomes a chance for healing through collective grief, with spaciousness for rawness and the honesty to truly come as one is. This container for even the most vulnerable expressions of what aches in the emotional heart is welcomed, letting these universal, intimate wounds heal in each other's reflection.

Even the more bitter experiences of human living earn their honor culturally, transforming in the soulful vocalization and communal witness—not unlike the bitterness of olives and their leaves in their power to heal us. These traditions ritualize loss as much as they celebrate land and livelihood, highlighting once again the centrality of collectivism, healing, and relationality as defining values, and reiterating the cyclical earth-based understandings that in life, loss and renewal are simultaneous and constant—a sacred duality to celebrate and tend within communal regard.

Part III

MATRIARCHAL MEDICINES: TENDING THE LIFE IN FRONT OF US

THIS SECTION RELAYS numerous ancestral reflections about feminine archetypal wisdoms from Cana'an, as well as our matriarchal and birth-tending traditions. I emphasize these themes with great respect to their centrality in our livelihood as a people and species, the immense intelligence for liberatory praxis they contain, and a reclamation of the sacredness within the feminine aspects inside all of us, regardless of gender and biology. This conversation also includes liminal and receptive realms familiar to many who live in the "in-between." Like birth, these intuitive thresholds are connected to the deep worlds of the everything and the nothing where creation takes form—the cosmic womb that is at once maternal and genderless, encompassing the fullest spectrum of existence and all its expansive expressions. This vastness is embedded in the mysticisms of the feminine, as I see them. I acknowledge the profound multiplicity contained within these themes, and the limitations of English and translated language to convey its fullness neatly across the various paradigms of experience, culture, generation, biology, and gender. Nothing shared here is meant to be prescriptive nor limiting within colonial and binaried conventions, but rather, a re-collection and continuation of ancestral knowledge that is being swiftly erased, and diminished explicitly because of its gendered associations with the feminine.

Everything in Teta's home was sewn by her. The curtains, her clothes, and even her underwear. Once, my cousin told her she could easily go to Walmart and buy her some cotton underwear for cheap, and my Teta replied to her, "If you were put on the streets right now with no means to live but your hands, would you know how?" My cousin looked at her with no response, and Teta replied, "I would. If the bank took my house right now and I had to live with nothing but my hands, I know how to grow food, and make my own clothes and even my underwear." Teta's words spoke for themselves: her ways are life-making ways. More valuable than reading, writing, or speaking English. More steadfast than university degrees and the "convenience" of capitalism.

The medicine of our matriarchs is powered by love and an unyielding devotion to life's affirmation, with every seed of possibility becoming a valuable resource at their hands. In our legacy, there is no medicine more encompassing than theirs. Both practical and spiritual, the cultural tools embedded inside our continuation are fundamentally made by them. Our matriarchs have prayed, stitched, and planted the intimate foundations of our livelihoods with unflinching care. They are the tenders of our beginnings, endings, and every spectrum in between. They grieve, hope, and mend constantly on our behalf. Humble and often understated.

This type of care was so natural in my family, so automatic that it took me a lifetime to truly see and grasp the immense depth inside what my matriarchs left me. For many years, my seeking mind looked endlessly from the lens of loss and fracture, my Western socialization waiting for some systematized version of cultural knowledge or linear wisdom to be transmitted in order to guide me. Some "complete" form of story or remedy passed down in a cohesive fashion in order to be sufficient somehow. But what my grandmothers embodied was a much deeper, older answer inscripted in their actualized ways of living; simply, their teaching was to tend the life in front of you.

Through imperfections and tribulations of small and severe kinds, my grandmothers and mother have persisted in servitude and guardianship of the life in their midst, without fearing that it will infringe on the dignity of their own. They have stewarded creation by nurturing the living in their own view, wherever they were and with whatever resources they've had available. This is the profound and prevailing mysticism of the earth and water inside of them, inside of us. It is the simplest and deepest practice that my eternal seeking seems to return me to over and over again—the steadiest, most reaching prayer and widest doorway to re-membrance, mutual liberation, and the integrity and beautification of our worlds.

To tend the life in front of you is a responsive relational correspondence with fluctuating cycles and circumstances that determine our daily realities. It is anchored by a fundamental respect for the life's sanctity and a practical commitment to its ongoing care. These matriarchal ways reflect an ingrained collectivist value and culture of generosity central to how we thrive. It involves no pretense or lofty philosophies and titles. Their remedies emerge completely from a responsibility towards the living kinships where they live and embody care consistently, defining the folk medicines that transmit our specific localized relationships to the beliefs and lands we come from as common people, and the plants, prayers, and customs that evolve to hold us together every day. All around the world, I have been greeted by the hearts of grandmothers who exude a similar devotion. The imprint of their love in action is what holds our worlds together and mends us when it falls apart.

And the power of who they and we are, all begins with birth.

Birth Is a
Sacred Threshold

BIRTH IS AT ONCE one of the most universal, mundane experiences on earth and one of the most miraculous and sacred. It requires incredible skill, reverence, and responsiveness to tend the tenuous threshold between life and what exists beyond it. It is a realm of knowledge and ritual care extended almost completely by and for our matriarchs in the context of Cana'an, and which has been safeguarded by them for thousands of years.

How a culture tends birth shows us something about how it honors life. How can we restore the dignity of our world if we do not respect life's very existence? How life enters and exits is a meaningful mirror into the paradigm and values of a people, and a direct reflection of how we treat the earth itself. Traditional legacies of birthwork rotate on the axis of ensuring life begins well, arrives safely, and with what care, nurture, and protections we need to survive and thrive forward as souls and bodies alike. It is how we steward life's sanctity.

In Arabic, the word "rahim رحم" means mercy, and reflects one of God's names and attributes: "Al Rahman." God, the Merciful. The word rahim also means womb. The maternal rahim is our first home. It shares God's name and essence. When someone dies or we want to pay honor to one's ancestors, we say, "Allah yirhamon," meaning may God have mercy upon their souls. My cousin teaches me that the mystical meaning of this phrase in our original traditions is "may their soul be returned to the womb of Creation." Our use of language lends layers into the relationship between birth, death, and the beyond, between the maternal womb where our creation begins, the divine where it returns, and the earth where both start and end. Our language weaves a sacred thread, a mirror between these realms and their mysticisms. Mercy is a state of profound grace towards another in their state of suffering or vulnerability. Such compassion is a divine aspiration in our cultural concept. The womb, in birth and otherwise, is a spiritual organ as much as a physical one in traditional understandings. It is a seat of the Divine, embodied. A place where mercy gives way to life.

In birth, the human body becomes a creation site, an origin story. And just like the cosmologies traditional peoples all over the world hold central and holy, inside these creation centers there lie keys, threads of divine and earthly power that shape how a people move through the world, make sense of it, tend it. Creation sites and their stories are sacred places that can heal and transform. They reflect and define unwavering universal truths that inform the whole lifeways of a people and their ways of relating to place and one another in sanctity. Birth mirrors this, and those who tend and perform it are at the very crux of its holy mysteries and our earthly sustenance alike.

In birth, the earth is our destination. From the embryonic waters of our infinite maternal lineages, our heads arrive from the rahm towards soil first. In birth, our very first relationship with the earth is realized. This arrival establishes the foundation of our kinship to place, to nurturance, to "home" and our own bodies, in a continuous chain that our ancestors have been cultivating since the beginning of time. Birth is the divine juncture where our unique souls become embodied, where past meets present and creates the possibility for more futures.

Where and how a life is welcomed into this existence encompasses everything. It sets the tone for one's decades to come as it is woven with all that came before it. To tend birth is to tend life in its full spectrum and memory of experiences. It is a portal whose imprints have the potential to heal generationally forward and back in time, guide and bless for a lifetime or many.

Birth is "the dot where everything else begins" (Al-Rawi). As these legacies of birth tending die, we eventually deteriorate with them. When they are forgotten, we lose a part of ourselves and the deeper scripture of our lineages and their generational guidance and protections. We sever codes of life-affirming possibility inside our contract and kinship with the earth, who becomes our mother mutually through this very same act of birth and its tending rites. To restore the sanctity of birth is an act of profound healing towards the integrity of our worlds. It is an ultimate re-membrance with the power to recalibrate our collective existence for generations to come.

Birth Tending in Cana'an

In the context of Cana'an, I am the first generation on both sides of my family to be born in a hospital. Meaning, every generation of my lineages before me—my parents, grandparents, and their parents and grandparents and on—have been born in village homes, tended mostly by the hands of aunties and grandmothers who lived amongst them. All across the region, I am met with stories about the local midwife and the practices surrounding a baby's arrival. The Arabic name for a traditional midwife is dayeh داية, pronounced "dayah" in some regions, or qabla قابلة in some Arabic-speaking countries, coming from the root word "to receive." These stories recalled seem almost nonchalant most times, so natural a part of our way that it was not unheard of for women in our village to birth with no midwife at all. A local uncle recounts to me about one elder who caught all of her own babies, well enough to be active again in her own home after just hours or days each time. Across our villages, I am met with similar stories of women who birthed by themselves while harvesting in the fields, with little external support or fuss. In the mountains of northern Lebanon, an elder named Domina tells me about a time when her neighbors sought a local doctor to support birth in their village instead of the dayeh. The doctor refused, insisting that in their dayeh's care, they were in the best of hands, as she was more skilled and experienced than him in tending labors by far.

It strikes me how recently this stopped being the norm in the context of Lebanon's villages and most of the broader region, and how starkly it has changed in such a short amount of time. Not only is home birth almost completely nonexistent and penalized legally in most of the region today, but the culture of modern birthing in Lebanon, for example, rarely even attempts natural processes in a hospital. Many of my generation schedule unnecessary C-sections months in advance with encouragement from their doctors that it is more convenient. While medicalized services and options for emergency care certainly have a place in protecting birth outcomes and mitigating risks when they are present, countless elders regionally note complications they never saw before hospitalized births became such a norm. From the mountains of Lebanon to the shores of Upper Egypt's Nile, uncles and aunties alike have reiterated stories of their daughter's lingering pain, debilitating menstrual and uterine disorders developed postpartum, and generally delayed healing after surgical births. Many of them attribute this to the "cold" nature of surgical instruments and the lack of immediate postpartum care typically tended by our traditional customs and remedies to support appropriate clearing.

Meanwhile, they seem surprised at the opportunity to share their honest reflections with someone of my generation. I have combed through dozens of villages hoping to meet these dayeh whose stories are still so present in the memory of local families. Yet these stories are usually followed up with "she died a few years ago," with no apprentice or persisting legacy to speak of—whole lineages of matriarchal intelligence gone within just two generations. It pains me that even when speaking to members of my own village and family who have played roles in the birthing and postpartum traditions of our communities, they are so accustomed to being dismissed that they withhold a great deal of detail in their sharing, presuming they are not helpful. Their skills have been made obsolete by the quickly modernizing world around them and younger generations who bypass their contributions as irrelevant, despite their own births being protected by these exact hands and ways.

The colonial influence on educational systems of Cana'an's cities starting in the mid-nineteenth century played a significant role in this eventual shift, changing the standard of medical practices and the role of the healer within them. Before this point, medicine in general was practiced in a more improvisational cultural manner,[1] anchored in our local plants, traditional understandings, and network of communal relationships. This remained the case for longer outside the cities and amongst women, where access to higher education and hospitals was more limited and the colonial paradigms that came with them were held at bay.

The few times I have been lucky enough to meet one of these endangered village birth tenders myself, I have witnessed the seamless ways they are integrated into the ongoing care of their communities and families. They were honored and loved by those they serve, but also humble participants in the colloquial networks of the community daily. They may be just as likely to have helped knead dough or prepare a meal for their neighbor's large family, as they were to offer a remedy or treatment when a child or family member fell suddenly sick. Midwives always played a significant role in the pre-colonial systems of wellness regionally, not only for birth and pregnancy but for care of any family member across life's stages. Their remedies often made up the first line of defense relied on by locals for any issue that arose. In an interview with Hiba Abbani for *Kohl* journal in 2019, the founder of the Lebanese Order of Midwives Nayla Doughane noted that the dayeh was so influential in villages that she could appoint or remove a mayor from office. She notes that everyone sought her care. Home birth was a collective act involving family members and neighbors, hospital birth delegated mostly to those who lacked these intact relational networks.[2] To be alone is seen as a misfortune in our cultural notions of wealth, so this was not likely an advantage in the eyes of locals. The mayor, or mukhtar مختار, in village culture was traditionally more than just an elected official. He was a respectable elder seen as a trustworthy person villagers shared common investment in and felt represented by. He not only managed practical affairs for the village's cohesion, but mediated social and interpersonal ones that included things like guiding conflict-resolution processes within shared cultural values and their corresponding laws. Doughane's statement speaks to the significant authority and wisdom the dayeh cultivated in the eyes of her community, surely reinforced by the deeply relational nature with which she worked and lived. It speaks to the underlying matriarchy of our actual organization as communities across Cana'an, dictated ultimately by the domestic spheres of care and influence cultivated by our matriarchs. Unfortunately, legally speaking this is not typically the case, men carrying not only family names but the deeds, citizenship, and authority in the material world of most of our region, despite our cultural deference to Teta in the daily affairs of our lives that matter most.

The roles of birth keepers was also not professionalized regionally before European colonial influence in our educational systems and institutions.[3] The traditional dayeh was an ingrained part of the life-affirming responsibilities stewarded out of necessity and a calling to tend the life in front of them, motivated by dutiful love and need. The service of these women was not for social status, and had no monetary wealth or exchange attached to it. Each of the women whose stories I was honored to receive, regardless of religious affiliation, attributed their contributions as foremost, a divinely guided service in God's name. While many of them mentioned learning these skills through inheritance and apprenticeship from mothers or in-laws, a few of them conveyed distinctive ways in which their role began as a more sudden spiritual calling they did not expect. They described unusual circumstances where they "just knew" their designated roles and how to perform them after specific dreams or embodied experiences when they came of age. Their tending roles were initiated by holy transmissions for the needed care of their communities, refining the skills through practice and communal exchange along the way.

The Way of the Dayeh

My maternal grandmother recounts her own labors per the traditions of her tiny village in the mountains of South Lebanon. Teta Renee, like many village dwellers of her generation, lived a very embodied, active life. Her body was strong, accustomed to lots of movement and physical labor, and the consumption of mostly seasonal traditional foods rich in nutrients from the local landscape. I asked Teta if she refrained from or added any particular foods or activities into her life while pregnant. She said maintaining a regular diet was important to acclimate the baby to a diversity of foods and mitigate allergies, and she emphasized plenty of greens, beans, and iron-rich foods. One should not skip meals, and should have snacks in between. Regional beliefs emphasize that all cravings and desires should be fulfilled during pregnancy. The surrounding community ensures those gestating life are well nourished, cared for, and protected from undue emotional stress as an embedded value. Beyond this, much of the daily routines continue as usual; pregnancy is treated as a natural seamless continuation of our livelihoods. Unless complications or circumstances determine a specific need, adequate vitamins and minerals are ample through customary foods, and physical preparation is aided by maintaining regular activities as long as it is comfortable.

In truth, refraining from the physical demands of a land-based life was not an option for my Teta and many like her. But the power inside this ongoing practice of strength and trust in the body's capabilities seems to endow a particular aid to ease in birthing for her generation.

Teta iterated the ease and speed with which each of her own children came, by the second major talq طلق, or contraction, she insisted, with no complications or prolonged stress. The dayeh would massage her abdomen gently with olive oil immediately after, encouraging the full release of afterbirth and placenta. Someone present would give Teta a cup of cinnamon and anise seed tea, which she would drink ongoing for the following days until her postpartum bleeding stopped completely. Teta reiterated the role of cinnamon in encouraging warmth, circulation, and release, and the importance of ensuring that there remains no stagnant blood or tissue in the uterus after pregnancy and labor. This reminisces the anecdotes of the earlier village elders, who warned against modern ailments caused by the "cold" stagnant nature of surgical processes and protocols employed in hospitalized birth.

Teta went on to describe a pot of warm water used to sponge bath her and the baby once the placenta was released, baby wrapped immediately after and brought close to her to prevent cold from entering. A grandmother named Domina from a village called Barhalyun in the northern mountains of Lebanon tells me she would help her relative who was the dayeh by washing the child in warm salted water followed by an olive oil massage, and swaddling well for the first three days after birth. Some Bedouin tribes of the Sinai refrain from washing the newborn at all for the first three days, due to an understanding that the amniotic fluids remaining on their body instill protective antibodies. On the fourth day, they too are washed with salt and lukewarm water.[4]

Teta demonstrated with her hands to me how the dayeh would measure four fingers' length of the umbilical cord to remain attached to the baby's navel. Teta and my mom would show me how to sew with these same hand measurements throughout my life, counting palms and fingers as a unit of length. The midwife would cut at this four-finger mark then tie a knot as close to the skin as possible, covering it with salt to help it dry and eventually fall off naturally. Teta Domina shared with me that when the umbilical falls off, local traditions of her village would have folks place it in the arena where you wish the child's purpose in life be fulfilled. For example, if you want your child to be a farmer, you would place it in a farm, or a hospital if you want them to be a doctor, and so on. It is necessary that it be placed in an elevated area, not anywhere that people will step on it or cast their shadow on it. She told a story shared by a Muslim man from a neighboring area who placed his daughter's umbilical in a monastery nearby; she converted to Christianity and became a nun when she grew up. Teta Domina put her children's umbilicals in the home above a high closet, and all her daughters grew up to tend families and raise children at home. In a similar tradition, my friend from the United Arab Emirates says that her communities place it in a location they want the child to maintain a close connection to.

The navel in my maternal grandmother's dialect is called the "zikra ذكرى," which comes from the word for memory or remembrance. This singular word conveys so much emotion, expressing the preciousness, power, and kinship within the act of being born and its relational imprints. Within this language, the navel is a remembrance of connection with the first home—the maternal womb—but also within this folkloric practice, it evokes a remembrance or a contract with a purpose and path on earth, fortified by this place of first nourishment and life made before even arriving earthside. I suspect that in times where our traditions were more cohesive, attuning to the purpose of a child and the appropriate place where the umbilical could offer its power and memory towards manifestation was revealed in the context of dreams, prayers, and rituals adhered by a whole community, rather than merely parental preference. I am told by a mystic of the area that our naming occurred with similar intention once upon a time, determined by a relationship with the stars in the seasonal sky of our birth, and an energetic compatibility with the names of our parents who are at the center of our earthly constellation.

Teta Renee called the placenta "beit il walad بيت الولد," or the "home of the child," also sometimes called "khalās خلاص," meaning "what remains at the end," or amongst some Bedouin tribes of our region called the "sister" (Palestine) or "sister of the baby" (shared with me by Atallah Bin Qattash of the Badia region, Jordan). These words again convey the respect, emotions, and cultural understandings of birth, the bodies and organs involved, and the many layers of relationship and endearment entailed. Teta said the placenta would be buried in the earth promptly after delivery, alongside all other remnants of the uterus shed during birth. Like our elevated dead, these parts may be wrapped in a thin piece of natural cloth before laying it deep in the soil. In some places in our region, aunties have told me they would specifically be buried underneath the front doorway or stone walls built around the periphery of the home. This is in part to protect the placenta from being eaten or dug up by animals, which is a bad omen for future barrenness for the new mother.[5] On a small island village in Nubia (Aswan, Egypt) an aunty shared with me a tradition in which if the mother wanted to have more children, she would bury the placenta near the front door, and if not, it would be placed in a clay pot and sent down the Nile. Amongst Bedouin communities in Palestine, cord clamping and burial of the placenta is delayed for a few hours so the baby can drink strength, blood, and remaining nourishment from the organ, while allowing the nafseh نفسة (title for a postpartum person) to rest after labor. It is some-times even left unclamped overnight if the baby is born after dark, as it is taboo to bury the placenta in the evening.[6]

These acts of burial mimic the rituals of mourning that we adhere to human life when it is complete. The placenta is a mother in its own rite, developing purely to care for the child's development in utero. To bury it close somehow honors the completion of this embryonic stage as it solidifies the child's arrival to a new home: "beit il walad" now becomes the earth, and the specific place upon it where they were born. Its "grave" ends up marking the sacred site of the child's origin story, which most typically was their own family's generational home. This ritual and the language attached to it become a poignant mirror of life's cycles on earth. As one thing dies, another begins.

Inside these traditions, there is implicit space for the integration of grief and transmutation inherent within birthing processes, even as new life is centered and celebrated. While the placenta's burial marks a new chapter for a child, it also becomes an embodied metaphor for the nafseh whose page has just turned as well—whose physical body, so recently full, has become suddenly empty. The earth aids in the energetic transmutations taking place through the subtle ritual of burial at hand. Some Bedouin communities in Palestine leave a few centimeters of the umbilical cord showing above the ground and pierce it with a branch of white broom plant (ratem, *Lygos raetam*) as a protective blessing. This is believed to appease the local angels and divert any negative harm cast by demons or malevolent spirits, which will be absorbed by the plant instead of the placenta. Other Bedouin communities bury the umbilical cord under the pole of the tent to ensure a spirit of closeness and loyalty to the family as the child grows up.[7] The ratem plant is a common antimicrobial desert plant, used in Bedouin weddings to usher fertility.[8] Again it reminisces the protection for one cycle's completion, while somehow ushering the blessings for future ones to be made.

Teta Domina shared with me a local belief about children born in the caul. They are considered to be blessed with luck. While every other remnant of the afterbirth and placenta is buried, she iterates that the caul of a child born in the sac is instead dried and preserved with salt, folded and put in the pocket of their father. It is believed to endow him with support, khair (blessings), and luck. My Armenian friend Kamee Abrahamian tells me a story about a similar tradition amongst Armenians living throughout Cana'an. In their family's case, this preserved caul became a lucky charm for the whole community, one neighbor borrowing it to support his success in court one day, while others would borrow it likewise in situations where extra blessings were needed. They unfortunately lost track of it during the civil war in Lebanon, where they lived in exile after the Armenian genocide. The dried caul has served as an amulet and a prayer across our villages, endowing the divine creative power and blessing of birth onto the lives of the family and community that usher it.

When I asked Teta Renee what she ate or how she cared for herself as a nafseh, she shared a personal ritual of food preparation she adhered to. Teta's own mother died young, and she was the oldest girl in her family. She became accustomed to caring for herself and her siblings early in her life, and developed strict personal standards of how she liked her food prepared in the process. While it was likely customary for others to do this preparation for most nafseh, Teta insisted on covering her own ground as she had grown used to. Teta would raise small baladi chickens specifically for her postpartum food. As soon as the earliest stages of labor began, she would butcher a few of these chickens herself, cleaning and removing their feathers to prepare them for cooking. When her contractions began to strengthen, the midwife or someone assisting her would put these chickens into a boiling pot of water. After the first boil, the foamy layer of zankha زنخة would be removed, water changed, and spices with bay leaves and an onion added to make a nutrient-rich broth. By the time the labor was over, it would be ready to consume. This broth was Teta's primary form of nourishment after birth. She said many others were encouraged to drink milk, believed to lend support as a galactagogue, but Teta never liked milk. Instead, she added pine nuts, walnuts, and almonds to her cinnamon and anise tea, often mixing in some of the broth. The nuts and herbs together encouraged the production of milk and the continued clearing of her uterus, while the broth replenished nutrients as her body healed. Versions of this postpartum tea across Cana'an are called aynar إينار, often including other milk-producing and circulatory herbs such as caraway and ginger, and served regularly in the postpartum period.

The role of food in the ritual care of a nafseh is so significant culturally that I once met a Syrian grandmother in Lebanon whose chin tattoo symbolized the traditional meal her village prepared for her after birth. Another Syrian friend from the village of Tal shared family stories involving a postpartum food ritual called sofrit il khalās سفرة الخلاص, meaning "meal of completion," involving special dishes featuring boiled chickens, broths, and meats. The tradition symbolizes how much the nafseh struggled during birth and how much blood was lost. A sheep liver is cooked with cilantro and given to the nafseh soon after birth, a special part of the meal which was typically offered to the village's new mothers by my friend's Jiddo. Sheep liver is dense in blood and iron, supporting replenishment after labor. Sheep are also a ceremonial sacrifice in our region, offered to celebrate and secure blessings through significant life events and rites of passage. Meat was not a daily meal in most of Cana'an's villages in my parents' and grandparents' generations. It was raised locally or at home and required resources and effort, usually eaten only once a month or at most once a week for those with more resources. The offering of a full spread of meat-centric foods for the nafseh highlights how special this occasion is and the prioritization of care, nourishment, and honor for the new mother and child. My friend's Teta attended many births in the village in Syria before their family was forced into exile. She recalled one of her own labors: she was working in the field and a big poisonous male snake called a hnees went under her leg. She went into labor. Panicking, she ran to her mother-in-law's house. Her mother-in-law assured her that this was a good omen that she would give birth to a boy. She did indeed.

One day I was driving down from the mountains in northern Lebanon and I stopped in the village of Tourza, where there was a small vegetable stand on the side of the road where I could buy a basket of figs. In the back of the store, I met a grandmother who was sitting in a chair with her legs propped up while she cracked fresh walnuts with a stone. She was shrouded in black clothing, a rosary around her neck. I began to talk with her and she told me her own birthing stories. She was eighty-one years old and gave birth to nine children in her lifetime: eight at home and one in the hospital due to complications after three days of labor. She said her children came so quickly that the dayeh never had time to arrive. She managed to receive them herself, her mother-in-law often present with her. Like others around Cana'an, her newborns would be bathed in salted water for three days, rubbed with olive oil, stretched and massaged in the traditional method, and then swaddled well. The placenta would be buried, and the umbilical that fell from the belly button hung on top of the front door. Like Teta Domina, she emphasized that the zikra should never be left in a low place where it can be stepped on. If so, she said, the child would never grow. By hanging them above the door, the divine blessings of their birth would bring goodness to the family and all who entered the home.

She demonstrated an understanding that the way a child arrives determines a quality in their lives as they develop. She shared about her son, the shopkeeper, who came out of her womb while she was standing up, insisting that to this day he can never seem to sit down and rest. He smirked in acknowledgment when he heard her. Like Teta Domina, this elder insisted that her one hospital birth was much more difficult and painful than the eight home births. When I asked her about the herbs used in her care, she emphasized anise seed for both her and her children. She said when they were sick as babies, she would give them some anise tea, bring their bodies close to hers and hug them tightly until they broke a sweat. This method proved tried and true for all their lifetimes. She recounted a story of her own mother's birth: her pregnant mother was at the top of a tree picking fruit when her labor began. The child arrived quickly in the field and she used the manjal (sickle) tool in her hand to cut the umbilical cord and tie it herself. She placed the placenta inside one of the stone terraced walls near the tree and continued on her way back to the house. Stories like this are shared all over the region amongst a generation of strong, land-tending matriarchs whose bodies remained active for a lifetime and whose births appear often as seamless and prolific as the land they tended. This made it difficult to find stories about the techniques employed by the dayeh when complications arose, though all these tetas emphasized that she knew where the limitations of her knowledge were and when intervention by a hospital was required. At most, a few of them described the dayeh's ability to turn the child through massage techniques if they were breeched (feet first).

Elemental Concepts and Traditions

In traditional birth-tending cultures, our matriarchs collaborate with the earth, our first mother, to facilitate our safe arrival. An understanding of the elements surrounding the process is harnessed and guarded against respectively to ensure well-being for both babies and birthers.

152

There remains in the region a whole plethora of herbal and ancestral wisdom rooted in Cana'an's matriarchal legacies for care through birth and beyond, and some basic principles that guide the protocols employed. Many of these principles are adhered across the traditional birth-tending practices of various communities on earth, and apply as equally to the postpartum period as they do to general well-being through the menstruating years. My grandmothers were known to light a candle and offer prayer for any journey taken by loved ones in any form, our births, conceptions, deaths and lifetimes complete with such light and power lent. In fact, there was rarely a moment in our lives that was not prayed on by them—no remedy, no blessing, no instant, however common or exceptional—absent of God's mention in our favor and guardianship. In birth, such prayers to Divine Realms merge with the elemental support of local plants, water, and soil itself to provide care through labor and beyond.

Unlike in hospitals, birth could happen in grounded and sitting positions as opposed to beds, literally harnessing the ground's strength as the body expands to make way for another. The earth's gravity helps draw the baby downward, welcoming the spirit home while anchoring the person in labor. One grandmother in my paternal village mentions a rock sat upon for birthing processes, though she herself did not birth at home to experience it. In her book about Iraqi traditions, Al-Rawi mentions a practice where soil is spread in front of the birthing mother to catch the blood and afterbirth, and two stones are used to ritualize the birthing process and harness the earth's support.[9] She also mentions cases in which ropes are secured to the ceilings or trees for the laboring person to hang on to while pushing. Warm waters, steams, and teas can also support the expansion of the body and its replenishment and healing. Sometimes the steam from a hot pot of water is used to support expansion and cervical opening in the early stages of labor. These principles of warmth remain a consistent theme in supporting expansion, protection, and healing throughout birthcare philosophies.

Two of the most important principles emphasized in labor and postnatal care relate to the elements of fire/warmth and its role in protecting against wind. In Arabic, there is a common concept of being ailed by wind. Grandmothers everywhere will caution you not to go outside with wet hair or allow a cold breeze to touch you after a warm shower. When you wake up feverish, sick, or stiff from being in an air-conditioned room after a ninety-degree day, or being exposed to a strong cold breeze after sweating in the field, they will say "safa'k il hawa سفقك الهوة," meaning "the wind hit you." Wind, especially when combined with the contrast of sudden coldness upon your warm body, explains a variety of ailments and associated symptoms in our cultural concept of illness. Warmth softens and opens us, making us more vulnerable to the pathogens of the wind and cold when juxtaposed suddenly. Furthermore, it is not uncommon to hear villagers commenting on the nuances and nature of different types of wind in the environmental landscape. While the hawa sharqi هوة شرقي, or eastern wind, brings gentle coolness and blessings, the shmeli شمالي (northern) wind is notoriously harsher with greater risks in the folkloric understandings. Wind and coldness combined become particularly dangerous in the postpartum body. Pregnancy and labor expand and soften the body more massively than any other human experience, making vulnerability to wind's ailments that much more threatening. Returning from this open state calls for extra protections both physically and energetically.

The stages of pregnancy mimic the cycles of life as a whole. Early life is mirrored by the prenatal period, characterized and supported primarily by the earth element. It emphasizes the needs of growing bodies. Getting adequate nourishment and rest, building the blood, supplementing minerals, and reinforcing the muscles and bones with strength and comforts as they expand are necessary through this period. Soil must be tended for seeds to properly flourish. This stage emphasizes the most foundational needs that ensure our material existence and continuation.

Labor culminates in the elemental power of water, harnessing the strength of the earth while riding the tides of an ocean that turns and transforms. It moves in cycles and waves as the body's contractions build surges of otherworldly power, liquids literally marking the beginning and end as the child emerges from a river of embryonic fluids to take their first breath. Labor requires a harmony with the hormonal cascade and bodily rhythms at work, and a level of collaborative surrender within water's less predictable currents. It is a primordial element that connects us to realms beyond just the material, calling the more receptive, instinctive parts of us in to support and respond to the mysterious threshold at hand. Labor is a portal and a bridge where the spiritual realms of the deep watery womb and its gestating undergrounds, meet the light and form of the physical earth for the first time.

Once this cosmic river has been crossed, the bodies involved have massively transformed in every way. First breaths—nafas—are taken for both. The birthing body has been broken open to make way for life's arrival. All the organs have been shuffled and shifted, the muscles and bones stretching and bending to make way for new selves to emerge. A space rests where the baby and placenta have been dwelling for months. It must be ensured that air and coldness do not become trapped in their absence. Life blood must be replenished, all remnants of the natal tissue completely released, and the body and spirit drawn back together in order to mend and heal forward. A majority of the protocols and remedies utilized traditionally reflect this purpose, the postpartum period characterized by fire revitalizing earth as does the sun, and ensuring the elimination of air/wind where it does not belong. Just as beit il walad is transformed by its arrival to the soil, the postpartum being enters a transitional state of simultaneous release and regeneration. The return to earth is a process of transmutation that requires replenishment, tenderness, and support as the new bodies and beings are realized, and old ones are put respectfully to rest.

9

Postpartum Protocols for the Nafseh

IN OUR REGION, the name of a person changes after they are initiated into parenthood. Once you become a parent, your name goes from "Renee," in my Teta's case for example, to "Imm Hanna," meaning the mother of Hanna. It is likewise for fathers, who become "Abu Hanna" or whatever the name of their child is. Typically this follows specifically in the name of the eldest son, even if their firstborn is a daughter. To be named "Imm" (mother) or "Abu" is an utmost title of respect in our region, considered the most polite and honorable way to acknowledge an elder. Our cultures emphasize relational roles to family and community over identities limited to the self. I resisted the gendered aspect of this tradition with a wise mountain elder in Lebanon, provoking an understanding of why one wouldn't be named "Imm Mariam" for example if their firstborn was a daughter named Mariam. He insisted to me that the deeper wisdom inside this is the power of women to constantly create and self-generate, rather than a suggestion that women are weak, less valuable, or intended to live in the shadow of born sons. In his philosophy, men need the relationship to their family to remain close to give them support, context, and purpose, whereas women carry the power to create their own families and re-create themselves constantly, and their name must remain their own for them to have the space spiritually to do so. Women are inherently autonomous by the virtue of this life-giving power, and their autonomy is preserved by the keeping of their own name.

The significance of names and titles after birth is also reflected in our designated title for the postpartum person. The fact that we have a word dedicated to the postpartum transition establishes how important the initiation of birth is in our cultural view. Their title is nafseh نفسة (pronounced "nafsa" in some dialects), coming from the word for breath, or nafas نَفَس in Arabic. The breath is a divine mystery that initiates our life on earth. To breathe is an ongoing ritual of renewal and connection with the elements of this living planet that sustain us, and the grace of the divine force that animates our own lives and essences. This evokes the sense of newness and "firsts" associated not only with the baby but specifically for the birthing mother or parent who is also being initiated into a new life, body, and role. The roots of this word in Arabic also carry meanings associated with nafs نفس, meaning spirit, sometimes also meaning the psyche, or the self. Nafisa نفيسة also means to be precious, valuable, or priceless. Together, these words infer the profound spiritual importance placed on the rites of birth and specifically the person who has performed it, and the immediate postpartum period in particular.

Moroccan birth tender Layla B. Rachid relays traditional cultural knowledge about the care of the nafseh from the midwives of her community. Their saying is that in the forty days after birth, the grave of the nafseh is still open.[1] The Moroccan saying speaks to a tenuous threshold between life and death that does not dissipate immediately once the child has arrived. There remain vulnerabilities, tender needs, and attention for extra support in these weeks immediately after labor. What happens in this period determines the longer-term wellness of those involved, both spiritually and physically. Forty is a sacred number and cycle of time in our traditions, dictating many of our spiritual calendars and ritual processes regardless of sect. It typically takes forty weeks for a baby to come to term. Across the earth, the notion of a forty-day care period after labor is adhered consistently by most traditional peoples. It takes forty days for the initial healing after labor, to establish new patterns and the relationships at hand, begin nursing and bonding with baby, begin adjusting to new sleep cycles, regulate digestive processes, and curb postpartum bleeding. This period is needed to transition spiritually and stabilize internally, to find balance as the hormonal roller-coaster of labor settles, and tend the raw body and spirits who have just come through its transformative threshold. It takes forty days for baby and nafseh to truly arrive back into their communities and initiate their new roles on earth. In Mexico, this period is called the cuarenteña. In the West, this is sometimes called the fourth trimester. In Arabic, it is called the arba'aeen أربعين, meaning forty.

This ritual period is traditionally marked by protective care: minimizing physical labor and domestic tasks, preventing exposure to the outside elements by staying home, guarding the spiritual and emotional energy from unwanted forces, and focusing on bodily rest and cultural ceremonies that reground, bless, and welcome new life in their transitional period. Postpartum healing and integration can take closer to nine months or a year, even longer, with various stages of development in the first few years requiring different needs over time. But forty days marks the most immediate and significant stage of care securing the nafseh and baby into their new lives and bodies. This is not dissimilar to the customs observed in regional mourning rites, adhering an immediate ceremonial tending in the initial three days, a period of communal care and prayerful withdrawal from day-to-day life in the first forty days, and a ritual acknowledgment of the soul lost once again at the one-year mark and annually after that.

It is worth noting that many traditional protocols encouraged for the nafseh are advisable for healing through all pregnancy outcomes, including miscarriage and abortion. Since many of these protocols are not just for physical healing but for spiritual integration, one may also benefit from performing them months or years after birth if they missed out on such care. In fact, many of these traditions are suited perfectly to supporting any period of potent healing, trauma recovery, or creative transformation in our lives. This is part of the intelligence in our matriarchal ways of care passed down: our lives are in constant cycles of completion and renewal, just like the earth itself, just like the birthing body, and these rites provide ways to honor and integrate them towards our ultimate expansion forward.

Herbal and Culinary Protocols

As the cycle of birth fulfills itself, we must replenish the earth of our bodies once again. The major digestive organs of the body are all still reorienting into place after labor, needing gentle restorative foods that replenish minerals and vitamins while not requiring too much effort to break down. An intense amount of body power is required for labor, and there is a significant loss of blood and fluids. Nursing can also be depleting and requires additional food and mineral supplementation. One of the primary tasks of this period is restoration of physical strength for both the nafseh and baby, which may happen through bodywork, ancestral foods, and herbal preparations that heal labor wounds and support energetic integration.

Nutrition in this period emphasizes warm, nutrient-dense, easy-to-digest foods that supplement iron and minerals, safeguarding against anemia and other deficiencies. Iron also plays a role in ensuring milk supplies, as does frequent nursing and eating generously. Like Teta, Layla B. Rachid emphasizes baladi chicken made into broths and porridges, which are comforting and gentle while providing adequate energy. This seems to be the most consistent regional postpartum food, as it has been reiterated to me by multiple grandmothers from across the broader region spanning from Cana'an to northern Africa to Yemen. Organ meats are an iron-dense food also encouraged for revitalization of the blood. Alongside chicken broth and well-cooked stews that incorporate these types of meats, the nuts, beans, and herbs incorporated into many cultural meals support milk production, balance electrolytes, and up energy intake while nursing a baby.

Iron- and mineral-rich preserves like carob, grape, or date molasses are also helpful aids in this matter. Tahini طحينة is another dietary staple rich in iron and replenishing minerals and fats. Traditional servings of dibis wa tahini—generous swirls of sesame paste into sweet molasses and served with bread—make an excellent, simple postpartum snack. Dates stuffed with nuts or nut butter, or some creation of "date balls" that incorporate these types of ingredients, are equally suitable. These sweet preparations can supplement needed nourishment in easy, low-maintenance ways. Whereas iron-rich raw greens and vegetables like parsley that feature in tabbouleh and other fresh salads could also supplement the diet in such ways, warm and well-cooked foods are typically preferred in the initial postpartum period. They are easier to digest, and their warmth contributes to the circulatory energetic quality strived for. Iron-rich leafy greens and vegetables in the form of soups and stews such as mlokhiyeh are preferable over their raw cold forms for the nafseh.

Traditional protocols for uterine health and balance nearly always encourage circulatory-warming spices to guard against uterine inflammation and stagnation. These kitchen spices serve multiple healing layers in the nafseh's body, encouraging circulation in the uterus to expel stagnant blood and tissues, releasing "wind" trapped in the gut, supporting digestive regulation, providing protective warmth to the inside of the body, easing inflammation and pain, fighting bacterial infections, and producing milk. They pass these medicinal properties to the newborn via nursing, simultaneously easing conditions such as colic and supporting their inflamed bodies in recovery from the intense passage of birth. These herbs are naturally incorporated in many of the meals and remedies prepared in our culinary traditions, including savory dishes.

In addition to the aynar tea recipes referenced in Teta's story, a rice porridge dish named meghli مغلي is ritually prepared across Cana'an to celebrate the arrival of a new child while supplementing the nafseh in this spirit. "Meghli" means "boiled," inspired by the consistent stirring of the pot required as this dish boils slowly into its thickened form. Meghli is a celebratory food offered to guests who come to lend their blessings to the new baby. It is served commonly on Christmas in the Eastern traditions, ritualizing Jesus's birth. Meghli is prepared from rice flour mixed with generous amounts of caraway, complemented with cinnamon, anise seed, and some sugar to sweeten. It should be mixed thoroughly in its dry powdered form, then placed in a pot of water and stirred constantly as it simmers into a thick caramel-colored porridge. Once complete, shredded coconuts and soaked nuts such as pistachios, pine nuts, almonds, and walnuts are added to the face of the cup served. Soaking the nuts makes them easier to assimilate, and the herbs are all carminative, warming spices that ease digestive processes, support circulation and cleansing of the uterus postpartum, and encourage the production of milk simultaneously. The dish can be served warm or cold, though it is advisable for the nafseh to consume it warm.

IRFEH | قرفة | CINNAMON | *CINNAMOMUM VERUM*

Cinnamon, known as irfeh in Arabic, is used in nearly every lamb dish prepared in Cana'an and is as helpful in the postpartum period as it is in the menstruating years more generally. Note that the *Cinnamomum verum* species is preferable over *Cinnamomum cassia*; it has a more subtle flavor and is considered generally safer in larger doses, due to its chemistry. They can be generally differentiated in their stick form by the many thin layers of light brown bark in the former, versus the singular thick bark of the darker-colored cassia more common in the Western hemisphere.

Cinnamon is a star herb in regional care for good reason. It is a warming, anti-inflammatory, hemostatic kitchen plant with analgesic properties. As a tea, wash, or steam, it has been used by traditional midwives in Lebanon and Palestine to restore warmth immediately after the baby's arrival, prevent hemorrhage, and encourage the complete release of the placenta and afterbirth to prevent lingering uterine congestion and its longer-term complications. Additionally, studies have been done documenting cinnamon's aide in reducing perineal pain, healing and minimizing vaginal tears during childbirth, as well as easing endometriosis and its associated pain, regulating menstrual cycles and delayed bleeding, and reducing insulin resistance in women with polycystic ovary syndrome.[2] It is uplifting, protective, and circulatory. It is indicated in our folk traditions as a tea for treatment of menstrual cramps, chills, coughs, rheumatism, and generally keeping warm and healthy through the colder seasons. It is also given to babies and elderly people to prevent excess slobbering.[3]

YANSOON | يانسون | ANISE | *PIMPINELLA ANISUM*

Whereas cinnamon seems most central in the birth protocols of South Lebanon and Palestine, anise takes precedence in the northern regions and mountains. Yansoon (anise seed—*Pimpinella anisum*) is amongst the most pivotal and common herbs used as medicine and food regionally for a range of maladies. It has a warm energetic quality which is sometimes classified as drying and other times as moistening. It is incorporated into numerous desserts and dishes, seeds decocted as a tea, and distilled into our famous alcohol drink, arak. Arak was one of my Teta Renee's go-to remedies for nearly any common condition—gargle when your throat hurts, rub on the gums of a colicky baby, and prepare yansoon seeds as a tea when your stomach hurts, you have indigestion, a cold, or cramps. Anise is antimicrobial, antifungal, antiviral, antioxidant, analgesic, carminative, galactagogue, diuretic, anti-inflammatory, and anticonvulsant. It features high levels of anethole, lending it a sweet licorice-like flavor and an estrogenic action. It is dense with fatty acids and protein. In addition to its milk-producing and digestive properties, it is used traditionally to relieve migraines, treat menstrual disorders, ease menopausal symptoms, balance blood sugar, treat epilepsy, and in some Iranian texts is noted to alleviate nightmares and melancholy.[4]

Anise has a number of additional effects on sexual health and the menstrual, birthing, and menopausal body. It is an aphrodisiac with pain-relieving and hormone-balancing qualities. It has been used to ease childbirth and can relieve uterine pain in the postpartum period, balances estrogen in the menopausal body easing hot flashes and depression, supports fertility, treats PCOS and alleviates menstrual pain.[5] It is also an effective remedy for easing anxiety and depression, with a generally uplifting energy.[6] It is common for spoons full of anise tea to be given directly to babies suffering from colic or fevers or added to their bottles across Cana'an. Additionally, it is believed in Lebanese folk medicine to repel the evil eye.[7]

Teta Renee notes that frightful experiences can block nursing, with emotional states determining physical ones in the postpartum period. As the vibrational quality of plants often follows their biological action, warming spices that aid the regulation and clearing of the uterus and blood also support in energetic release for the nafseh who is integrating birth and whatever emotions and wisdoms it has opened. These spices contain protective qualities for the emotional as well as the physical, enlivening and lifting the nafseh while supporting the energies present to move along and transform as a new version of the self is emerging. Warmth ushers movement as well as comfort, and nourishes a quality of connection to our inner fire and vital source that keeps dimness and death at bay while strengthening our spirits and bodies.

Similar cultural and culinary herbs that feature in the postpartum reper-toire of our region and foods include fenugreek hilbeh حلبة (which also acti-vates the thyroid, so be cautious if you are vulnerable in this area), fennel shomar شمرة, caraway carawyeh كراوية, and habbit il barakeh حبة البركة or black seed (Nigella sativa), translated as "the seed of blessings" in Arabic, and often incorporated into desserts, breads, and cheeses in our traditional cuisine. These kitchen plants are all milk-producing and carry antibacterial and antiviral qualities, further protecting the healing body from infection as labor wounds are mended and energetic transitions take place.

HABBIT IL BARAKEH | حبة البركة | BLACK SEED | NIGELLA SATIVA, NIGELLA DAMASCENA

Habbit il barakeh is a sacred herb in Islam, known to treat over forty different illnesses. The Prophet Muhammad said that seven seeds could cure "everything but death," indicating its tonic use for sustaining the health of the body. The sacred herb's earliest use is documented in Khemetic Egypt over 3,000 years ago, where its oil was found in the tomb of King Tut.[8] These holy seeds are a powerful panacea that treats nearly every organ in the body, central to the traditional medicine of peoples ranging from Morocco to Ethiopia, Egypt to Syria, Sicily to Armenia, India, and Pakistan where various local species are pressed into oil, honey, or their seeds are ground and incorporated whole in foods. The honey made from their pollen is also common regionally, utilized as a medicine in and of itself. The seeds are carminative and astringent, with a warm and slightly stimulating energy. Amongst their plethora of uses, they are implemented as an aid for fertility, depression and anxiety, memory impairment, thyroiditis, and treatment of hemorrhoids, which are common after birth. In Palestine and Iran, the seeds are also used as an emmenagogue, an aid for labor, and regulation of menstrual cycles.[9] I once found myself in the old souq (marketplace) of Saida, Lebanon, where the charming old baker offered me a special dessert made specifically for the nafseh. It was a diamond-shaped biscuit that was black in color due to these sacred seeds being their main ingredient.

Nigella is also antidiabetic, anticancer, immunomodulatory, anti-inflammatory, antimicrobial, antispasmodic, antioxidant, neuroprotective, antihypertensive, cholesterol lowering and anti-atherosclerotic, a bronchodilator, acts against kidney stones, is protective to the liver, heart, and stomach, and so much more.[10] I have used nigella's medicine for treating everything from eczema to ear infections and colds. It has been used to effectively treat antibiotic-resistant infections, and some very impressive studies have been done documenting its potential treatment of various cancers, including antitumor action and the mitigation of metastasization (spreading of cancer in the body).[11] Its potent anti-inflammatory and immune-modulating action has made it an exceptional ally in the treatment of various autoimmune disorders, and the fatigue they sometimes cause.

My relationship with this plantcestor has been particularly evocative. When I first began to research more deeply about its medicine, nigella began to reveal itself in my physical environment in a compelling way. I was preparing for a workshop in Huichin, Ohlone land (Oakland, California) with a group of students from the diaspora of the Crossroads. I had planned for us to do a number of things that included grinding these seeds into honey for a home remedy. In the meanwhile, a friend of mine invited me to co-host a flower essence workshop in someone's local garden. We invited the group attending to soften their senses as they silently perused the landscape, collectively attuning to reveal which flower beckoned our group to work with it. Unbeknownst to me at just that moment, it was a species of nigella that appeared for this task, calling us into its potent prolific universe. As I was still in the midst of gleeful learning about its seed, the spontaneous invitation to work with it as a flower left me in utter awe. It felt like a ceremonial beckoning, a call and response between us, letting me know the plant's spirit was receptive to my efforts and guiding them along. Whereas the seeds of the *Nigella sativa* species are most sought for their biochemical potency, it was *Nigella damascena* flower, its native Canaanite cousin, who revealed to us on this day, making the personalized resonance of this invitation yet more visceral. *Nigella damascena* seeds are used for similar purposes medicinally in their native bioregions; I also took this cue as a signal from the plantcestor to embrace its medicinal attributes in greater wholeness through developing a medicinal relationship with its flower; its healing aspects demanded attention beyond only its seeds.

This flower is one of the most powerful essences I have ever worked with. Whereas the seeds address the needs of our bodies in extensive ways, the flower's energy anchors it in something differently expansive, cosmic even. If you have ever seen this flower, you may not be surprised by this suggestion. It's either white or an ethereal shade of blue that deepens as it matures, with stamens that reach like antennae towards the sky. It has wispy green hairs that surround its petals, which make it look like it's almost glowing. This probably has something to do with its common English name, "love-in-a-mist." Its seed pods are prolific and round in shape, resembling the head of an alien. The flower took our group through a journey of deep unveiling, working profoundly in the realm of our dreams to encourage greater discernment, integrity, and strength to reckon with the difficult decisions and delusions of our waking lives. On the other hand, it facilitated majestic journeys through ancestral sacred sites of diaspora and homeland alike. This plantcestor worked so spiritually across time, without bypassing or separating us from our earthly engagements. It evoked for me Stevie Wonder's epic song "A Seed's a Star," lyrically enchanting us within ancestral wisdoms of the Dogon people of Mali, Africa in their honoring of our mutually sacred star, Po Tolo, aka Sirius, known for "spirit travel."[12] The song speaks of the ways ancestral wisdom is passed down from the stars since the beginning of time, who are like the seeds of plants and trees that bloom amongst us with ancient mysteries to bring spiritual "light." How the tiniest thing on earth (a seed) contains the fullness of life and all its keys.

Nigella's black seeds and ethereal flowers enchanted me personally within some mystery of revelation between the stars and their cosmologies of life on earth. Not just plantcestors, but actually, plantce*stars*. It is no wonder these particular seeds also have such a role in the insurance of fertility, safe labors, and nurturance during the postpartum period; these themes of "stars as seeds" are just as deeply reflected in the mysteries of our birthing human bodies—the dark expanses of sacred mystery our own lives are born from. This flower essence, though not considered psychoactive, took me on multiple dream journeys while I slept, ushering a "spirit travel" of its own rite. It transported me through cross-cultural cosmological scenes some nights, and the marketplaces of diaspora the next, weaving an understanding of the earthly worlds and the spiritual seeds it emerges from, from the purview of my own bed.

Our Plantcestral Re-Membrance for the People of the Crossroads workshop took place at my Oakland house only a couple weeks later. Naturally, I heeded the call to share this flower essence with the group. I had just moved in a few months earlier, and frequently spent time in the garden tending my plants. Yet this morning, as I walked around collecting flowers for our class altar, I found a small spontaneous stand of . . . you guessed it—nigella flowers I had never seen there before! Growing inconspicuously against the periphery of the garden, their synchronistic appearance once again felt no less than magical. Another cue of playful confirmation from this beloved mystical plant, who showed me simply that the ancestors and their legacies are even closer than they seem—beyond time and space, across the universe even, beyond diaspora and the limitations of the body. The plantcestors have an incredible power to usher us homeward through our infinitely multiple worlds, and through the miracle of our own bodies. Undoubtedly, the barakeh (blessing) they hold for life is one held for the realm of "homeward" arrivals signified by birth too.

ZA'AFARAN | زعفران | SAFFRON | CROCUS SATIVUS, SPP.

Saffron, known as za'afaran in Arabic, is another powerful cultural kitchen spice with potent implications in the support of the nafseh and beyond, and one of my personal favorites. It is antispasmodic, aphrodisiac, carminative, diuretic, sedative, tonic, emmenagogue, antidepressant, antianxiety, and stimulant. As with other herbs mentioned earlier, Bedouin communities of Palestine mix it with honey and take it every morning for a week to ease cold-induced inflammation in the uterus afterbirth. It is also used by them as a sedative during labor, and to treat menstrual disorders, constipation, and sexual impotence.[13] Saffron has been used across our ancient civilizations for the treatment of sexual disorders, neurological imbalances, and beyond.[14] In Cana'an, not only the stamens but the leaves and flowers are used as a tea for the treatment of depression, impotence, and infertility.[15] Various species are collected by women across Lebanon and Syria to treat menstrual disorders including abnormal bleeding as well as delayed bleeding.[16]

Saffron is my star ally in the treatment of postpartum and menstrual-related depression and anxiety, uplifting the mood and activating the senses while supporting hormonal balance and relief of pain. Even when not clinically depressed, a nafseh's postpartum period often includes layers of complex emotions, sometimes birth trauma or generational memories, and often disorientation as the body and spirit have transformed so massively. This passage often benefits from support to emotionally and somatically integrate. Incorporating saffron into meals, drinks, and intentional meditations may support not only mood balancing but reacquainting with the new body and sensual aspects of the self for pleasure, expression, and healing. It is used regionally and has been backed scientifically for its effective relief of premenstrual mood disorders and pain, and treatment of mild as well as severe menstrual disorders such as polycystic ovary syndrome and endometriosis.[17]

FEYJAN—SADHAB | فيجن—سذاب | RUE | *RUTA GRAVEOLENS, RUTA CHALEPENSIS*

Body care in the postpartum period is also extended in the form of massages and hands-on bodywork. Olive oil is used to support massage and healing for child and nafseh alike as physical needs arise. It can also be infused in supportive herbs to aid the healing taking place. My personal favorite is rue (*Ruta graveolens*), known in Cana'an as feyjan or sadhab, a powerful aromatic plant used across the world for spiritual protection and healing. Rosemary or mugwort could be an excellent alternative where rue is not available or suited to one's constitution.

Rue is native to Cana'an, parts of Northeast Africa, the Balkans, and the whole of the Mediterranean Basin, where it is used in various culinary capacities as well as for medicine and ritual protection. However, it has traveled across continents and been naturalized and domesticated across many parts of the Americas. This plantcestor has supported relationships of soul-level healing for both displaced and Indigenous peoples across this planet, who fiercely regard this plantcestor as their kin and have incorporated into their own respective traditions of practice. I myself first became acquainted with rue in the context of diaspora, taking me on a roundabout journey to find myself back in our mutual homeland eventually. But the main message anchored through rue's traveling journey with me was that what we need to heal is usually closer than we think. That "home" travels with us, and is reclaimed from an internal source of power. Rue embodies an ethos of reclamation and re-membrance at its very core, and anchors us in the fundamental power of these states as an ultimate healing and protection.

Medicinally, rue has an affinity to the nervous system, the spirit, and the uterus, known for clearing stagnation of blood and wind. It relaxes smooth muscles and is warming and anti-inflammatory. One of its uses locally is for easing pain in the joints and other such rheumatic complaints, one uncle in my dad's village recounting his father eating sprigs of it when his arthritis acted up. It is as helpful in the treatment of sciatica, reducing inflammation around the nerves. In other parts of Lebanon, rue is noted as a venom antidote, a treatment for "hysteria," an emmenagogue, a carminative, an expectorant, and a treatment for colds, colic, and other "cold" conditions.[18] It is also used for headaches, earaches, and its flowers infused in wine for an eyewash.[19] In Algeria, the seeds are powdered and made into a paste with honey for treatment of spleen ailments, and the leaves used for fever, syphilis, and medicinal smoke baths.[20] It features in a number of culinary blends, sometimes eaten fresh or pickled with olives. It is also one of the herbs in the mansaf spice blend of Jordan, and the berbere sauce of Ethiopia.

Rue infused in olive oil and a bit of castor oil is one of my personal go-to remedies for all kinds of pain, menstrual discomforts, and regrounding from intense experiences that cause emotional and spiritual distress. The warm, blood-stimulating herb is commonly incorporated into remedies for inducing menses and abortion, effectively clearing stagnation, tension, and inflammation in the uterus. It is suited ideally for the postpartum nafseh as both a bodily and energetic aid. Abdominal massages of rue encourage continued clearing of afterbirth while providing protective warmth and spiritual reinforcements to the body as it is still closing. It can be similarly used in hip and leg massages to alleviate pain and inflammation in the nerves, joints, and muscles after labor's expansion. Note that it should only be used after birth or before conception—not during pregnancy, due to its stimulating properties. Rue has been noted as a folk remedy in the north of Lebanon to induce abortion after rape.[21] While many plants have the ability to induce bleeding and abortion, its energetic application in addressing the traumatic wounding of violation makes it a prime choice for multi-dimensional layers of support in these particular circumstances. Using it in the postpartum period offers appropriate aid for comforting the body, while protecting new life and ushering new selves at once. It may be particularly helpful in instances where birth, sexual, or medical trauma have been elicited.

On the other hand, rue is also used regionally to support fertility. One Bedouin remedy to heal a "closed womb" involves a vaginal steam of feyjan leaves, bay laurel leaves (ghar غار, *Laurus nobilis*), and madder (fuwwa فوة, *Rubia tinctorum*).[22] Spiritually, I learned from Sephardic herbalist Dori Midnight that rue's use as an amulet to protect pregnancy and newborn babies is specifically indicated in the Jewish tradition, who know this wonderful plant as "la reina de las yervas," or the queen of all herbs. Palestinian physician and ethnographic scholar Tewfik Canaan shared ways that sprigs of this plant have been hung on the caps of children in Cana'an for protection likewise.[23] Part of its esoteric healing quality is related to the five-petaled shape it grows in, evocative of the kaff كف, or hand, a common cultural amulet of protection.[24]

From the Jewish traditions of Spain to the mountains of Mexico and the villages of Cana'an and the Crossroads, rue is most esteemed for its powerful ability to clear and repel the evil eye and release fear and trauma from the spirit. A friend in Palestine tells me that they plant it in front of their front doors to repel shaytan شيطان, or evil spirits, as well as other forms of negativity.[25] Italians use it similarly for cleansings and protection of the spirit, for which it was known across the old-world civilizations of the Mediterranean and beyond. The curanderas of Mexico and Meso-America consider rue a master plant for ceremonial cleansings known as limpias, and the treatment of susto (a form of traumatic fright). It is also used to repel nightmares, simply placing a sprig under your pillow, and to aid processes of (self-) forgiveness. I once learned from a Mayan wisdom keeper from Guatemala who shared their traditional preparations of rue as the primary plant aiding effective recovery from traumatic stress amongst even the most severe torture victims in their community. Bedouins of the Sinai and Palestine use it in a number of remedies for healing from emotional and spiritual disturbances likewise. It is used in the Naqab region (Negev) to treat "khof خوف," meaning fright, which refers generally to all types of anxieties and intrusive fears.[26] In Iraq, this herb was given to warriors to imbue courage.[27]

Rue's ability to support the spirit and body is complemented by a quality of freedom it embodies. It has a truth-telling kind of energy that seems to repel some with its sharpness, but this quality is also what helps us vibrationally recalibrate to our own axis of integrity, vitality, and agency. Rue is world-renowned for its ability to ward off malevolent spirits, break "bad medicine," and protect spiritual and dream states from attack. One of rue's associations is with the snake, whose venom it has also been used to treat in Cana'an and across the Old World.[28] I believe that its connection to this animal is deeper still. While snakes are sometimes perceived as a negative omen or a sign to watch for an enemy in our cultural understandings, their symbolism is also embedded in healing, fertility, life, and regeneration in the ancient mysticisms of our region.[29] The way this plantcestor grows reminisces the shedding and renewing qualities of a snake. Its branches wind a bit as they grow, and it seems like there is always some part of the plant turning yellow and dry while another part is already coming back to life with fresh green. It also makes the nesting place for swallowtail butterflies, who eat its leaves and spin their cocoons inside its branches. I have often sighted them coming back for pollen after they metamorphosed too. In so many ways, this plantcestor imbues the possibilities of transmutation from old selves, both protecting the threshold of its vulnerability and becoming, while also facilitating the courage it requires.

Note that this powerful plant has a particular constitution not suitable for everyone, evoking strong reactions and repulsion from some for its smell, and causing skin rashes for certain individuals when exposed to the sun. While rue is favored as a colloquial relative and consumed regularly across the Crossroads and Global South diasporas worldwide, contemporary sentiments in Western herbalism typically discourage consumption of this plant and its possible reactions. Working with rue is a good opportunity to pay attention to the personal relationship between your unique being and that of rue, taking time to listen and heed the sentiments and cues of your body and connection before diving in full force. This alone is an indication of rue's teachings and the potent medicine contained within; this plant is all about restoring agency and alignment.

KHARWA'A | خروع | CASTOR | *RICINUS COMMUNIS*

Castor (*Ricinus communis*), known as kharwa'a in Arabic, is anti-inflammatory, circulatory, analgesic, and deeply moisturizing. It is believed to support absorption beyond the epidermal layer, allowing herbal components and moisture to more deeply penetrate the body. It is a native plant across Cana'an used since ancient times as a medicine, particularly in cosmetic and hair care. Alongside nigella oil and others, it is one of the star ingredients in traditional hair oil blends, used to thicken hair and relieve scalp irritations, while locking in deep moisture. Its pounded seeds are used as a poultice to treat abscesses and draw out infections, and its leaves for dressing sores and wounds.[30] Traditional midwives worldwide use the oil as an effective remedy to induce labor. My Syrian friend's stepmother from Damascus says that she would take castor oil before labor to "clear the stomach," and also used it as a remedy for her children when they had stomach issues. Bedouins of Egypt and Palestine use it as a purgative, to treat kidney infections and stones, syphilis, and to remedy infertility. A piece of cotton or wool is soaked in the oil, heated, and then used as a uterine suppository. It is inserted for one hour before removal. It is used to induce menstrual bleeding, and seeds prepared as an internal medicine for use as a contraceptive.[31] Similar hot castor oil packs are used contemporarily amongst folk herbalists and uterine health practitioners worldwide as an abdominal poultice. Soaked in oil and then placed on the abdomen with a heat pack on top, castor packs help ease dysmenorrhea and uterine stagnations. Applied regularly, they can even support the breakdown of uterine fibroids and cysts, heal a variety of menstrual disorders, and support fertility. They are a common remedy for menstrual pain. Added to a rue-infused olive oil for postpartum massage of the legs, abdomen, and hips, castor is well suited to support the circulatory release of afterbirth and stagnant tissue, ease swelling, pain, and inflammation, and deepen the action of olive oil and rue in healing the body. It also aids skin repair from stretch marks and other irritations. Its leaves are used as a wound-healing agent.[32]

Castor plant grows invasively across the city of Los Angeles where I was raised. Its seeds float down the LA River, planting itself across the local habitat where native species are in a struggle to strive in their midst. Generously harvesting their California seeds to produce therapeutic oils could provide a mutual service to healing practices and the native ecologies in removal of a highly invasive plant whose presence infringes on local species.

UTUN SHARQI | قطن شرقي | LEVANT COTTON | GOSSYPIAM HERBACEUM L.

While castor is perhaps the most common plant used for inducing pregnancy amongst modern Western midwives, amongst the dayeh of Cana'an the inner root of the local cotton plant utun sharqi, or "eastern cotton" (*Gossypiam herbaceum* L.), were a more widely applied remedy for inducing childbirth, as well as abortion, particularly in the wealthier urban centers. The English word "cotton" actually has its roots in the Arabic name for this plant, which is utun/qutun. The plant has been used in Lebanon for a variety of additional sexual health and reproductive remedies: its seeds a sexual stimulant, roots helpful for treating impotency, low doses used as an emmenagogue and aid for various menstrual disorders and as a galactagogue, while high doses have been used to break down tumors (also not unlike the castor aka kharwa'a plant).[33] This species of cotton is native to the semiarid regions of Africa and the Arabian Peninsula. It was first domesticated in Ethiopia or southern Arabia and spread around the world for cultivation as a textile from there.[34]

The history of the cotton genus is intimately tied up with colonial violence and forced labor to make this important textile material profitable and useful all around the globe. Particularly, it evokes the chilling realities of the transatlantic slave trade. I am immediately called to reflect on the multilateral violence and vile exploitation committed by European settlers in the American continent my own family eventually settled in, but also the fierce resistance, cultural continuation, and determination of African and Native peoples who masterfully navigated unfathomable circumstances to survive. I recall stories shared with me about the legacies of Black midwives and their descendants, whose forced labor cultivating this familiar plantcestor simultaneously elicited its medicinal continuation in birth tending and healing for the survival of their own communities and beyond. Its root was used amongst Native tribes and enslaved Africans alike to ease childbirth, stop hemorrhage, promote contractions, relieve pain, treat painful menstruation and uterine fibroids, promote milk production, and induce abortions.[35] European settlers benefitted from this knowledge and the midwifery skills of Black "Granny Midwives," whose traditional know-how protected birth in both white and Black communities for generations.[36] But what sticks with me most of all was cotton's use as a defiant self-reclamation in resistance to forced reproduction by the plantation owners who exploited, raped, and abused African women and their children and families.[37] Enslaved women would chew on the root bark as a contraception while working the fields or decoct it alongside seeds to induce an abortion, insisting on bodily self-determination in whatever ways they could.[38] It is impossible to think about cotton's medicine without acknowledging these complex legacies and the power of plantcestral redemption within. Despite the forced nature of relationship between African peoples and the cotton plant in the Americas, this plantcestor was ultimately theirs to know and be aided by. Both African, both displaced and exploited for profit, both thick with generational knowledge and the medicine to protect, steward, and care for life in its ultimate dignity despite the direst of odds.

What's less commonly known is the relationship of empire to this plant's cultivation in the Crossroads, and its direct relationship to the American legacies of slavery and its abolition. In Cana'an, the growing of cotton for export to Europe existed as early as the tenth century and expanded alongside Egypt in the Ottoman era (early to mid 1800s), when its demand multiplied severely.[39] The textile industry was a major factor in Europe's industrialization and colonial expansion. While Egypt was the primary hub for cotton export in the Crossroads, Cana'an had a role which varied in degree of significance to European nations in the tenth to eighteenth centuries. The regional production of cotton was managed through a consistent relationship between the rural plantations, manufacturing factories, and trading posts between Nablus, Beirut, and Damascus. Much infrastructure was created by the Ottomans, and later the British, to facilitate these efforts, critical to their accumulation of wealth; dams, railroads, and the like all had their own impact on the local ecologies of Cana'an and Egypt, just as the monocrop plantations slowly degraded those they grew within.[40] The British and French leveraged their relationships with the Ottomans, who massively expanded cotton production in a type of serfdom throughout Egypt to fund their military and capitalist aspirations.[41]

In the late eighteenth to early nineteenth century, a French entrepreneur named Louis Jumel partnered with the Albanian Ottoman ruler of Egypt, Mehmet Ali, to scale up production and export across the Nile. Jumel imported American and Peruvian seeds to create a hybrid variety that became the famous "Egyptian Cotton," leading to one of the "most efficient exploitation of the resources of Egypt since Roman times," says historian Jason Thompson.[42] As the American Civil War came to, the abolishment of slavery in the American South eroded the system of forced labor through which "King Cotton" reigned. Egypt was strategically positioned by European colonists to take its place in cheap production for the global market.[43] It was merely a couple decades later in 1882 that Egypt officially became a British colony, allowing the Brits to further monopolize this cash crop by exploiting the lands and people whose labor it depended on. They also gained control over the Suez

Canal, a major passageway for trade, which allowed them to further leverage their power and control globally, and more quickly access the other limbs of their cotton pillaging empire in India.[44] The ravaging effects of their colonial policies on the economy and livelihood of Egyptians eventually led to the revolt of 1919;[45] cotton was just as central a culprit in this process that led to independence in 1922.[*]

This cotton plant, whose fibers still touch and swaddle our bodies daily, who has facilitated the births and reclaimed the bodily agency of our matriarchs across continents of violence and oceans of empire globally, connects us vastly in these stories of duality. It insists on our reckoning with the destructive systems that define our modern world, and somehow still whispers into the unexpected pathways of resistance within which we manage to reassert our lives from under the thumb of those who oppress us; redemption comes through connection with the earth it embodies, that ultimately powers every one of these possibilities at hand.

Herbal Steams and Infusions

In her book *Revive Restore Reclaim: Traditional Moroccan Wisdom to Heal the New Mother in the First Forty Days*, Layla B. Rachid shares a postpartum vaginal steam protocol used by the Moroccan midwives in the traditional hammam, or communal bathhouse. The nafseh is encouraged to sit over a steaming pot of the herbs to aid healing. The warmth of the steam and herbs provide circulation and clearing of the uterus, much like Teta's cinnamon, as well as anti-infection, wound-healing, and analgesic properties to help mend the labor wounds and provide

---

[*] It should be noted that the British didn't surrender control of the Suez Canal until they were forcefully ousted by Egypt in 1956. Furthermore, the imperialist trajectory that established the modern nation-state rearranged our region in profoundly destructive ways—culturally, ecologically, geopolitically, economically, and in every imaginable way. "Independence" is very contextual considering this fundamental imprint we are still reeling from, and the colonial system it ultimately obliges us to keep relating within.

relief. The aromatic oils provide ease to the nervous system and spirit simultaneously, and the ritual allows the nafseh a chance to recenter in her body as a pause of care is taken. Rachid's recipe includes lavender, apple mint, pennyroyal, and myrtle, and is followed by an olive oil massage of the feet next covered with socks, then being tucked into a warm bed swiftly.[46] Other herbs that can support postpartum steaming protocols similarly may include warming aromatic plants such as sage, rosemary, rue, za'atar, wormwood, or mugwort to support clearing the uterus while fighting infections, plus herbs such as yarrow or rose to ease inflammation, mitigate excessive bleeding, and tonify the uterus and heal wounds, and chamomile or cinnamon to balance the astringent drying quality of the other herbs while encouraging similar healing. Moistening herbs like cinnamon and chamomile ease irritation of the mucous membranes, calming inflammation discomforts. Many of these herbs also support healing from painful hemorrhoids common in the postpartum body and endow protective and comforting qualities to the spirit as they calm the nerves and bring ease to emotionally distressed states. They can be used alternatively in a bath in the weeks after labor. Traditionally, our region has also used such protocols in a dry steam or "fumigation," sitting over the smoke of the dry herbs for similar therapeutic qualities.

Herbal tea infusions of nettles, oatstraw, rosehips, and roses can be used to replenish and support the body internally alongside these protocols, rich in minerals and vitamins while gently supporting the bodily systems and nerves without any threat to nursing. Versions of this combination are perhaps the most common folk herbal remedy utilized amongst herbalists and midwives to support pre- and postnatal nourishment. Where many use red raspberry leaf to support uterine tonification, I lean on rose petals for a similar action. Vervain tea can help encourage milk production, ease nervous distress, and support hormonal balancing. Lemon balm, lemon verbena, or chamomile can aid sleep while supporting emotional and digestive regulation. All these herbs grow natively or are used culturally across Cana'an and the Crossroads region. Many of them are also readily available across the Western hemisphere, where these folk herbal remedies are shared and common amongst herbalists and birth tenders.

Rituals to Close, Bless, and Protect

Teta Renee recounted in detail the sewing technique employed by the midwives to make long pieces of fabric into a wide belt, then wrapping it around the nafseh's belly a few times over to "gather her back together" after birth. It was to be worn until the bleeding stopped—for Teta, exactly four days—but she reiterated that it could take up to forty for others. Teta Domina on the other hand insisted that to be wrapped or constricted in such ways may be less supportive for those with natural births, recounting a story in which one nafseh in her village was feeling ill until Teta Domina helped her cut the fabric from her belly. She insisted on the other hand that it was necessary for those with surgical births. Her stories about the birth traditions of her own mountain village reminisced a consistent sense of how natural birth is, and how minimal intervention should be—including with herbs—until and unless a problem indicates a need for them.

Rachid elaborates on the knowledge hinted in my Teta's care, describing the Moroccan closing ritual called el shedd الشَدّ, meaning to pull or tighten. This ritual is one I also learned in the diaspora from Mexican and Indigenous curanderas (traditional healers) who share a parallel custom of "closing the bones" of the body after birth or traumatic wounding has occurred, using a thick loom woven scarf called the reboso as a chiropractic tool to heal and mend the body "back together," as my Teta phrased it. Rachid describes the use of long scarves or cloths placed under the nafseh's reclined body to wrap from head to toe as two people gently tug from either end to apply comforting pressure.[47] The body and spirit are supported to "close" again, re-membering themselves back to center after a major expansion. It is followed up by massaging the hips and legs with olive oil, relieving lingering pain and tension in the joints and muscles and supporting the bones and tissues to reel back inward as they resume a non-natal shape. Rachid, like many of the Mexican and Indigenous curanderas I have learned from, noted that this postpartum tradition was sometimes used to support healing for other traumatic wounds, such as in warriors on the front lines of violence. The intelligence in this ritual provides physical adjustments and relief, while somatically supporting the spirit to return to itself and reground after the upheaval of intense experiences like birth and war.

As the baby gets swaddled constantly, these rituals of wrapping the mother back together envelop the nafseh in similar care and tenderness as rebirth takes form and new roots in the body have to find their ground once again. After opening and expanding for months, the body, like a flower or plant, must contract again for some seasons to replenish its life force—but only after its cycle has been properly completed. There may be many mixed emotions that exist in this transition simultaneously, and sometimes even trauma. These practices, herbal and nutritional protocols, and the forty-day care period allow space to honor these layers of what is present, while supporting the body to integrate and move through them. Life constantly mimics this cycle of departure and return, death and renewal as we heal through its stages and evolutions, perhaps most potently demonstrated in the act of physical birth and reminisced in these traditional ceremonies.

Across villages everywhere in Cana'an, the bathing of babies in salt water and then rubbing with an olive oil massage and swaddling is believed to protect them from the harshness of the elements as they age and restore healing warmth to their bodies. It is often accompanied with a set of stretches performed, sometimes by the midwife herself. Taunt Violette was not a dayeh but had a role in natal care and gave birth to all her own babies herself. She was a beloved aunty to all the village children, her hands having blessed the bodies of newborns in this traditional chiropractic massage aimed at strengthening the baby's body after birth, and reinforcing it for a lifetime of growth to come. She would utter her prayerful wishes and repetitive rhymes over their body as she stretched and circled their limbs to aid their body in its expansion and arrival from the womb. For some children, this practice happened consistently through their earliest months of life, accompanied with the olive oil massages. She also at times incorporated baths of myrtle leaves and other herbs if skin sensitivities or funguses developed after labor. My cousin swears that his near career as a nationally sought professional soccer player was due to her steady treatments through his early life. Even though many modern mothers tend to dismiss the relevance or validity of such practices, there was not a baby in the village who did not receive at least one of these treatments from Taunt Violette before she died, though their parents may be squealing at the sight of their newborn being confidently flipped and stretched in her hands with her full security and prayerful care.

These folk practices are typically complemented by more formal ceremonial rituals like baptisms and naming ceremonies intended for the spiritual guardianship of the child, which vary based on the family's ethnic, religious, and familial lineage. Additionally, amulets of protection for both baby and nafseh are not uncommon in our traditions. It is customary to pay congratulatory visits to the nafseh and newborn, often gifting the child with gold or jewelry, sometimes carved with religious inscriptions for protection, engraved with their own name, or turquoise stones to repel the a'ain, or evil eye. This reminisces the famous visit of the biblical three wise men, who brought gold, frankincense, and myrrh to bless the holy child for his lifetime to come. Metal and gold are seen not just as an omen of wealth but as protective. In my visit to Hormuz island in the south of Iran, an aunty shared with me their customary effort to surround the nafseh with metal jewelry and objects in the first forty days, believed to deter unwelcome spirits. She noted that they would also sometimes leave offerings of food and sweets outside for these energies to appease them away from the nafseh and baby. In Cana'an, a similar tradition is adhered to involving the use of metal jewelry and amulets believed to protect the fetus, and even placed at times in the water of a nafseh's bath or on the baby's body for healing as needed.[48] Many of our traditional jewelry adornments serve this purpose likewise.

Plants are also employed for protection after birth. One such ceremony called the mawlid مولد, coming from the word for "birth," occurs in the north of Palestine where Jesus himself was from. A newborn is laid on a bed of sage leaves while the nafseh sips on its tea. The community is invited to witness and celebrate as the Sheikh reads Quranic blessings over the baby. A lamb is sacrificed as an offering and fed to all the guests, who also take home sage and barley from the ceremony to burn as a protective blessing in their own families.[49] Our local sage is a protective plant seen to safeguard against the evil eye and malevolent spirits, as well as against various types of disease and illness. Sacrificing a lamb is a common gesture across our region to mark and bless life milestones such as new babies, new homes, and marriages. Surrounding the nafseh and baby with protective prayers and elements are naturally incorporated into our cultural way through these gestures, which are integrated within our Abrahamic religious practices; both are natural continuations of our relationship with land, place, and spirit since the beginning of time.

I learned from Dori Midnight that rue pinned to the newborn as a protective amulet is traditional in the Sephardic traditions. My friend who lived in Yemen, tells me about "haflet il wilade حفلة الولادة" (party for the new mother), a traditional ritual that happens during the several days after birth. Alongside feeding her the most nourishing, purest, baladi foods, the nafseh's bed is put on an elevated platform and her head is crowned with protective herbs and flowers placed in her hair by community visitors who come to celebrate her. They surround her with dance and song meant to uplift, celebrate, and bless her during the vulnerable and venerable period of transition. Layla B. Rachid describes similar celebrations of ritual dance and song for the nafseh. Such celebrations not only support protective roles but affirm purpose for the nafseh and baby as they are initiated into new lives and recognized by their communities who celebrate, witness, and honor them.

The care provided to nafseh and baby in the postpartum period are meant to fortify them for a lifetime, both physically and spiritually. The passage of birth is traditionally treated as a sacred and tender one that requires care and support, and is graced with immense love from the surrounding community who welcome them back into society with respect and blessings. Most especially, the prayers, meals, and hands of our matriarchs who have safeguarded the passages of our liveli-hoods from beginning to end, that they may continue infinitely. While deeper relationships to the whys and hows within many of these rituals seem to have faded largely in recent generations across Cana'an, some of them are still maintained in varying degrees or for tradition's sake. Their impact is observed and felt in the generations who were anchored by their presence. So many of the keys to modern people's sense of dis-placement and disconnection are naturally remedied by these simple traditions practiced generationally and safeguarded by our Tetas and elders. To start in these ways establishes an imprint in our foundational sense of self, spirit, value, and belonging as we develop in the world. Our cultural ways embed us naturally in the land, its wisdom, and each other's care, where we may find every answer we need, and re-member who we are.

IO

Raqs Baladi: A Spiritual and Somatic System of Health

Another day came when my grandmother called me. She sat on a bench in the garden, one leg folded under her, the other resting on the ground.

"Anchor your feet to the earth and balance your weight on both legs. Now shift your pelvis to the right and then to the left, as if you were drawing a shell. Every time you reach the furthest outward point, stop, balance back to your middle, and then to the other side. Now come, make the same movement with the chalk on the board: ب. Does this shape remind you of something?"

"It's the second letter of the alphabet, grandmother, but the dot underneath is missing."

"The dot is the beginning," she explained. "The dot begets all the other letters. The dot is the below and the alif in between: ب. Together, they form the word أب (father), one of the names of the Divine. When you whirl or when you circle your pelvis, you are drawing the dot, the origins. From this shape, all other movements are born—they all stem from this dot, from the navel in your belly."

—ROSINA-FAWZIA AL-RAWI, *GRANDMOTHER'S SECRETS*, 5

I AM AN OCEAN of primordial beginnings. A wave of tides crash and recede through my body, moons and their infinite cycles transcending time inside of me. In the undulations of my abdomen, my organs are massaged and softened through earthen energy filling me from the soul in my feet. The serpentine rhythms simultaneously regenerate and unhinge me, flat footed and soft, swaying pelvis tethering me to the earth while my limbs express freely from exactly that same core. Water-like and round, sensual and infinite. I am at once anchored and fluid, without constriction. The circular movements draw me from and towards my own center, insisting I acquaint with what is present, aching and joyful inside of me. I return to myself despite myself, suddenly held enough to feel, to know clearly because of how the shapes themselves contain me, connect me. I embody expression from this intimate place of personal communion first. This movement way unsticks me and revives my ability to feel. To receive and surrender. To find my place in what ails and blesses me, what surrounds and fills me. To let go and become, to release and create. To reflect and reclaim, circulating blood as vital energy moves along my spinal axis. Waking all my nerves and organs as breath returns to each cell of my body, this way regenerates me. Re-members me as it anchors me to the earth's loving source, to the ocean and its night sky lover conversing inside of me, to myself as a central axis. My body awakens the grace and power of my ancestors, their rhythms inciting my sway, revealing the medicine that persists inside the intimacy of this dance as a way.

"Raqs baladi رقص بلدي" translates as "dance of this earth" or "local/folk dance." Raqs baladi evokes a folk dance that comes from the earth itself, and our specific place and culture upon it. It is the matriarchal dance lineage of Cana'an and the broader Crossroads region, and the root of more common popular expressions known in the world as belly dance, or raqs sharqi رقص شرقي, which means "dance of the east."

Traditionally, raqs baladi is a matriarchal form of movement medicine practiced ritually by, with, and for women to prepare, support, and facilitate bodily healing and spiritual wisdom for feminine rites of passage across every stage of life, including the tenuous threshold of birth itself. The movements of this dance are anchored in the pelvic/abdominal center of the body, which determines our gravitational relationship to the earth and personal creation centers not only biologically, but energetically. This dance, like birth itself, connects us to the creative mysteries inside life's very making, and the threshold of universal wisdom and revelation that resides within.

The shapes of this dance heal us while re-membering a first language, repairing the compass of the sensual and feeling bodies and recalibrating the expansive realm of deeper knowing, bodily power, and elemental attunement at once. Intuitive, integrative, and fortifying in every aspect, these primordial movements and matriarchal ways of embodiment teach flexibility, connection, and graceful aptitude for navigating the practical and mysterious passages of life, while toning the strength of our bodies and organs. They harness the creative wisdom inside the earth of our bodies as an extension of the land, activating its primordial elements inside of us to provide vitality, balance, and insight from within our own personal axis. While other dances express in large motions across spacious physical stages, raqs baladi is often more subtle in the power it harnesses, its widest stage being the inside of the body, encouraging intimate engagement with the interior worlds for the dancer to emote, understand themselves, and connect through.

In her book *Grandmother's Secrets: The Ancient Rituals and Healing Power of Belly Dancing*, Iraqi writer Rosina-Fawzia Al-Rawi shares her inheritance of this dance as passed down by her mystical grandmother and practiced throughout her upbringing. She encapsulates the ways this tradition connects us to a primordial universal essence and the mysticisms of the Crossroads region, describing its varying expressions across the Arabic-speaking world to this very day. She shares rituals of passage, including one where first menstruations gather aunties and grandmothers to celebrate in a circle of this dance together, their shape creating a sacred container to lend experiential wisdom while supporting the coming-of-age process. Henna adorns the hands and feet of those present, representative of the red blood of life now flowing through their young bodies as they express through earth-connective sensual movements and engage in the transmission of generational knowledge.[1] Henna is a plantcestor that continues to accompany our cultural ritual adornment, imbuing blessings and protective energies to weddings and other celebratory customs while evoking this same wish of vitality, fertility, and prosperity to its wearers.

Raqs baladi is also a bodily invocation of these abundant energies, mimicking creative movements from whence our own lives arose and re-anchoring our connections with each other and the earth. The dance has been used traditionally to aid fertility and support conception. My experience is that its movements not only activate the prolific creative energies inside us but physically support the proper placement of the uterus and regulate its corresponding biological cycles, not unlike traditions of uterine massage and vaginal steaming practiced in various parts of the world to aid reproductive and holistic health. The movements perform an internal massage of the many human organs residing in the abdominal area, simultaneously assisting digestive balance and toning the general function of our bodies. In pregnancy, this circular dance aids proper positioning of the baby in a similar sense, expanding the space between the hips while easing pressure and pain. Al-Rawi describes the traditions of raqs baladi during birth across parts of the Arabic-speaking world. Traditionally, women would gather in circles around the birthing mother with undulating movements that mirror the contractions and pushing motions of labor. Their hypnotically dancing bodies serve as a force of power and solidarity, and an energetic conduit to encourage, uplift, and draw forward the bodily strength and movements conjured by the laboring mother to birth her child earthside.[2] These rites emphasize once again the relational centrality of our cultural legacies and every expression of our medicine and healing practices—even in the most intimate passages of our lives.

In her program Embody Birth as well as her book *Dance of the Womb: The Essential Guide to Belly Dance for Pregnancy and Birth*, Maha al Musa shares stories and practical techniques for the medicinal practice of this ancestral tradition.[3] Maha is a Palestinian-Lebanese birth educator living in Australia whose work retrains communities in the use of this dance to prepare for and support natural birth specifically. I have been thankful to relearn alongside her. Maha emphasizes the self-determination inside this dance and its capacity to support the prenatal body while deepening relationship to our instinctual primal knowing. She notes how these movements reconnect us with the parts of our body, brain, and memory most active during birth, while gently massaging expanding bones and muscles as the body makes room for a child. She demonstrates its role in regulating our nervous systems and psycho-physical orientation so that we may reattune to the internal centers of power and wisdom that guide us spiritually, and reinforce an innate compass for navigating the biological rhythms and uncharted specificities of one's own unique labor. Maha's teachings emphasize bodily self-determination within laboring processes. She educates about the ways this dance tradition naturally supports the physiological and hormonal cascade of a birthing process. She also indicates how it stimulates our vagus nerve, helping regulate trauma responses and recalibrate us emotionally through birth preparation and labor, shown to have an effect on birth outcomes.[4] In a societal context where both sexual and medical trauma are common, this aspect of its benefit should not be undermined in its potential to mitigate impact and duress during birth and beyond, potentially transforming these experiences into reclamations of agency and healing rooted in the body.

Whether biological or otherwise, I experience the power in this dance to aid not only the preparation and act of birth, but the integration of new selves that come as a result of life's most transformative initiations. Its serpentine form endows somatic secrets of transmutation, embodying the constancy of shedding and rebirth as we move in connection to the underlying worlds where new life gestates and decaying things transform. Through whatever evolutions and renewals, the human experience constantly requires anchors and avenues of integration and reconnection. This dance recalibrates us to the earth and our expression as a part of it. It provides a somatic mirror into the dark fertile places of our most interior landscapes and allows its articulation in communion with the land where we are. It awakens the cyclical wisdom and strength of the earth, allowing us to harness its reservoirs from within our own depths.

This dance is soulful by its nature, a deep practice of call and response that begins and ends internally, even while it connects communally. It is the only dance I myself have never been able to tolerate as choreographed learning, as it seems to defy its own emergent epicenter. Rather, it is a fundamental essence of shapes which incite spacious and authentic expressions that heal through their own revelation. Like most aspects of our cultural intelligence, it is practiced through relational communion that provides witness and reflection. A circle forms, sometimes mirroring one another in unison, while other times holding one person in the center with full attention and vocalizations that encourage and embrace. It is a concentric circle that begins at the dancer's own navel; their innermost sensations become the axis and wellsource of embodiment through which connection with others is born. The power inside raqs baladi's form embeds the mysteries and intelligence of the circle itself—the dot where all life begins, the rahm we emerge from and return to.

These movements are meant to be shared with reverence and practiced in joint intimacy. In its contemporary form across Cana'an, these movements are most common in celebratory festivities such as weddings and social gatherings, sometimes also in the more performative-style belly dance traditions made popular in the media of 1960s Egypt and mimicked across the world. Today, everywhere we are gathered, people of all genders connect and heal in the sensual practice of this dance, whose primordial shapes re-member us homeward in joyful union.

II

Wayfinding

OUR PEOPLE, LIKE so many other traditional folk around the world, are anchored in poetry and story, symbol and metaphor, keen to read the cues between the lines to glean wisdom. Engaging with the unseen and unspoken layers of communication surrounding us is part of the navigational system our elders have leaned upon to support life. "Tibseer تبصير " comes from the root for "basar بصر," meaning to look or see, to understand, perceive, discern, or gain insight. In Cana'an, tibseer, or divination, occurs in a plethora of forms. These are amongst the ways our ancestors have illuminated the crevices of their lives, and navigated the passages we can "sense" but not quite touch. The state of being human is so often characterized by existential mysteries, our lives a balancing dance of surrender, and the wisdom to act and foresee. These traditions are part of the way that realms beyond the physical have been stewarded for greater attunement and deeper clarity through the unknown. They have been part of our ongoing "call and response" with life.

Common traditions of tibseer in Cana'an and the Crossroads include reading coffee grinds, palms, or faces. More elaborate traditions of geomancy known as a'alm el raml علم الرمل, meaning "knowledge of the sand," are practiced in some of the more esoteric Islamic enclaves in our region; they use a system of markings revealed through patterns made by tossing sixteen cowry shells. Even interpreting playing cards, reading tarot, and casting astrological charts are common new-age practices that have been appropriated from ancient roots of practice in our region. I myself remember my aunt pulling a deck of playing cards to "read" on my grandma's dining table as a child. Our people can divine just about anything, and have. Once my cousins told me about a woman in our village who was reading the lead from bullets. These tools are merely a mirror, the art of attuning to how what is "above" is reflected in what is "below," the ways that what materializes around us is in conversation with what is going on within and beyond.

There is an engrained keenness of "sight" integrated into the colloquial baselines of our people and the ways we connect, beyond formal divination forms; because health in our ancestral concept has always entailed the body as an extension of the spirit, these traditions of knowledge gathering from less visible and verbal worlds are naturally embedded in our ways of life. To look beyond the immediately visible involves a constant sensory attunement, and surveying of body language and patterns to detect unspoken energies. Information is as present in the lines of one's face or cup as it is in the cues of nature, our dreams, or the "how" in which our prayers get answered. This is why we also converse through story and song, archive in improvisation and poetry, adorn in embroidery and symbols, heed omens with conviction and trust. Our ways of being are deeply relational and sensory, and the spirit, though unseen, is always operating in and through us and the environment we encompass.

In the marketplace, our eyes scan those surrounding us for information that is signaled in the tone and body. We are notorious for shameless staring. People in our region "look" so intently that they will rarely forget a face, even if you return somewhere after years of absence or only went there once. Last summer, I was sitting with an elder at his shopfront in the mountains, and a woman joined us. We offered her a cup of coffee as she chased her young children running amok. When she walked away, my elder said to me, "She is in a challenging period right now, but she will be fine. Didn't you see she had wijeh khair وجه خير (a face of blessings)," pointing his finger towards his own forehead and eyes to indicate to me where he detected this quality. His tone of assumption suggested this is something I too should know. My mother used to study faces like this naturally with the friends I brought home as a child, almost always correct in her intuitions no matter how much I resisted. My mother is the most practically minded amongst us, yet she remains the first to consult me about a strong dream or omen. She goes on a walk thinking intensely about my brother. She passes a snake and then a hawk en route, and returns to tell me about her hopes and concerns for his well-being based on this sequence of events. These are barely messages sought actively, but rather heeded as natural extensions of an ongoing conversation with life's layers, and an embedded respect for what they may offer. Minding them is as practical as anything else.

Despite these intuitive instincts, many of our formal divinatory practices have become nearly extinct or simplified over generations in our region. These days, practices of tibseer are frequently dismissed as empty folklore and superstition, engaged more for entertainment than sincerity, or worst, considered "haram." Haram حرام is a cultural and religious concept rooted in blasphemy and shame, and whose lines seem to morph alongside social acceptability politics with each shifting empire and expression of dogma. Haram is increasingly used to attack and punish cultural practices of healing and spiritual insight deemed as deviations to the socially sanctioned religious orders and their supposed laws and leadership. It is commonly directed towards the older earth-based folk and syncretized Abrahamic rituals still expressed in our villages, and other highly localized cultural customs carried down from pre-colonial generations. This conservatism has become more present in the imperial influence on both Islam and Christianity in varying degrees across our region, actively contributing to the erasure of ways that were until recent generations, seamlessly woven within them.

Haram is one of the primary tactics used by both internal and external dominating forces to assimilate and homogenize the vast ethnic expressions within our communities, eroding the pluralism integral to our region, and stripping what's left of our indigeneity in the process. It has alienated many of us from these religions all together along the way—particularly those within marginalized identities that draw further attention to our difference or "deviance." Reclaiming the earth-based essence of these Abrahamic legacies on our own ancestral terms is a re-membrance worth some attention, if for no other reason than a consideration of their centrality to the lifeways of our majorities and the technologies of resilience inside our recent lineages. Ultimately, their localized expressions are a continuation of our spiritualism born from the land itself. Realms of practice in the more private spheres of our matriarchs are, per usual, amongst the last remnants of such localized wisdoms to give out. But even they are becoming more taboo and stripped of their depth over time, if not dismissed for their actual power.

Regardless, to attune to the environmental and symbolic cues around us is deeply embedded in our customs and our essence as a people. No matter how much the forms change over time, this reading beyond the linear also connects us to the original language of plants, land, and water, of the senses, the body, and spirit—the holy preverbal place where we ourselves first began, and the earth continues to express.

AHWEH | قهوة | COFFEE | *COFFEA* SPP.

In the late morning, the house clears out as most go on to begin their day. But the aunties and grandmothers' work often resumes in the kitchen once the routine has settled. We gather at the kitchen table with a fresh rakweh of coffee on the fire, simultaneously picking through vegetables or rolling grape leaves or whatever that day's meal or domestic tasks call for. This is by far my favorite time to commune with the women in my family, and to drink alongside them. In this phase of the morning, the motion of bodies working with their hands in unison evokes a particular chance for reflection and intimacy, the softening of feeling and memory. I tip my cup over the demitasse plate once the liquid has finished, rotating it three times towards my heart as my aunty once taught me. Thick grinds from the bottom percolate for a moment in the dark, coloring the sides of the cup with shapes and all their secrets. As the cup turns upside down, the realm it conveys also transforms. Some moments pass before I lift it, allowing its insides to dry before someone peers into it. The ease with which it removes or suctions to the plate is already a sign, khair خير (blessings) if it sticks or lingers. If it doesn't lift at all, some will refrain from reading it altogether, so fortunate it is complete as is. But most days, it will be passed to someone in the room to look into more deeply for cues. They scan its walls for patterns, threads, symbols. Sometimes animals, sometimes letters, whatever reminisces a feeling or meaning to draw about the life of the drinker.

The cup becomes a mirror, a womb—its black grinds like soil, littered with seeds of what is sprouting and yet to arise. It mimics the realm of the everything and the nothing where life first becomes. This oracle lends a glimpse into the internal worlds and the spiritual ones where things are planted before they manifest. I ask my great-aunt Lucia for her wisdom in how to read. She reiterates that this is not a way that can be taught. Sure, there are symbols with common meanings, techniques that support the art, but to "see" is ultimately to feel and know from someplace deeper; this way is enshrouded in an ancient language that speaks constantly in the embodied and elemental worlds inside and around us, for those receptive enough to interpret. To look is not to tell a fortune, rather to attune to what is and heed its unveiling and meaning. To steward the path with greater consciousness and care, and bring light to what may need caution or a remedy likewise.

The tradition of coffee divination has grown less common over the years, taboo even amongst many. Still, these intuitive cultural forms can be found across kitchen tables from Anatolia to Cana'an and Egypt. It is a colloquial practice and lends a chance for those present—usually women—to speak and seek candidly. Here they listen deeply and reflect wisdom through a disarmed connection with one another that goes just beyond the surface most daily cultural interactions encourage. Just like raqs baladi where our shapes emerge and emote from within, the cup draws out what is underlying, obliging us to attune to the same primordial dialect to glean insight from the energies operating through our lives at that moment.

Coffee is by far the most foundational ritual in my own family, and an honored tradition across the Crossroads where black coffee served in demitasse cups is considered a fundamental respect to guests and during ritual celebrations and honorings of every kind. The coffee plant is native to the Kaffa region of Ethiopia, where around 850 AD it was found by a goat herder named Kaldi who noticed its invigorating effect on his sheep. He tried some and took it to a local monastery for deeper exploration. The monks there ate the red beans, noticing the alert effect it lent to their night of prayer. It retained its reputation as a spiritual aid when it traveled across the Red Sea to Yemen, where Sufi communities began to use the plant to support long nights of prayer and zikr during the holy month of Ramadan, popularizing its form as a drink. When the Ottomans invaded the Arabian Peninsula, Cana'an, and northern Africa, they adopted the drink and developed their own variations of preparation. Under their empire, the first coffee houses in the world were opened all across the broader region, initiating coffee's inception as the colloquial drink we cherish globally today. From our corner of the earth, the drink was eventually taken by Europe and traveled across the globe from there.[1]

There are many unique preparations of coffee throughout the Crossroads cultures still today. In Ethiopia, its grounds are roasted and brewed alongside the burning of sacred frankincense resins that bless and cleanse, reminiscing its monastic beginnings. In the Arab Gulf, spices of many varieties are added to the brew, such as cinnamon, cardamom, or ginger. Amongst our Bedouin communities, it was traditionally pounded in a tall wooden mortar and pestle, sometimes within a soulful percussive rhythm and song, and then roasted in the hot embers of desert sands. Hosts serve three cups in a row to honor a guest, offered in a shared cup passed from guest to guest until all have partaken. But in the rest of Cana'an, the most common preparation is in the Anatolian tradition, roasted typically dark or medium and then ground into a very fine powder and brewed either plain or with cardamom.

Coffee is quite stimulating, though the darker roasts and combination with these other spices is understood to curb and balance its acidity and intensity—another culinary formulary geniusly interwoven into our daily cuisine. While my nervous system is more sensitive than my mother's—who drinks coffee three times a day without question—she encourages me to do so at least a couple times a week to benefit from its incredible antioxidant benefits. For her, coffee is the ultimate medicine. Studies prove as much, indicating the ways that regular consumption of coffee in moderate doses can help protect the heart, prevent type 2 diabetes, strengthen the brain and DNA, support the liver and digestion, mitigate depression, guard against colon cancer, dementia, and more.[2]

The spiritual origins of its usage in the Crossroads region certainly emphasize a deeper layer of its possibility for healing and guidance in our lives. The energy of this plantcestor embodies an oracular quality and sacred association contained in the beans we still drink every day. For the Sufis, it featured as a part of the prayers that lent to mental focus and revelation in the deepening of union with God through zikr (re-membrance), and for our grandmothers and aunties, the practice of gleaning intuitive wisdom and divine messages to support the passages of their personal lives. These practices are amongst the tools our cultures have cultivated towards deeper clarity, connection, and elevation through the passages of our inner lives.

The A'ain (Evil Eye)

It is still possible to find a skilled reader now and again whose ability to "see" comes with the tools to repair some of the common maladies that appear in our cultural paradigms. A most common of these ailments is the a'ain العين, or "the (evil) eye." The a'ain can be detected by the shapes in a cup as well as by the feelings and responses in the body of a reader, often indicated by incessant yawning, tearing, or other somatic cues in various contexts that indicate the presence of an unwanted energy. At times, the release taking place in the body through these forms is itself considered a liberation from these energies as the reader—usually a woman—harnesses them and stagnation or concentration of the energy is broken. The a'ain can also be detected beyond divinatory forms all together. Physical eye ailments, sudden misfortunes or barriers, "bad luck," or general malaise may all cause concern that you have caught the a'ain. Its suspicion is often raised as a potential source of feeling generally "off," and is sometimes confirmed only through the process of the rituals to clear them.

The a'ain is a very ancient ailment recognized by our region's earliest ancestors and adhered by many traditional peoples all around the world. Its earliest documentation is from 5000 BC in Sumerian tablets of Ugarit, Mesopotamia, where several incantations against the evil eye are noted as remedies.[3] The angry eyes of the gods and goddesses also feature as a theme in their various cosmologies and stories, in which the power of the wrathful gaze can throw the natural world into chaos and imbalance.[4] Symbols of the eye are many across the eras, two of the earliest appearing in Khemetic Egypt: the Eye of Horus and the Eye of Ra.

As you will see in the sections that follow, there is an inherent duality in the eye and its power, on one hand capable of vexing us when anger and wrongdoing is present, and on another hand, lending deeper vision, protection, and healing. There is also power in our own eyes, and the responsibility we carry for the potency and impact of our energy and creative force. "A'ain," after all, simply means "eye" in Arabic, and the eye is what allows us ourselves to see, to read as we do in these cups—a portal for wisdom rooted in the senses of the body and what's beyond it. The eye and its potential to both vex and protect continues throughout every iteration of our region and belief systems, present even in the current Judaic, Christian, and Islamic traditions and their sacred books.

Causes

The evil eye can have collective impacts as demonstrated by the mythologies mentioned previously. But more commonly today, its interpersonal impacts are emphasized in our folk beliefs and rituals to remedy it. The a'ain can be caused by a number of sources. Sometimes purposefully by a person with explicit malice, other times unconsciously when the people around us carry jealousy, anger, or envy in their hearts, and at times even as a result of too much admiration or attention, even if it's from people with positive intentions towards us. Simply, if the energy and emotion of someone in our midst is strong enough—especially in women, it can be projected onto us from the eyes, disrupting our spiritual integrity and resulting in the loss of good fortune and health. One example of the less malicious intent of this phenomenon is amongst newborn babies. They receive so much attention for their purity and beauty as a new life that the focus can afflict them with its intensity. If a child seems fussy or unexplainably disturbed suddenly after being around others, it may be suspected that the a'ain is the cause. This is part of why they are surrounded by charms and amulets to safeguard them from it. Brides are another example of this in our region's tradition, typically adorned with henna, gold, and other protective garb for this reason.

Treatment

A variety of folk ways are used across the region to dispel the eye and other similar disturbances once they have occurred. It is customary in our traditions to follow any compliment of someone's beauty, prosperity, or blessings with phrases like "mashallah ما شاء الله" or "smallah إسمالله," meaning in the will or name of God, or even "yikhzi il a'ain يخزي العين," which means to shame or disgrace the evil eye. Words are amongst the first and most powerful vessels of creation, healing, and guardianship in our region's legacy, offered as incantations and evocations in numerous forms of ritual and day-to-day practice across sects, eras, and borders. These words are common prayers that refocus the intent and energy of praise to the Divine's graces and protection, endowing the compliments offered with a spirit of protective humility and respect. This type of language is uttered constantly in our conversations and interactions every single day.

In the spirit of prayerful words, another common treatment involves praying over the body and head of the affected. An elderly or spiritual person reads verses of the Quran or Bible or other Holy Passages to clear the energy, sometimes via laying of the hands on the head or body while calling in divine support in whatever lineage is familiar to them. My friend who is half Lebanese and half Palestinian shares a tradition of such a'ain removal from her own grandmother from Reineh, Palestine. Her Teta Badia caresses the person gently with her hand while saying the phrase "min a'ain immik wa abuki wa a'ain li hassadouki من عين أمك و أبوك و عين اللي حسدوك," meaning "from the eye of your mother and your father and the one who gazed upon you with envy," followed by recitation of the Hail Mary prayer in Arabic. Her tears would start falling like when a person yawns, releasing the energy and indicating that the a'ain was being cleared. My mother recalls a similar tradition passed down to her mother by their Muslim neighbors in Beirut, who offered Teta Renee a specific verse of the Quran to aid in the energetic clearing of this common ailment. In the Islamic tradition, specific verses exist to clear a number of such ailments and evoke specific protection. This tradition is known as ruqya رقية.

Another form of clearing involves special bowls inscribed with prayers from sacred texts, and filled with water to bless and heal the individual from a variety of specific maladies, including the a'ain.[5] These bowls are contemporarily associated primarily with Islam, made of brass or bronze, and customized for the person to whom they belong. Sometimes they also feature zodiac symbols and various other sacred shapes and forms. These bowls are often used to protect pregnant mothers and babies.[6] They appear to be connected to a much older practice in which Jews, Zoroastrians, and Christians used a clay version of inscribed Aramaic bowls for healing and divination, bringing the power of the word and the water together.[7]

Water and the Portals of Becoming

The word "a'ain" in Arabic is also the word for a spring of water, central to livelihood all across our villages. Many of the towns in Cana'an are named after their life-giving springs, with the common prefix "a'ain" (or "ain") familiar on our maps. A spring resembles an eye in that it is a circular hole in the earth from which water emanates. But a spring is also a sheer miracle, life emerging seemingly from nowhere, blessing even our deserts with oases of fertility and possibility. Again, the vaginal imagery and miraculous possibilities of birth are evoked. More than one version of creation stories in Egypt involves the emergence of human life from the tears of the gods, lending a hint to the deeper mysticisms at hand. On one hand, our tears and grief are so sacred they can transmute and create; this is part of their purpose. On the other hand, the eye, like the womb, is a portal of power and creation where the not yet manifest can become.

Water is our very first medicine, the primordial element that imbues us with life and has the potential to correct every imbalance with its memory. In Islamic texts the Prophet Muhammad explicitly notes water as our origin. He advises against the evil eye's impact and suggests that a bath in water is precisely what has the power to dispel its negativity for the afflicted.[8] All of our religious traditions continue to regard water as a holiest vessel, so receptive and potent it can transmit prayers, cleanse, and recreate us with its power. Water alone has been used for healing of infinite kinds in our region since the beginning of time, be it holy water blessed by saints, prophets, religious leaders, or our grandmothers. Basins for ritual bathing are found at the healing shrines of Astarte and Eshmun, the Canaanite god of healing, in the temple at Saida, Lebanon, where people would petition the deities for miracles of healing from ailments of numerous spiritual and physical kinds. The collective bath, or hamam حمام, is a place where cleansing of the body always involved a purification of the spirit. Just like we distill our flowers in water to alchemize and access their purest essence, so does the ritual of the hamam distill our own beings to our purest forms, removing all impurities and malevolent debris picked up along the way. "Cleanliness is next to godliness." Muslims wash before they pray. Christians bless their heads with sacred water, perform baptisms of initiation, Jews perform mikvah. Arabs, Zoroastrians, Armenians, Canaanites, Mesopotamians, Nubians . . . There is no belief system in our region that does not honor the primary sacredness of this element that makes life.

Protection

Amongst our ancients, all orifices of the body where openings exist were simultaneously vulnerable and powerful. They are the places in our body where energy can enter and exit, for better and worse, and they also connect us to our senses and their embedded intelligence: we hear through our ears, our eyes have the power to perceive and to vex, our mouths utter words that pierce or transform, consume what either ails or nourishes, our anus and urethra expel what is toxic and unnecessary, and our vagina creates through both pleasure and birth. These orifices, like a'ain in the earth, are spiritually endowed with their own power.

The stories of the eyes of Ra and Horus exemplify the sacred power of the eye. The Eye of Horus is a protective and healing symbol that emerges out of the story of Isis and Osiris. After Isis re-members Osiris's body to resurrect him, their son Horus goes on to avenge his father's murder and restore peaceful ruling to the people of Egypt. He enters a battle with his greedy uncle Set to do so, in which his eye gets injured. Horus has to retrieve and restore his eye back into wholeness. Its depiction becomes an amulet, adorned by the royal blue stone lapis lazuli.[9] The Eye of Ra is born of an earlier era, in which the elder god Ra, who represents the sun, becomes disrespected in his kingdom. Ra was the creator god, the people of Egypt born from his golden tears. In his old age, the people developed disregard for him and devised a plot to overthrow him. But Ra is all seeing, and he knew of this plan before it was executed. Enraged with betrayal, he summoned a council of the gods in secret to determine how best to respond. He summoned his eye, embodied by a lioness goddess of war and healing, Sekhmet (who in parts of this myth evolves from Hathor, a goddess of life and fertility), to go across the lands and correct the wrongdoings on Ra's behalf. She prowls loyally through the villages and cities, consuming every human

202

in sight until the deserts become filled with blood. Her taste for it continues and grows, becoming uncontrollable, until Ra realizes that soon he will have no people left to protect and lead. He devises a remedy to appease Sekhmet with a brew of beer and red herbs that resembles blood, which eventually settles her killing spree and rage.[10] Sekhmet's raging river of blood is not just corrective in the sense of retribution for human transgressions; it simultaneously evokes the life-giving possibility of menstruation, and marks the annual flooding of the Nile, which blessed its shores with fertility and abundance for Egypt's farmers. This story again demonstrates the duality in feminine archetypal energies as a mirror of the earth and its cycles of regeneration, as well as the protocols and behaviors that can ensure its balance and continuation.

Our facial adornments—be they tattoos or makeup—originally emerged in part to protect these open places on our body, as well as our palms and the soles of our feet where our nerves collect and we connect with and gather information about the world. This is also part of why henna is especially used on the feet and hands to this day. Starting as early as 6000 BC in Egypt, all genders used kohl and green or blue shadow on the eyes to adorn and elicit the protection of the gods Ra and Horus against the a'ain, while also diffusing the brightness of the sun and harsh desert elements.[11] Desert dwellers of all genders in our region still practice this today. Red lipstick likewise was first used to repel the evil eye and malevolent spirits from entering the body, as were markings with henna on the body, and of course protective jewelry made of stones and metals. These practices were as common in Sumeria and across the ancient civilizations of the Mediterranean. The minerals and plants used to create these makeups carried their own sacred and healing properties as well, even minerals considered toxic by modern science eventually being proven as effective protective remedies for deterring physical ailments and disease, such as conjunctivitis,[12] which to this day is associated with the a'ain in our folk belief systems.

Many of the historical amulets to repel the a'ain also resemble an eye itself. The "eye" is what we protect ourselves against as well as what protects us or reflects the gaze back away from us. The glass blue nazar eye (meaning "to gaze or perceive," in Arabic) is perhaps the most popular and familiar symbol of this still common across the Levant, Anatolia, and Greece, and increasingly appropriated in commercialized forms across the Global North. As the initial energy of one's gaze is often the strongest, the nazar's bright colors and shape are meant to divert the intensity of attention and capture some of the energy to diffuse it. Whereas other eyes or protective eye-like symbols represent and evoke the "Eye of God," in a similar spirit to the ancient ones associated with Horus and Ra. Beginning with Ra, blue is the most common thread between these eyes. They occur alongside other common symbols such as the kaff كف or khamsa خمسة (meaning "five," referencing five fingers of the hand/the palm), also known as the Hand of Mariam or Fatima, especially popular protective icons within Judaism and Islam. Various crosses or four-pointed signs and stars, contemporary religious symbols or inscriptions of the name of Allah, the wearing of silver or gold sometimes in the form of amulets or containers that can hold written talismans, and protective geometrical shapes found in the embroidery of our clothes, rugs, and adornments have infinite expressions across our daily lives for this same purpose.[13]

In the south of Iran, I saw hanging cowry shells in belt-like textiles in a small shop, where locals told me that it was traditional to include one or two cowry shells in these adornments for each guest at a wedding, their eye-like shape protecting the bride and groom from any negativity or envy that may be cast in their direction. The belt of cowries would be placed on the animal that the bride enters the procession on. In Nubia, Aswan (Egypt), some elders from one of the islands gifted me a bracelet with seven cowry shells in a similar spirit of protection. The shells simultaneously represent fertility as their shape also resembles a vulva, and their origin is from the abundant realms of water where life emerges.

Amongst the matriarchs of Palestine, the legacy of cross-stitched traditional dresses called thobe ثوب continue to be made as a powerful living archive of identity, memory, and belonging to place. Full of protective and descriptive symbols of endless iterations, each village

204

has its own lexicon of colors and shapes. Wafa Ghnaim of the Tatreez and Tea art initiative is a Palestinian based in the US whose work is dedicated to the preservation and practice of Palestinian embroidery as passed down by her own mother. In a workshop our community archive, the Ancestral HUB, co-hosted with her in January 2021, she shared about the amulet symbol coming out of the Galilee and Khalil regions, represented by a triangle with various forms and details. Wafa recalled stories shared by her mother about ways these amulets were used for healing from the evil eye and other forms of negativity in Palestinian folk traditions. This protective shape is particularly interesting, as it is the modern thread of an old tradition in which written prayers were folded in a triangle shape and carried for safeguarding by our ancestors.[14] The triangle itself has become a signifier of these prayerful enchantments in the hands of Cana'an's stitching grandmothers, where even our adornments and clothing become medicine to heal and bless. It also reminisces the folded triangle of the amniotic sac of babies born in caul, whose luck is carried by the community in that similar triangular form. The number three is sacred in our region, and the trinity formed by this triangular shape repeated in our regional healing signs evokes suggestions of a sacred energy conjured in specific association with the number's mysticisms.

The amulet shape is only one of many protective and healing signs in the tatreez تطريز (embroidery) traditions of Palestine and Cana'an more broadly. In addition to the symbols evoked, colors are used to protect and potentiate their qualities further. In Palestinian tatreez, white thread may be used to encourage mother's milk, and red (the most common color traditionally used) to encourage healthy blood and circulation and safeguard against hemorrhage during menstruation or childbirth, whereas light green thread may be employed to protect against the a'ain.[15] More generally, shades of turquoise and blue are commonly used in our traditions to evoke protection against the evil eye, including the turquoise stone known as fairuz فيروز in Arabic. A kharzeh zar'a خرزة زرقاء, or singular blue or turquoise stone bead alone, represents a protection against the evil eye, evoking the lapis lazuli origins of Ra's Eye and the reflective hue of water at once. They can be worn alone or sewn into jewelry and other forms for this purpose. I once bought a string necklace of such beads threaded with cloves in between from a Kurdish street vendor.

The commonality and continuation of these endless symbols and colors repelling the a'ain in our culture today is a testament to how integrated these philosophies and charms of protection remain, even unconsciously, in our colloquial traditions. Whereas many scoff them off as empty superstitions, they are amongst the most lingering remnants of folk-healing practice otherwise severely eroded by era after era of conquest and erasure.

HARMAL—ESFAND | حرمل—إسفند |
SYRIAN RUE | PEGANUM HARMALA

As mentioned in various earlier passages, there are also many regional plants such as rue, anise, and others that are utilized for their protective and healing powers against the a'ain and similar spiritual afflictions. Many of them include those burned for their aromatic smokes, which are believed to call in holy energies and sanctify space, like the tree resins coming from frankincense, myrrh, cedar, and pines. There are countless types of incense made for ritual purposes across the Crossroads region, each country and town with their own blends. Alum is a mineral that often features within these uses or in combination with these other plants used for sacred invocations through burning.

One of the most powerful smokes used for remedying the evil eye and protecting from unwanted energies is Syrian rue (*Peganum harmala*), known as harmal in Arabic and esfand in Farsi and Kurdish. This is a plant that grows in more arid desert-like environments and has a strong fragrance when burned, used more commonly in Iran, Anatolia, and amongst Kurdish communities than it is in Cana'an. I do however have a Lebanese aunty who, after identifying the evil eye in a coffee or card reading, would remove it from the home and person by burning harmal and garlic peels on a specific day of the week after sundown. The seeds

206

make an intense popping sound when placed on hot charcoal or fire, believed to break the power of the negative energy's grip. Tala Khanmalek shared on our Ancestral HUB archive a similar practice in which her Iranian grandmother would sing the words "esfand o esfand dooneesfand 33 doonebetarake cheshme bakhil, hasood, o bigane" ("esfand and esfand seeds, may the eye of the jealous and vexing people pop") while circling the burning seeds of this plant mixed with cardamom to cleanse her from the evil eye, encouraging her to breathe in deeply to ensure the aromatic smoke touched her.[16]

In Tala's ancestral city of Yazd in Iran, I saw these seeds hanging as tassels on decorative four-pointed diamonds woven with red, yellow, green, and white yarn as a charm for repelling the evil eye. In Anatolia, where it is sometimes strung and worn as a necklace for protection similarly, I found it growing all across the ancient goddess site of Cybele, the Great Mother, at Catal Huyuk, interspersed with black obsidian and fossilized stones, dwelled amidst by ancestors who inhabited the site 9,000 years ago.[17] I have often seen this plant growing in sacred sites across the region, whether it was the destroyed temple of Anahita in Eastern Kurdistan (occupied by Iran), or the trails of the Sinai where Moses realized the ten commandments.

The Quran names the harmal plant, stating that "every root and leaf of harmal is watched over by an angel who waits for a person to come in search for healing." It can be found in blends and remedies all throughout the Crossroads as an incense for both physical and spiritual medicine. In addition to its mystical properties, it is cardiovascular, neurologic, antimicrobial, insecticidal, anticancer, gastrointestinal, antidiabetic, galactagogue, carminative, diuretic, emmenagogue, and analgesic.[18] The seeds and leaves have been used as traditional medicine for treating a variety of infections, heart, respiratory, and neurological conditions, and pain of various kinds, as well as to induce abortions. Its active components contain the alkaloid harmaline, which is a common constituent of ayahuasca, a sacred vision-inducing plant used ritually by Indigenous tribes in the Amazon for healing,[19] and increasingly appropriated for use across the Global North. Some theorize that this plant was the burning bush where Moses received his prophetic visions.

Note that while this plant shares the common name "rue" in its title, it is a completely different species than the feyjan plant also known as rue (*Ruta graveolens*), though they carry similar qualities in their potent capacity to protect the spirit, as well as some of their physical attributes.

HENNA | حناء | *LAWSONIA INERMIS*

In numerous regional contexts, henna imbues blessings of fertility, vitality, and protection by virtue of its life-blood and soil-hued associations, and its proficient ability to dispel excess heat. Earliest records of its use in the Crossroads are in Egypt (3400 BC) and early Bronze Age Ugarit—a Canaanite city in modern-day Syria.[20] Our cosmologies document the warrior goddess Anat adorning herself with henna to celebrate victory over the enemies of the principal deity, Baal. At that time, henna's growing range included Cana'an and the Mediterranean.[21] It was used in the mummification processes of both Saida (Cana'an) and across Egypt, as well as ritually, medicinally, and as a dye agent for hair, nails, lips, and textiles. It was ubiquitous across Jewish, Christian, and Muslim wedding rituals of Cana'an, where it is still common as a dyeing and healing agent.[22] Today, it grows predominantly in eastern and northern Africa, South Asia, and the Arabian Peninsula, where it has numerous significant ethnobotanical applications.

Henna is associated with rites of passage, honoring the sacred within transitional thresholds; it is a holy plant of life's "in-betweens" that protects, blesses, and heals through reinforcing our connection with the earth and its creative secrets. It especially adorns our feet, hair, and hands—the connection points of our contact with the earth, our ancestors, and each other, respectively. Reminiscing the goddess Anat after war, my friend from the United Arab Emirates tells me henna would be placed on the feet of her uncles when they returned from military service, restoring coolness and re-affirming life-affirming connection to the earth and their responsibility towards it as they transition from a realm associated with potential trauma and violence. In Morocco, it plays a similar role in mourning rituals and the transition of babies and nafseh, protecting them from jinn (unwelcome spirits) while helping them arrive earthside.[23] Henna is sanctified in the Islamic tradition and mentioned in the Bible a number of times. It remains central in wedding rituals across the region, preceded by a women's-only celebration to adorn the bride and her companions. Prayerful wishes are delivered through celebratory songs as ornate protective symbols are drawn on their bodies. This is more common for Muslim communities in contemporary Cana'an and across the Crossroads, also maintained amongst the Jewish and Indigenous communities of northern and eastern Africa, where the plant remains abundant.

Dreams

My paternal grandmother, Hind, was very good friends with her doctor. She never shied away from the medications or treatments she required to be well. Simply, whether it was herbs or pills, if it worked, she would engage it all. In all cases, Tetitna's medicines never worked alone. More than most, she exemplified the power of spiritual practice to manifest healing in our physical lives. She was so known for her skill in this arena that the other village mothers would come to solicit her prayers for their own children. Of everyone in our family tree, she was the cornerstone of "heart-to-heart" care and counsel; there was rarely a time I could walk into her room without finding some cousin or relative spilling their beans to her for wisdom and comfort. She was my own confidant and friend likewise, always curious and intimate with a fullness of presence. Her power to aid us was usually fortified by what happened after we left the room: a devotion of prayers or a rosary in our name. Even the most secularly inclined people in my family have admitted it's probably her prayers securing their good fortunes. Tetitna taught me much about the art of prayer, including its relationship to the realm of our dreams. Once, she shared a story of the time she had a surgery scheduled to remove some kind of growth from her eye. She lit her candles and prayed ferociously to secure her healing. The night before the surgery, she had a dream that a saint-like figure with a long white beard reached his arm out to her with something in his hands. She looked, and found a white cotton ball with blood on it. When she awoke, she prepared herself to go to the hospital, but there was no growth left to remove. Even the doctor concluded that there was no rational explanation—she had seemingly been healed by the saint conjured in her dream. This happened to Teta on more than one occasion in her life. Both sides of my family are full of such stories of dreams and miracles.

Dreams are amongst the most intact practices of oracle and revelation still active in our region's descendants. In our dreams, the threshold between the past and future, the seen and unseen, the spiritual and the material all collapse. This realm is one where the seeds of what begins in the heavens can manifest towards a reality on earth. Whereas some dreams come spontaneously to offer guidance, warning, or insight, others are called upon by the dreamer and their prayers. The earliest documentation of dream-incubation practices originate in Mesopotamia around 3100 BC with the Sumerian peoples.[24] Dream incubation is a process wherein dreams are explicitly requested by a person, oftentimes accompanied by offerings, fasting, and prayer rituals of various kinds, to usher the guidance of the spiritual realms. While the common relationship to dream incubation has changed in the context of Abrahamic norms, these realms remain a significant arena for prayerful connection and fulfillment regionally, as demonstrated in my grandparents' stories. Our contemporary traditions still heed the dream world as one of gravity and direct connection to the spiritual world, where our ancestors, angels, prophets, and saints can speak and influence our lives. They are a realm capable of prophecy, healing, and guidance customized and specific to the dreamer where they land, and sacred by way of their intimacy.

This understanding is the continuation of our ancestors' healing legacies. Our earliest ancestors understood all physical illness to be rooted in and connected to the spiritual and environmental.[25] Healing always required a rebalancing of all these worlds to be secure, and illness often indicated a violation of said balance. In Khemetic Egypt, Sumeria, and Cana'an alike, dreamers and their interpreters had a highly respected role. People of all strata in society paid great attention to their dreams and the suggestions therein, and people of higher social strata often hired special mediums, usually women, whose ability to interpret dream meanings was consulted on a daily basis.[26] A dream might offer insight to a great blessing or a major danger to one's life that was yet to come, or a solution to a problem or health issue whose root was not consciously known. Oftentimes the dreams would require a particular action on behalf of the dreamer in order to manifest favorably. Dreams were used as primary tools to maintain balance and well-being for life on earth, and offered a direct compass and opportunity to ensure that the people were living in harmony with the cosmic forces that governed their quality of life.[27] In Tetitna Hind's case, the dream realm was so powerful it became a place for the actualization of physical healing and miracle with the aid of beneficial spirits.

Dreams are a direct connection to the places and people we come from and the ones yet to arrive—of intuitive cultivation from our deepest source that cannot be broken or taken easily. A dream is a place of internal power, so intimate and boundless, it is unreachable even by the weapons of colonial displacement and occupation, imprisonment and war. Even when we are restricted from our agency in the mundane world, our dreams travel with us as a source of guidance, a lightpost of power. The sacred texts of our ancients are not the only places wherein such potencies and prophecies live. I am reminded of these ways passed down by diasporic legacies of Black Liberation in the continent of my birth. Harriet Tubman's dreams revealed to her the Underground Railroad she would use to liberate her people from slavery.[28] During Assata Shakur's political imprisonment for her role in the Black Liberation movement, her grandmother interpreted a prophetic dream of her escape, which soon after manifested despite all odds.[29] Whereas my own family's stories highlight the personal healing inside dreams, these stories reiterate their sheer power to support self-determination and community freedom even where it is most scarce, and the ways this skill has been continued by matriarchs across continents and cultures, in the service of life. In the colonized paradigms of the modern world, the dream realm is one repeatedly diminished and forgotten for its power to guide and heal through even the most severe tribulations life poses. More importantly, our abilities to effectively cultivate and interpret this realm have eroded severely.

But to wake up and discuss the visions in our most lingering dreams is still a common occurrence in my family and amongst my peers of diaspora and homeland alike. Gathering with others to heed the intelligence in our collective dreams was one of the first ways of re-membrance that initiated my own communal work, and has been a consistent compass for thoughtful action, insight, and healing in the pursuit of this path both individually and in unison. In my experience, consistent stewardship of the dream realm yields greater clarity, discernment, and access to its wisdoms over time. It is a realm that elucidates with cultivation and practice, and obliges us to humbly listen as we attempt to resurrect the symbolic fluency once second nature to our elders. In our Plantcestral Re-Membrance Circles, we gather communally for embodied learning with our plantcestors and their legacies, taking time to "listen" deeply as we rekindle kinship with each one. The dreams have been a fertile place of understanding and collective retrieval, a rich arena of conversation with the plantcestors and their stories that push us to deepen our ways of thinking and connecting to the transmission of knowledge, while we wayfind through body and time. In the dream world, there is nothing completely "lost" to time and its systems of erasure and impact.

Because this threshold is so powerful and intimate, what happens in dream space can also warn and open us to misfortunes, and must be protected and treated with care likewise. This is why plants like rue and other such amulets often reference safeguarding these spiritual realms. This is also why historic examples of incubating dreams nearly always involve offerings and invocations to one's patron gods. While legibility in the common lexicon of interpretation has become more scarce, my aunties and grandmothers had their own understandings of certain kinds of dreams, and practices of care around "bad dreams" in particular. One of my aunts advised to spit immediately in the toilet upon waking from one, reminiscing an Armenian tradition shared by my friend Kamee Abrahamian to visit a running river and tell the water your bad dream. The purifying qualities of the water in both instances aid in spiritual purification and washing away the nightmare's energy. My Teta Renee advised to speak them aloud to a trusted person in the morning to dispel their power, but never after sunset. In fact, she advised not to speak of dreams after dark in general, suggesting an unspoken understanding of the relationship between the darker realms of the nighttime, where dreams themselves manifest, and their power to directly impact our material lives; the respect for potentiality within this threshold reminds me of the dark layers of soil where seeds also germinate in the earth, or hidden uterine universes where seeds become life in the quiet of our bodies. Darkness holds its own sacredness as a threshold for becoming, and this beckons careful intent. This in itself is bound with the mysteries inside dreams and their power per our regional understandings.

As my Tetas' experiences also showed, consistent spiritual cultivation is a primary way to aid and bless the dream space as one of manifestation and protection, which also builds our own receptivity to its wisdoms. For them, the dreams were a place where prayers get answered. In my Tetas' cases, this happened primarily through affinity with the saints, because they were amongst the most primary spirits they cultivated generational guardianship with. Teta Badia of Reineh, Palestine, shared a protective ritual in this vein: the placement of bread with the picture of a saint under your pillow case when suffering from bad dreams, to protect and guard against malevolent energies during the night. Bread evokes the life-affirming properties and beliefs of wheat as sacred in our region, and presumably acts as an absorbing agent for any negativity directed towards the dreamer during sleep. Wheat signifies the regeneration of life, its nourishment, and continuation forward in our cosmologies and our day-to-day lives. In Egypt, the name for bread is a'aish عيش, meaning to live. In another sense, the bread also acts as a type of offering to the saint for its guardianship, a reciprocity to fortify their needed presence.

There are many themes of visitation and warnings lent from the dream realm that still demand attention in our communities, and especially across our kitchen tables. Sometimes they are also delegated to the wisdom and expertise of mystics or clergy for added support. Across sect and affinity, the dreams gain importance as a ground by which the divine and ancestral forces speak clearly to and through us.

Whether one believes in these wayfinding practices or not, they demonstrate the interconnected nature of regional paradigms that emphasize an integrated relationship between the seen and unseen, internal and external, personal and relational worlds. They highlight an attention to the power and consciousness of one's own agency to impact and be impacted by the living network we live in. On one hand, we are enough a part of the earth and what's beyond it to tune in to its signals and messages through a shared language. On another, we can afflict and be afflicted by one another within it. And lastly, we have the capacity to heal if and when we are afflicted, typically by leveraging the aid of these same realms and the kinships at hand to restore integrity and balance.

12

Holy Archetypes of the Mother and Their Plantcestral Legacies

THE MOST FAMOUS birth and mothering story of our region (and possibly the world), is that of Mariam il a'adra مريم العذراء, the Virgin Mary. Mother Mariam is an icon of the feminine divine archetype indigenous to Cana'an and revered in the Islamic, Druze, and Christian lineages across the Crossroads region and worldwide. People of all religious backgrounds from all over the region and country flock to her shrine at Our Lady of Lebanon in Harissa to petition for her blessings, where a massive statue of her towers over the central coast of Lebanon on a mountain top, visible from miles away. Despite the typically reductive ways that Christianity has been reinterpreted to promote puritanical agendas by the colonizing forces of the Western world, many of the older mysticisms and rituals in the Eastern traditions still echo the land-based nature of our roots and remain in practice to some degree in our region.

In Cana'an, these original denominations of Eastern Christianity are predominant, including a number of Orthodox, Syriac, Armenian, and Catholic sects. These lineages heavily center the worship of the Blessed Mother, and have a long history of resisting Western colonialism and assimilation to latinized religious standards via the various empires which have attempted conversion and erasure since. As a direct result of these efforts, Copts, Maronites, Assyrians, and others have at times also maintained ethnically specific attributes within Christianity and the broader region. The Maronite church of my paternal lineage still performs liturgy in a local dialect of Aramaic-Syriac to this day—a ritualized version of the language spoken by Jesus. This dialect contains inflections of the original Canaanite languages of our ancestors, though ultimately was spread under the Persian and Assyrian empires in the first century AD.[1] It is one of the disappearing languages in our region, its colloquial dialect spoken only in small enclaves of Syria.[2] It was eventually replaced by the administrative usage of Arabic in the seventh century, for some communities not colloquialized until the eighteenth to nineteenth century.[3] The Arabic native to Cana'an is dialectical and unique, with particularly strong inflections from the earlier predominance of Aramaic and earlier Canaanite languages.[4] Our ancestors have necessarily evolved with the fluctuating influences dominating our region for thousands of years, weaving some degree of continuity and a testament of our embedded pluralisms even from one village to the next.

The Maronite church makes up the largest Christian community in Lebanon, followed by the Orthodox, whose presence is more predominant in the rest of Cana'an. The Orthodox honor Mother Mariam on August 15, and the Syriac churches dedicate the entire month of May to her veneration. A repetition of prayers, songs, and rituals are made daily in her name during this time of year, and the color blue is worn often in her remembrance and evocation. Each evening, a portrait of her is carried to a different neighbor's house where communal prayers take place. While the story of the Maronites has become associated intensely with modern state building and its inherent injustices in recent history, the origins of this denomination begin in a small refuge sanctuary built on the remains of an old shrine to Astarte, a Phoenician goddess of sexuality, love, and war, still visible from within the church. Saint Maron, a Syrian monastic and healer, found his way there in exile from religious persecution that persisted and was resisted for many years by different forces. He carried with him one item that has remained intact from that era: the ancient icon of Our Lady of Ilige (named after the Phoenician temple), a rare Eastern image of the Blessed Mother and baby Jesus, with no hint of Byzantine influence.[5] Mary is shrouded in a royal blue robe signifying divinity, with a star on her forehead and one on her shoulder representing the sun and moon, as she does the earth.[6] Jesus wears deep purple robes signifying royalty—a continuation of our Phoenician ancestors' legacies of murex dye. They both have plain gold halos and hold symbolic Syriac hand gestures. Faces of two angels with large Afros are perched in the upper corners. All the figures have dark hair and pronounced brown eyes, with ethnic features typical of our region. The background is a rich terracotta orange, evoking the color and spirit of fertile earth. This icon was covered in layers of paint that attempted to modify and Europeanize its image over the years, its true character finally revealed through restoration in the 1980s. The church is still active today and has been dedicated to the Blessed Mother since its early inception.

Undoubtedly, a lot has also been lost, diluted, and manipulated in our religious traditions, political, and ethnic self-conception over the past many generations of colonial intervention and nationalist projects. But the centrality of Mariam remains—amongst Christians and Muslims in our region especially. In the Islamic tradition, Mariam is considered the most highly regarded woman on earth, honored with affection as deep and steady. What I see in Mother Mariam's story and her worship retains some seed of our underlying essence, and lends a more expansive and liberatory message as a clear continuous thread to the older cosmologies of our region and their goddesses; most of all, the holiness of the mother, the earth, and our own matriarchs as her reflection.

In our village, there is a small outdoor chapel in her honor near the cemetery, where a weekly vigil takes place under the oak trees, and all the tetas gather and pray in her spirit. For them, every day is in her legacy. My grandmothers invoked her and prayed to her constantly, especially when the most trying situations involving their own children would come about. Be it a colloquial mishap where my baby cousin trips and my Teta utters "ya a'adra! يا عذراء" before he falls, or a tisa'awi-yeh تسعاوية—a nine-day devotional rosary prayer to the Blessed Mother regarding a specific problem or intention. Both my Tetas seemed to find closeness with Mother Mary as a primary spiritual affinity and support, next to the Lebanese saints. Mother Mary is the anchor of our family's tradition and the deliverance of each prayer laid down by our own matriarchs. She ties me to them, as much as she does to the earth itself.

This is not a surprise, considering her story. Mariam is the mother who has suffered and endured, the mother who has loved despite all costs, and found grace in the most unimaginable strife. She is the mother whose pregnancy before marriage was seen first as a scandal, likely marking her with a scarlet letter in her own society and obliging her to find faith and trust in her own soul to go forward. She is the mother who lost her son to state violence on display, and the one who prayed and mourned him back to life as Isis did to Osiris. She is a Jewish mother revered as lovingly in Christianity as she is in Islam, and the one whose life most resembles that of grandmothers all across this land that she herself called home. This is why she is understood to be the most receptive to their prayers, delivering possibilities for healing and strength in their day-to-day lives. Especially as mothers of this land who also raised children in eras of war, exile, and loss, in eras of displacement and migration, like her.

In my view, even the immaculate conception is a story about spiritual wholeness and the creative power of the feminine essence as a mirror of the earth. The story of a baby conceived and born inside his mother's body with only the Divine's grace suggests the completeness and wholeness, the expansiveness already entailed inside the feminine that yields creation itself, God-like in fact. Not that there is no masculine entailed or that sex itself is impure, but rather that the feminine Mary represents contains it inside of her already, and every spectrum of the living in between. As a mother, alone, she gives birth to a son who is also a holy divinity—an artisan and herbalist who harnessed the divine energy in the earth and its elements to heal people, who resisted oppression and harmful conventions for a lifetime, dignifying the life of even the most downtrodden around him. Holy and masculine and divine also because he comes from his mother, and hence contains the grace of her nature as equally. The story speaks to how complete we already are. How expansive. To how creation and its power emerges from inside this place of multitudes, our mothers and birthers divine and all-encompassing with every component needed naturally to create and sustain, like the earth we all breathe and drink daily. It is no wonder that all around the world, where colonizers took our religion to oppress, dominate, and erase the Indigenous of the lands they sought to exploit, it is Mother Mary who became the lap of refuge. It is her lap where grandmothers tucked inflections of their own ancestors' Indigenous prayers to survive and carry on for generations forward. In Islam, the story of Mariam's birth begins with how her own mother prayed upon her arrival and protection for a lifetime, in a moment of incredible political danger and struggle in their world, and after struggling to become pregnant herself. Her sacredness is ushered through the prayers of her own mother in this sacred life-yielding chain. Mariam represents the Universal Mother, whose power transcends religion and touches the very soul of our earthly existence, and the very origins of our pre-Abrahamic goddesses and our own stories as equally—the "womb of mercy" as a realm of everything and nothing—the lush darkness of soil, stars, and seeds—the love where creation itself begins, and every spectrum of its divine expression on earth emerges and resides.

In Cana'an's botanical traditions, there are several plants named after Mary or otherwise associated with her blessings. The cultural affection towards Mariam and her healing herbs offers telling mirrors into sentiments about motherhood, birth, and beyond through our cultural lens, connecting us to archetypal wisdom about the earth and the significance and nature of "the feminine" from our earliest civilizations.

TAMR—NAKHLEH | تمر—نخلة | DATE PALM | PHOENIX DACTYLIFERA

There is perhaps no plantcestor more significant than dates in the legacy of birth medicine and our matriarchal legacies regionally. In the Quranic version of Mary's labor, the Virgin Mother walked into the land by herself once her labor pains intensified. Alone, she settled at the trunk of a palm tree, tired and unsure she could endure the birthing pains any longer. She wailed into the sky of her suffering and exhaustion, her desperate desire for it to all be over. Her pain was as universal as any mother's in birth. The Divine heard her and graced her with a blessing. The tall date tree bent its neck, angels in its boughs where she reached dates to nourish and strengthen her forward. A spring spouted from beneath the tree just near her, refreshing her with water. She was revived, baby Jesus born safely to this earth.

Dates are a sacred food and versatile medicine for birth and beyond, with an ancient history in the traditions and medicinal repertoire of the Crossroads regions. These resilient trees provide necessary nourishment, with the capacity to grow in arid desert bioregions that contain minimal water and very few other trees for shade and habitat. Every part of the date palm tree has been used for practical, medicinal, and ritual purposes across the Crossroads region for thousands of years. In addition to medicinal uses for everything from blood sugar regulation to treating colds, fibers, baskets, and sewing needles have been made from their trunk to weave and build with. We use their pollen, eat them fresh or dry, and make them into molasses and syrups to use in our foods. These trees have multiple traditional uses for reproductive health specifically and are thick with mysticisms related to the cycles of birth, death, and resurrection in our cosmologies across the ages.

Scientific research has confirmed much of the ancestral knowledge surrounding dates in our ethnobotanical repertoire. Various studies have confirmed the potential of their flowers and fruits as effective fertility treatments across the sexes.[7] Their pollen is used for similar purposes across the region. Science has also corroborated their potent support in pre- and postnatal health, echoing the intelligence in the Virgin Mother's Quranic story. In addition to providing ample fiber plus minerals and vitamins galore, dates act as a powerful uterine tonic. Researchers have found that women who ate six dates a day for the last four weeks of their pregnancy were much less likely to need medical interventions to induce or expedite labor, they endured shorter first-stage labors, and had more intact membranes and better cervical dilation.[8] Other studies found that regular consumption of dates in the four to six weeks before labor and immediately after birth minimized postpartum hemorrhaging more effectively than oxytocin injections.[9] It is also a galactagogue, supporting milk production when eaten regularly after birth. These accessible fruits are underrated blessings in the protection and aide of birthing processes across the board, and are believed in Islam to endow a graceful merciful spirit onto the children born with their aid, per the example of Mary and Jesus.

Today dates are primarily grown in and associated with the deserts of the Arab Gulf countries, Jordan, and across northern Africa. However, in the Old World, it was the coastal territories of Phoenicia aka Cana'an that were referred to as "land of the palms" and were the largest traders of dates. Some theorize that this is how the tree earned its Latin name, *Phoenix dactylifera*. The significance in this name alone lends insight into deeper themes embedded in the date tree myths, including and preceding the story of Mary and her resurrected son. The phoenix is a magical bird with origins somewhere between Arabia and ancient Egypt. They are strongly associated with the sun and element of fire. Phoenixes live a singular life in their species, only one existing on earth at a time. After hundreds of years alive, the bird was said to fly to Phoenicia where it built a nest of herbs to set itself aflame in a ritual of death. From its ashes hatched a new phoenix bird.

Some suggest that Phoenicia itself was named after this bird's story, Lebanon's capital to this day carrying a reputation as a city that eternally "rises from the ashes" of destruction and loss to be rebuilt again, for better or for worse. This bird's power is one of renewal and resurrection in the unrelenting fire of life and its destruction. This is not unlike the date palm itself, which brings fertility, nourishment, and the possibilities of life in even the harshest desert sun where few trees know how to survive. Where date palms grow, there is a promise of water, a blessing of life for the whole habitat. Some suggest that the date palm is the tree in which the phoenix performed this ritual of death and rebirth, the boughs of the trees turning a shade of yellow and red resembling fire at the end of its reproduction cycle. This story reminisces the ritual of eternal life that Isis herself performed on the prince of Byblos when she came to Phoenicia to retrieve Osiris's body. Every night, she would immerse the boy in incantations and fire to endow him with eternity.

Till this day across our region, dates make up the primary ritual food associated with our religious holidays across sects. Most notably, ma'amoul is a buttery date-filled wheat cookie that is customary in the Eid holidays of both Muslims and Christians alike. Dates themselves feature an important role in Ramadan fast-breaking meals, replenishing the body with nourishment and medicine alike during a season of prayer. In the Eastern Christian traditions, ma'amoul is specifically prepared to celebrate the resurrection of Jesus on Easter, continuing these rebirth themes and ushering the beginning of spring as the earth's flowers also return to life. Date palm crafts and prostrating the church with palm branches wrapped around lit candles are common rituals of the holy week, followed by the sharing of ma'amoul on Easter day. Both wheat and dates are symbols of rebirth and renewal, death and resurrection, whose imprint was carried into the Abrahamic traditions of our region from much more ancient times. Both are associated specifically with the feminine divinities of fertility, sexuality, and harvest, but these themes as transmitted in our cosmological legacies are by no means one-dimensional.

Like Mary, Inanna is an expression of the feminine divine archetype in our region's legacy. She is the embodiment of Venus, and a divinity who represents the earthly and heavenly forces of life alike.

She is associated with fertility, sexuality, with the bounty of the earth and grains, war and the duality of destruction and creation, chaos and order, sacred and mundane inside everything in both the cosmos and the earth.

A creation story of the date palm tree features in the Sumerian telling of Inanna's rape and retribution:

A raven was delegated by the creator god Enki to create a garden plot through sacred incantations and materials that he alone specified. From these instructions and the raven's heeding emerged the date palm tree, tall and majestic unlike any other. A young man named Shukaletuda was delegated to install a well and care for this plot of plants where this date palm had grown alongside others. But instead, nothing survived; every single plant was ripped from its roots and destroyed by him. He looked over towards the eastern lands of the gods where he recognized Inanna sleeping under a poplar tree. Inanna, Queen of Heaven and Earth, wore a loincloth of the Seven Divine Powers over her genitals as she rested. The boy approached her and coveted them while she slept, removing the sacred cloth from her sacred genitals, raping her and kissing her there before he returned to his garden plot.

When she awoke, Inanna was enraged by the violation she discovered, determined to find retribution. She asked, "what should be destroyed" because of her genitals being violated? She filled the wells of the land with blood, irrigating all the plants and waters of the land the color red and embarked on a search for the man who was responsible. He went into hiding so she would not find him, but Inanna would not discontinue her search until justice was served. On her second day, she mounted on a cloud and conjured a dust storm of terror as she kept seeking. On the third, she blocked every highway of the land so people could not move freely. Yet still, she did not find him.

Inanna went to Father Enki, enraged and insisting on reparations for what had happened to her. She refused to continue her sacred duties until the man who raped her was found and brought to her for justice. Life on earth would be halted in her strike. Father

Enki agreed to help her. She turned her body into a rainbow, stretching herself across the sky and earth where Shukaletuda made himself small but could no longer hide.

When she faced him, she cursed and berated him. She interrogated him for his guilt. He confessed to his crimes, repeating them exactly as they occurred. He told her about the garden plot that would not grow, the well he did not build, the tree he violated her under, the hiding he later sought. She listened carefully so she may judge the fairest consequence.

Inanna determined his destiny would be death. And what would she think of it? Nothing at all. He earned no importance, none of her mourning. His name would however be remembered in the songs of shepherds to sweeten them, she said, and sung in the King's home. Yet his home would not be near the places where these sheep graze and sing the sweet songs of his name. Upon death, his home would become the "palace of the desert," scorching and bare. This was the justice she deemed.[10]

In this story about Inanna's retribution, a young man who cannot respect the life of garden plants is as quick to violate a goddess in her place of sacred rest. In violating her, he disrupts all life and the natural order of the whole universe until it is corrected and atoned again. The story suggests a sacred relationship between her sexuality and vulva, where her Divine Powers dwell, and the integrity of life on earth as a whole. Inanna is the representation of a woman who is a representation of the earth itself and its life-giving abundance. Life cannot continue without her, but her violator can be forgotten while life flourishes in his wake. Contrary to the modern context, Inanna bears no shame for her violation in this story. Rather, she is entitled to her public rage, and she contains the power to disable business as usual until reparations are ensured. She demonstrates the aspect of the feminine that can and sometimes must destroy in order to create and protect life and the land that ensures it. That wreaks havoc in defense of her own life's respect and the righteous pursuit of justice. Her rage is not destructive for the sheer power of it, like the boy who uproots plants he was delegated to care for; it is corrective and dignified with purpose. Even the blood that fill the fields reminisce the cycles of menstruation which may yield creation, as much as they represent its end.[11] But her agency, as well as her pleasure, is as central an aspect of its insurance.

I am reminded of an old ritual shared with me by my friend Muhammad Abu Jayyab who is a farmer raised in Gaza, Palestine. He tells me of a story he read about old women of a Palestinian village gathering in their fields at the end of the annual wheat harvest, engaging in a lamentation rite of sorts as they cried over the empty fields. While the harvest itself is typically cause for celebration, these matriarchs acknowledge a simultaneous grief in the absence of their recently full fields. Their tears nourish the land with the water of their bodies, as though a promise and prayer for another season of life yet to return—an invocation of eventual rain as they honor the cycle of completion and absence that will soon make their bellies full. They replay the rites of mourning present in these ancient tales quite strikingly. Specifically, the story of Inanna's descent into the underworld, in which she emerges back to the earth as a "Queen of Realms," only to find her lover Tammuz (also known as Dumuzi) has not mourned her at all. So, she sends him back to the underworld in her place. Tammuz is the god of vegetation, death and resurrection, and the agricultural cycles, particularly associated with wheat. He is akin to Adonis in the Canaanite pantheons and shares some similarities to Osiris in the Egyptian. His delegation to the underworld marks the start of the dry season in late summer across the Fertile Crescent. "Tammuz" is still our name for the month of July, in which the harvest and this ritual of grandmotherly lamentation take place. Inanna's story goes on to recount her people baking sweets to offer and reveling in her return, while simultaneously crying tears for Dumuzi's absence. Inanna herself mourns his loss, despite it being her own act of retribution for his disrespecting her. These tales demonstrate the incredible nuance and duality in our existence and within the feminine archetypal mysticisms specifically, depicting a capacity to embody multiple truths at once as we grieve and celebrate life simultaneously, as we destroy with fierceness and create and heal with tenderness at once.

There is constantly something dying and something being born in the earth and inside of us, and these stories offer customs to honor and harness the sanctity inside of this. Muhammad and I reflected on this story within a consideration of the postpartum state in particular, and what insight these matriarchal rites may offer in supporting the layered transformation of human birth, as the nafseh experiences absence in her once full body, while celebrating the arrival of a baby and the initiation in her own new realm of being. The traditional rituals of "closing" the body, the burial of the placenta, the immersion in blessings and herbs that support physical release while ritualizing the energetic transmutation occurring with appropriate time and supports in place, all gain deeper purpose and wisdom alongside these ancestral stories about our primordial matriarchs and our ancestral expression of the local land's cycles.

The date tree is associated with Inanna as it is with Mother Mary, illuminating multiple aspects of the feminine multitudes per our cultural legacy and its continuation within our own lineages. These stories about the date tree also demonstrate ancestral relationships to the earth itself, and ways it is mirrored by or contained inside "the feminine" in its various expressions and mysticisms. They narrate the local cycles of land, life, and death, and demonstrate ways of relating that can ensure and regard its ultimate integrity; the role of grief and mourning, the nature of justice, and the centrality of relationship and mutual care in the task of life's stewardship are all a part of it. Inanna's stories warns of the patriarchy and its dangers and desecration, and suggests alternatives for what life-affirming stewardship could better look like, or what downfalls systems of negligence to life and its safekeepers may ultimately create for the collective forward. All the while, these sacred tales feature wisdoms about our own souls, and the spiraling cultivation of our nature as spiritual beings on earth. Be it Isis, Inanna, or Mary, the threshold of transformation embodied by our matriarchs is often an intimate bridge between descent/the stewardship of loss and pain, and the sheer miracle of (re)birth/the reclamation of life's sanctity, for the longevity of all.

REMMAN | رمان | POMEGRANATE | *PUNICA GRANATUM*

Another medicinal tree whose cultural stories are associated with feminine archetypes and dualities is pomegranate, known as remman in Arabic. Native to Iran, Armenia, and the Western Himalayas, the pomegranate tree has been cultivated in Cana'an since at least the eighth century BC. Because of its abundant seeds, blood red color, and crown-shaped head, it has been associated with royalty and offered to deities of fertility and earthly abundance across the whole of Mesopotamia, Cana'an, and the Mediterranean. It also appears as a Tree of Life in places such as Assyria,[12] and as an icon of eternal life and fertility in the rituals of the Zoroastrians. It is a prominent symbol across Armenia, with similar representations of fertility, abundance, and the persistence of life. Across the ancient sites and temples of worship of Cana'an, pomegranates have been found at altars for Ishtar and Astarte, sometimes made into the shape of libation vessels for making ritual offerings. They also appear in representations of other maternal goddesses including Inanna, Tanit, Cybele, Aphrodite, and Athena.[13] They are equally featured in funerary sites and the decor of tombs, often associated with resurrection and immortality. Later, in the Abrahamic texts, they are associated with Mother Mary and with Jesus's resurrection, and mentioned as a symbol of fertility that bears the power over both death and life amongst Jews and Christians. Some have even theorized that this was the "forbidden fruit" of the Garden of Eden.[14] They feature similar associations to the blessing of life in the Quran.

Similarly to dates, pomegranates embed a layered symbolism of the life-death threshold, and its association with the feminine archetypes of fertility, birth, and sexuality, as well as the natural bounty of the earth and its all-encompassing cycles. It speaks not only to the life-affirming qualities of the mother, but also its endings and transgressions. In a parallel story to Inanna's underworld journey, the pomegranate features in the Greek tale where Persephone gets kidnapped from her mother Demeter by Hades, who rules the underworld. He fell in love with her at first sight, capturing the young girl to make her his wife. While her mother works to bring her back, Persephone eats four pomegranate seeds from Hades's realm. This binds her to remain there for four months of the year. These four months represent the seasonal cycles of winter, when life on earth goes dormant. The pomegranate in this case becomes associated with barrenness as opposed to fertility, and with the loss of innocence. In other stories, the fruit is evoked in stories of rape not unlike Inanna's, adding complex layers to the symbolism represented in this holy fruit.[15]

These stories lend to a more dynamic reality about the maternal and feminine archetypes, articulating the loss within our transitions through various stages of life. Even within the power and blessing of sexual maturity and the creative possibilities it ushers, there is grief, violation, and potential danger. Within the transition from girlhood to sexual maturity, there is a reckoning with pain and the world's desecration. Within the bounty of the earth, there are transgressions and a balance that requires protection and care. There are natural cycles of loss and renewal happening constantly that demand our regard. Pomegranate speaks into the transitional states of these experiences and the more complex emotions and energies they evoke, including the contrasting dualities within.

The pomegranate quite resembles the womb itself, containing seeds that either are shed through blood or nourish the vitality of a new life who arrives and ends at the earth. Fertility is a possibility more than it is a promise—a cycle that contains every multitude and choice. Within birth's threshold, death looms, and within death's, the soul is reborn as the body is returned to soil that grows onward. This is what the feminine mysticisms of our cultural legacy ultimately define and represent—the all-encompassing expanses of the creation cycle and every experience of life and loss, rage and beauty, pleasure, violation, destruction and possibility in between. This lends wisdom beyond merely biological reproduction. Our own agency, as Inanna insists, an abiding part of the justice within it all.

Every part of the pomegranate can be used medicinally and contains similar accounts of duality in its potential actions on the body, while also supporting a return to balance.[16] Since antiquity, pomegranates have been used as a remedy to cool the body from heat and help treat infections and fevers of various kinds. Their astringent qualities make them a supportive remedy for treatment of hemorrhage and diarrhea alike, helping to restore and regulate the digestive system and treat inflammatory conditions such as colitis. The rinds and fruits all together can be juiced or extracted for this purpose. Equally, they may balance heavy menstrual bleeding or prevent excessive postpartum blood loss. Yet pomegranate has also been used in other ways to induce menstruation, and in the Old World was applied as a paste on the sexual organs as a contraceptive, despite its association with fertility and its aphrodisiac qualities. A decoction of the root was used in Egypt to release tapeworms and can be used for treating other intestinal parasites.[17] In Lebanon, its powdered roots are used for a similar purpose, and an infusion of their bark is used as an antispasmodic, their dried flowers as a tonic for the stomach, and a remedy for diarrhea or sore gums.[18] Their high vitamin C and rich antioxidants make their seeds and juice an excellent aide to the immune system during colds or flus. They are highly anti-inflammatory and also make a wonderful contribution to cosmetic health. They help tonify the skin while nourishing it with vitamins and minerals.

Regionally, in addition to medicinal extracts, teas, and decoctions of its various parts, pomegranate is consumed as a food, a juice, and prepared into a molasses we call dibis il remman دبس الرمان. A Palestinian friend of mine insists that this molasses be included in any first aid kit for the treatment of digestive bugs and diarrhea. It is a potent plant with a powerful ritual history in our region as well as a wide scope of medicinal action for multiple organs of the body. I include different parts of the pomegranate in my skin care products, my remedies for sexual health, digestive and immune support, and postpartum healing.

My mother prepares a simple dessert including pomegranate seeds with a splash of orange blossom water and the option to add soaked walnuts or pine nuts. It is a common garnish on eggplant dishes such as mtabbal متبل or salatet el raheb سلطة الراهب, which both feature smoky eggplant cooked directly on the fire. Mtabbal blends it with tahini and lemon juice, while salatet el raheb (meaning the salad of the nuns) chops it into a salad with raw onions, tomatoes, and parsley with olive oil and salt. Pomegranate seeds can even be added to tabbouleh, a traditional salad made with parsley, bulgur (cracked wheat), onions, mint, and tomatoes. Pomegranate molasses often features in lamb dish preparations, sometimes even on the popular street food sandwiches known as shawarma. Their tart-sweet flavor complements the tangy taste so many of our dishes feature. There are also multiple kinds of pomegranates, some deep red with more sour tastes, while others are yellow with more sweetness. Each carry different aspects of the medicine mentioned, and offer their own pleasurable contribution to the culinary palette of our traditional cuisine. This ritual food offered over the ages to the goddesses and imbued with their stories and wisdoms, is one of the seasonal pleasures of day-to-day life in the fall seasons across Cana'an.

MARAMIYEH—OWAYSEH—QISA'AIN |
مرمية—قويسة—قصعين | SAGE | *SALVIA FRUTICOSA*

Sage is known as maramiyeh in Arabic. Other names for this plantcestor regionally are owayseh, qisa'ain, maryamieh, and marmariyeh. An ethnobotanist from northern Lebanon once told me a story of how this plant earned its name:

> There was a young boy who was severely ill. His family took him to doctor after doctor to discern what was wrong, but none of them could help him. His mother remained diligent in her prayers. One night, she had a dream that the Blessed Mother Mary came and guided her to the sage plant for her child. The next day, she collected sage and began to administer it to her son. He healed, thanks to its blessing. In memory of this miracle, the plant became named Meramiyeh in the Virgin Mother's honor. Now each time its name is spoken, her healing energy is evoked once again, supporting the potency of this generous plant.

For my grandmother from the south, this plant is called owayseh. In my father's northern village and most of Lebanon, the plant is known as qisa'ain. Tant Mariam from his village says to me one day, "We call her Imm il Hanoona أم الحنونة," meaning the tender mother. She didn't even know of the plant's story or regional name associated with the Virgin Mother when I told her of it. She simply shared this title as an endearing testament to its steadfast ability to provide both healing and comfort in our own village. She went on to speak of sage's ability to ease an aching tummy, the most fundamental of childhood aches we run to the comfort of our mother's lap to relieve.

Maramiyeh is one of the most common and beloved plantcestors of the household apothecary across Cana'an. Its Latin name "salvia" means "to save" and speaks to the reputation of this plant to heal and protect. Biblically and across old-world traditions, sage is associated with purification and longevity.[19] In Palestine and Jordan, its leaves are drunk almost daily as a tea or to flavor and dress black tea. In Lebanon, it is commonly distilled into a water extract aka hydrosol kept in the home apothecary for first aid.

Our most common local species is *Salvia fruticosa*, which grows generously all across the coasts, hills, and valleys of the region. The aromatic mineral-rich plant is antiviral, antiseptic, antifungal, nervine, antispasmodic, stomachic, antitussive, and hemostatic. It is wound healing, gum healing, and helpful for skin infections while acting as a tonic on nearly every system of the body. Fresh leaves are chewed by Bedouin communities in Palestine to heal mouth sores, and applied as a poultice on the skin to heal wounds.[20] It has a dry energy, helping clear damp conditions. But it also has an incredible ability to move and heal the waters in the body; I use it often in formulas for lymphatic support. My grandfather used to collect the plant late at night when he was kept up with heartburn, or after eating a heavy meal. It is a common remedy for digestive distress, treating coldness and "wind" in the stomach, relieving indigestion or irritable bowel syndrome, and tonifying the digestive organs when taken regularly. It is one of my personal favorite nervines for treating anxious, depressed, and irritable states. I often reach for it in formulas when people are grieving and experiencing other forms of loss. It is a nervous system tonic that helps restore balance and grounding to the emotions and spirit while enabling a deeper presence.

In South Lebanon and parts of Palestine, the plant was burned traditionally during funerary rites.[21] Aunties I have met in Jordan have likewise advised me to burn it alone or with salt to cleanse the home as well as repel unwanted critters such as mosquitos and fleas. In the north of Palestine, it is likewise burned on ceremonial occasions such as weddings and family gatherings to bless the space and repel negative spirits as well as the evil eye. It is grown on graveyards and offered at sacred places and saints' tombs for similar purposes, its fragrance said to attract angels to the spirit of the dead. Maramiyeh has an important role in both birth and death in these communities. As a newborn baby is laid on a bed of these leaves in the mawlid ceremony, dead bodies are also laid upon them in preparation for burial.[22] Maramiyeh blesses and protects all of life's passages, not unlike Mother Mariam herself.

Sage supports clarity of mind and thinking, aiding circulation in the brain. It has been used as a neurotonic for supporting memory and preventing dementia. My maternal grandmother utilized the plant to ease heart palpitations, and as a general heart tonic for those with cardiovascular vulnerabilities. Used as a tea or steam, it is an excellent plant for treating respiratory colds and sinus infections, easing inflammation and congestion while drying up boggy conditions. Its essential oil was found by the American University of Beirut to have anti-inflammatory and tumor-suppressive qualities in the potential treatment of cancer. It is used in Lebanese folk medicine to treat liver diseases.

Maramiyeh is commonly used as a gentle hormonal balancer in our region's medicine. It is drunk consistently to regulate menstrual cycles and is a folk remedy to ease premenstrual syndrome. It is used as an aid for fertility. It can likewise be helpful in cases of adrenal exhaustion, acting as a gentle adrenal tonic. It is an excellent ally in the relief of hot flashes, insomnia, and night sweats commonly associated with menopause. It has blood-moving qualities that can stimulate delayed periods, and hence is typically contraindicated during pregnancy. However, some traditional remedies regionally use it to support tonification of the uterine muscles before and after childbirth. Maramiyeh is useful in weaning nursing children, as it helps to dry up excess milk, though it is also utilized in some traditional remedies for milk production. Its aid in steams or baths postpartum can support healing birth wounds, easing hemorrhoids, supporting expulsion of lingering blood and tissue, and alleviating pain and nervous distress. Amongst Bedouin communities in Palestine, it is used to support those recovering from miscarriage, and ease nausea and vomiting.

Mild but effective hormonal tonics with comparable qualities to sage can be found in a number of our most common aromatic plants and traditions of folk medicine regionally. Chamomile (especially wild varieties, of which there are several), roses, anise seeds, and za'atar follow in this tradition, helpful especially in regulating menstrual and uterine disorders and often reached for first by elders across the villages of Cana'an for hormonal balancing and reproductive wellness. Each of these plants has different energetic qualities and strengths, which can be catered to different bodily constitutions and symptom profiles. I lean often on the combination of rose and sage in remedies for emotional and hormonal support for those who bleed, are in menopause, or simply are having a hard time in their lives. I include this combination in tonic teas for everyday bodily reinforcements with great success. A combination of za'atar and chamomile may be an alternative with similar effects for a different constitution, treating menstrual and hormonal imbalances or nervous system distressors alike.

Sage is hands-down one of the most important and familiar herbal remedies across the whole of our region. In fact, each of these flowers and herbs mentioned is profound in its versatility, yet incredibly common, generally safe, and accessible in our kitchens and gardens. They are colloquial plants nearly everyone in our cultural context has seen and tasted before. They are much like our matriarchs in this sense, the closest, most unsuspecting medicines often our most powerful and miraculous.

Unfortunately, maramiyeh is just as likely to be taken for granted. This plantcestor is amongst the many who have been improperly and overly harvested regionally for commercial export with constantly increasing demands. My cousins tell me how they used to return home from playing outside covered in the smell of this sage. It is still common in the village trails, but in not nearly the same volume. Once a man in a neighboring town told me he has seen people with truckloads of the plant leaving the northern coastal villages. My cousin once caught a man harvesting bag-loads of it from our village early in the morning. When he saw my cousin pulling out his phone to take a picture, he got afraid, dropped the bag, and ran. When my cousin looked in the bag, he found hundreds of sage plants ripped out from their root carelessly, likely to be sold by this man in monetary desperation. The UN Development Programme conservation guide marks it as "near threatened" as a result. Sellers not only over-harvest but negligently collect the early shoots of the plant without regard for its reproductive cycle. Urban growth and the expansion of industrial and agricultural lands are also diminishing the plant's native habitat. Increasing frequency of wildfires due to climate change are an additional concern for the plant's longevity.[23] Restoring traditional harvesting knowledge and adherence to sustainable collection and propagation practices for native medicinal herbs across Cana'an is a necessary factor in protection of these medicines and ecosystems forward.

This is not dissimilar to the threats endangering ceremonial white sage in my diasporic Southern California home. New age trends have capitalized on popular demand for this sacred cleansing plant, appropriating its use as a spiritual smudge practiced for centuries by local Indigenous tribes within their own private rites. Mass over-harvesting to meet the demands of commercial trends has contributed to soil erosion in the ecosystems that depend on it, while diminishing availability of this plant for the Native communities whose traditions have cultivated profound relationships with it locally for thousands of years. Meanwhile, new-age buyers consume these exploited plants in the name of "spiritual wellness" with no regard for the desecration within its practice, people, and the lands from which it was stolen carelessly. A ritual sought in the spirit of healing becomes wrought with colonial violence and earth desecration instead. In these instances, we see explicitly how capitalistic and colonial paradigms ride on each other, reinforced by our own displacement and the negligence it creates. To protect and continue the knowledge and relationships of our Indigenous ancestors to the places we dwell on earth is directly tied to the practice and preservation of land-based medicine and the integrity of this planet forward. We cannot truly heal without either.

WARD | ورد | ROSE | *ROSA* SPP.

Rose is a holy plantcestor I associate strongly with my matriarchs and the underlying healing of grandmotherly energies that hold and pray our world together. I consider this plantcestor a relative, both my grandmothers born to women named Rose/Wardeh. My Teta Renee insisted that roses of every color and variety be present in her garden. While most of her crops were lovingly cultivated for consumption, rose had a sentimental and spiritual place in her tending, surrounding the shrine of Mother Mary that guarded her plot of medicinal weeds at the front door. She insisted to me once that for as long as her Florida house existed, whether she lived in it or not, a Damascus Rose must grow there in her memory. "So it will always be known that, once, your grandmother who loved roses lived here." It was an honor to be able to deliver this dream to her myself the second year before she died, passing down one of the beloved plantcestors tended from my garden to hers for a change.

While rose has become consumed with cliche tropes and commercialized symbols of love, it remains potent in its applications as a medicine globally in the hands of grandmothers and beyond all across this earth. I have met curanderas in Mexico who exclusively heal with roses, understanding their energetic capacity to purify and elevate the spirit. In the Crossroads, the rose carries special associations to the Venusian goddesses of ancient times and the purity and holiness of the Prophet Muhammad and Virgin Mother Mary. In fact, rosaries used to pray to the Virgin Mother were traditionally crafted from the flowers of this divine plant, hence their name. Rose's documented use as a medicine is noted in Mesopotamian tablets aging over 5,000 years old. A fossilized rose over 35 million years old has been found, with suspected origins in Iran.[24] Imagine, this plantcestor records memories of our region on earth for over 35 million years. In addition to the many healing attributes of rose discussed in earlier chapters, it is a mineral- and vitamin-rich aphrodisiac, a uterine tonic, an emmenagogue, analgesic, and anti-inflammatory, with important usages in the realm of menstrual, prenatal, and postpartum care.[25]

Roses are used as a gentle but effective plantcestor for restoring hormonal balance and regulating menstrual systems, as well as aiding the menopausal body. They ease premenstrual syndrome and dysmenorrhea, help relieve menopausal symptoms such as hot flashes, anxiety, and depression, and generally endow balance to the reproductive system when utilized regularly.[26] Their cooling astringent petals can help in cases of hemorrhoids as well as hemorrhage, and have been used in the postpartum context via baths and steams to both bless babies and protect postpartum bodies from excess blood loss. They are also pain relieving, and when used topically as an oil have been found to effectively relieve lower back pain associated with pregnancy, and their aromatic oils as a birthing aid to relieve both anxiety and pain during labor.[27] They also help tonify and moisturize the skin, retraining our cells to hold the right amount of moisture. This has made them a globally favored remedy in facial products, but they may also support menopausal discomforts in which hormonal fluctuations lend to more dryness vaginally and elsewhere. It is not uncommon to find a bottle of rosewater on the bathroom sink of tetas all across Cana'an for use as a facial toner. My great-aunt used to add a dash of lemon and vegetable glycerine to her bottle for added benefits.

Roses are deeply healing to the nervous system and spirit, helping ease mood disorders and restore deep internal balance.[28] They can bring support through low times of depression, constricting states of stress, irritability, and anxiety, and hot emotions like anger and rage. In addition to supporting the nervous system on a physical level, they carry an energetic quality of softening, creativity, and connection. They embody a vibrational wisdom that heals and emphasizes the sanctity of relationship and its various and central impacts on our lives. This makes rose a foundational ally in my own practice for the reconfiguration of relational and traumatic wounding of many kinds, especially that which occurred in the context of intimacy such as sexual trauma, heartbreak, familial conflicts, betrayal, or other painful ruptures between loved ones.

Healing traumatic wounds centers around repairing relational integrity, restoring security with the self, if not with others. As these intimate parts of the body and spirit are activated, I have found roses equally helpful in recovery from birth trauma or postpartum integration more generally. Roses cool and mend the energetic body, helping us reclaim lost and suppressed parts of the self, supporting the expression and digestion of authentic feelings, and helping us process strong emotions within their gentle embrace. They are also an aphrodisiac, reconnecting us with our capacity for pleasure and the power inside our bodily senses. They may help restore the bridge between our bodily senses, our emotional expressions, and our creative joy, spacious to the multiple layers involved with healing and re-membrance from life experiences that have jolted us profoundly. Rose plants are as tenacious as they are sensual—blooming delicately as their petals unfurl, thorny and rugged enough to withstand dry and hot environments with minimal care. Their dynamic spirit and aromatic beauty reconnect us with the fundamental creative capacity and wellsource unique within each of us. Their power reminisces a deeper intelligence of our interdependent earth and the loving web of our life-tending matriarchs in all their resilience, grace, and grit alike.

KAFF MARIAM | كف مريم | "MARY'S PALM"— ROSE OF JERICHO | ANASTATICA HIEROCHUNTICA

The deserts of our region feature their own "rose" of sorts, a majestic plant with tiny white flowers that grows in shallow gravel surfaces in early spring. As it dries and goes to seed, it is harvested from its root and disseminated across the apothecaries of the Crossroads region, specifically sought for its magical use in birth. Kaff Mariam is a visual amulet and physical medicine to aid the birthing process. Its shape is round, with a head of woody stems that curl inward as they dry to form a ball, with one bare taproot underneath. Upon looking at it in its dry form, one can immediately recognize its resemblance to the placenta, a sacred organ dedicated exclusively to sustaining the life of a child in utero. As active labor begins, this dry desert plant is immersed in water by the midwife. It slowly begins to open alongside the laboring person, expanding like a rose as life returns to it. They dilate and transform in tandem. The midwife offers sips of the liquid to the birther to aid them with pain and provide nourishing minerals, evoking the plant's medical constituents as well as its unfurling spirit to smoothly encourage the birth forward.

It is believed that Mary clung on to this plant for strength while giving birth to Jesus. The name "kaff Mariam" simultaneously evokes this memory and the protective hand of the mother who safeguards spiritually while providing physically. The kaff كف, meaning hand or palm, is an ancient symbol in our region evoked to repel the evil eye and associated forms of negativity. It has been syncretized to maintain relevance in the Abrahamic traditions, associated most commonly now with figures of the holy feminine archetypes such as the Virgin Mary and Fatima, the daughter of the Prophet Muhammad. Birth is at once understood as a holy act and a vulnerable one, where one body becomes two, and must completely break open and change form in order to do so. Spiritual aids become as important as physical ones in ensuring both bodies arrive and transition safely. This plantcestor plays a role in both aspects.

"Anastatica" is the Greek word meaning "to resurrect." This plant's almost magical ability to restore its living form once reimmersed in water has earned its name as the "resurrection plant," further alluding to its power and blessing upon the act of birth and its participants. The initiation into motherhood/parenthood is one of rebirth and new life for all involved, as old roles, bodies, and concepts of the self transmute and evolve to meet new ones. A metaphorical death occurs in the journey to deliver a baby earthside. To be safe on the other side of this transformation is a divine grace and victory not taken for granted; it is rather surrounded with prayerful evocations and protective aids to bless the transition homeward for birther and baby alike. The initiation into new life requires multidimensional attention as the bodies and souls involved are built back in a novel form.

In addition to its role in birth, kaff Mariam is used as medicine for various conditions. Bedouins of Palestine pound the seeds and mix it with butter for use as a poultice to treat hemorrhoids. Its cold infusion is used to treat infertility, resolve uterine disorders, and prevent miscarriage.[29] It is also used as an amulet alongside other plants in the treatment of mental illness.[30] Across North Africa, it is noted for its antidiabetic activity and is taken as an infusion or mixed with honey and oil to treat colds. In addition to minimizing labor pains, it is employed to prevent uterine hemorrhage and as an emmenagogue to evoke menstrual bleeding. As an infusion, it is also used to remedy sterility. In Egypt, the crushed plant is taken with sugar as a purge for jaundice, followed by a milk diet.[31] In other contexts, it is sometimes burned as an incense to support the birthing process.[32]

This plant has a North American sister, *Selaginella lepidophylla*, which is sometimes used to conjure abundance, fertility, protection, and luck in the Black American Hoodoo traditions and other Afro-Diasporic lineages of spiritual and folk practice across the Americas. It is much leafier than kaff Mariam, with green leaves returning as it unfurls. It shares common names and some similar properties in its amulet-like usage but is not in fact the same plant. Note cautiously that it may or may not carry the same physical healing attributes if you intend to utilize it. Also note, across the Crossroads region, the name "kaff Mariam" may be delegated to a number of different medicinal plants. Be sure to identify the plantcestor properly before using it for the listed purposes, as their properties naturally vary.

BAKHOOR MARIAM | بخور مريم | "INCENSE OF MARY"—
CYCLAMEN | *CYCLAMEN* SPP.

Cyclamen has many names across Cana'an, several referencing its appearance such as asa il ra'ai (staff of the shepherd) or arn il ghazal (horn of the deer). But in my village, the name for the fall blooming flower is bakhoor Mariam, meaning "the incense of Mary." I recently learned from a Palestinian social media account called metras_global that this name originates from the use of its tubers as a sweet-smelling incense in the Eastern churches.[33] The flowers have likewise been used to symbolize Mother Mary's humility and grace, the heart-shaped leaves and bowed flower head referencing her grief over the body of Jesus after he was crucified. In Cana'an, its tubers are used in coastal areas as a bait for fish, stunning them as a strategy for hunting. A few species of cyclamen grow natively across Cana'an, including a couple endemic ones. They grow in patches under my grandfather's olive trees in late fall, with light pink or white flowers that have a faintly sweet smell and an ethereal quality to them. Their presence evokes softness and grounding at once, and when I spend time near them, I feel almost transported into a fairy-like realm.

The heart-shaped leaves of this flower are stuffed for food in some parts of Palestine, replacing grape leaves at a time of year when those vines have gone dormant. A decoction of the leaf and bulbs is used to treat ear infections in Lebanon,[34] as well as skin infections across Cana'an. The tubers have been used as a form of soap root, rich with saponins that create a cleansing lather, in remedies to heal broken bones, digestive distress, and menstrual pain.[35] Their tubers are mashed and applied to ulcers for healing, and sometimes mixed with honey and olive oil to dress the umbilical of a newborn baby.[36] They are highly anti-inflammatory and antioxidant and used for various infectious diseases, including treatment of cancer. Ancient Greek doctor Dioscorides recorded its usage to induce abortions and speed up the delivery of babies, as well as to make hair regrow and heal wounds and boils. Ancient Romans used it as an aphrodisiac. Hippocrates employed its "purifying and dissolving" qualities in a number of uterine conditions. Its roots were added into vaginal suppositories to induce menstruation, as well as to ease inflammation and uterine residue after a miscarriage.[37] It is associated with Venus and the goddess Hecate, and utilized medicinally as a contraceptive. It was also used as an amulet and believed to ward off evil everywhere it grew. The flower has been associated with the cervix due to its shape and downward-facing direction, and so its flower essence is implicated contemporarily in supporting any conditions involving the health of the cervix and birthing/creative processes, and associated by modern practitioners with the integration of themes associated with feminine archetypal wisdoms.

Part IV

SOUL MEDICINE AND THE RITUAL OF BELONGING

Our Feminism of Soil and Soul is grounded in amal *[hope] as the abiding force, the core, that continuously calls on us to return to it to invigorate our search for and action towards liberation but also our recognition of the ways in which we are already free. Amal in Arabic follows the form of* fa'al فَعَل *meaning "to produce/to put into action/ to accomplish." Amal is a form of longing towards that which may not be in sight. It is a form of* rajaa رجاء *[return]—a hopeful expectation, but also a request. As such, in Arabic, the concept of hope does not hold the possibility of negation. There is no such thing in Arabic as hope-lessness or loss of hope. Amal is a longing, an action, and a request, knowing what we hope for may not be attainable but what makes it seem attainable is a state of faithfulness to the desire, a state of belief in the worthiness of the asker and a state of faith in the omnipotence of the giver. An oft-repeated Hadith of the Prophet Mohammad says:* Ia'aqal wa Tawakkal اعقل وتوكل. *This translates to "use reason and entrust to God." It urges us to consider all the issues surrounding the desirable outcome, take all action necessary to understand and address them, while simultaneously surrendering to and accepting all outcomes with faith that even when our longing is not fulfilled, then* la a'alahu khair لعله خير *(perhaps it is for the good).*

—*Raghda Butros, 2022*

13

Rouhaniyat: Mystical Traditions and Elemental Healing Lineages

IT WAS UP to only a couple years ago that I could ask any local elder about my grandfather and their memory of him would be delivered through a narration of his poems they knew by heart and continued to remember and recite even after his death over forty years earlier. The elders within our more traditional communities still transmit the life of our lineages through each other's proverbs and poetry, meet each other with songs of call and response to express a feeling or story that arises while together; they live within an ethos that everything with a soul lives on. Even their most banal tasks become animated and healing—the baskets they make for gathering or drying herbs become a purposeful expression of symbols, our traditional clothing a colorful vessel for archiving personal and communal stories, watering the garden turns into poems and songs of homage to the soil and its fruits and flowers.

Whether in the solitary act of one's own duties or the communal efforts of labor, daily tasks of our village legacies naturally transform into soulful improvisations that channel healing to the lives of its members. These integrated lifeways are our most potent remedies. Our traditions of togetherness, culture, and craftsmanship allow our body to move, touch, and feel, while our spirits express and digest. They are a method of emotional integration and articulation that reinforces life not only practically but spiritually, emotionally, and bodily through the fulfill-ment of our wide spectrum of senses as we live through even the grav-est tribulations. They ritualize the moments of our life into an archive of feeling and memory, each one when it's honored, able to move on with deeper grace and wisdom. Simply practicing culture carries profound possibilities of healing.

There is a whole realm of wounding beyond our bodies that beckons attention. Emotional and generational traumas damper life and cloud its essence and possibilities of beauty and deeper belonging. These inte-rior landscapes are often hardest to articulate and find adequate care for, yet they massively determine the quality and capacity of our daily lives and relationships. How have our ancestors and traditions negoti-ated the invisible wounds of life? How did they find a way through the treacherous passages of pain and loss that their own stories of exile are full of?

Increasingly, it seems that these are the terrains that most afflict us as modern humans; our colonial displacement becomes spiritual displace-ment, all the fragmentation it creates landing in the utter disruption of our mental health. I have witnessed this repeatedly in my personal life, my family, and broader communities. In my travels across Cana'an and the Crossroads, I have often asked traditional elders what their approach for this layer of healing entails. Though the question seemed unfamiliar to many of them, I found a consistent answer everywhere from Nubia to the highest mountains of Lebanon: heart-to-heart con-versations with someone who the person feels comfortable, respected, and understood by is the foundational support towards emotional healing. Once more, relationship is the heart of what keeps us intact, reflecting our fundamental cultural value and way of navigating life. Religious leaders and spiritual practice also play a significant role in mitigating such wounding.

In parts of our region, ceremonial healing happens through rituals like zar, still practiced in places mostly across northern and eastern Africa, the Arab Gulf countries, and Iran. Zar is an Afro-Arab tradition that utilizes polyrhythmic drums and chants to evoke trance states and spirit possession, whose messages are then interpreted by a trained ritualist who discerns and negotiates what is needed to appease the spirits revealed through the ceremony. In my time visiting the island of Hormuz in the southern Gulf of Iran, the family I stayed with recalled their own stories involving the zar for reconciling severe emotional states and imbalances, believed to be caused by jinn جن, or spirits. The whole island was filled with colorful sands considered sacred, and corresponding songs and stories of the jinn with whom they interfaced and lived amongst. Such traditions are also common in northern Africa, where similar practices of spirit possession through dance occur for ceremonial healing, such as the Gnawa of Morocco. I once talked to a Moroccan healer who insisted to me that zar was once predominant in Cana'an, so much so that their jinn often came speaking in Assyrian by way of our region. The practice of these ceremonies has largely declined in Cana'an since, perhaps no longer existing at all. And throughout the broader region, is increasingly delegated to the realm of haram, where it persists in the secretive underground of our rarest communities, or takes on more performative and celebratory roles stripped of their full ritualistic or healing aspects.

Part of the restorative intelligence inside these ceremonial healing traditions lies in their multidimensional and multisensory approach, embedded in the nature of cultural practice more generally. On one hand, it is built on the axis of the interconnected impact between the spiritual and the physical worlds, which is at the crux of "mental health." On another hand, in the absence of contemporary theories about trauma, our ancestors already understood that healing emotional ruptures begins with the body. Every aspect of our ceremonial cultures joins the intelligence of the earth and elements (through burning sacred plants, the use of water, oils, etc.), the senses of the body (through movement/touch, song, smell), connection and emotional expression (through expressive communal practice), and spiritual partnerships to negotiate the mysteries beyond and inside it all. Where many systems of these cohesive spirit-healing practices have dwindled or changed in recent decades, these aspects still persist in some form through most of our social and cultural rituals—our dances, crafts, food, ways of gathering, and praying, each leveraging layers of what we need to heal. Our traditional crafts are more than just practicality alone, more even than just beauty; they are altars at the foot of life, and their way can heal us too. To create and to tend is to mirror the divine in the earth and the beyond, the source of all this life, after all. Our traditions and the willingness within their making are full of understated rituals and love that persist in their power to aid and transform, more often than not in collaboration with the bounty provided by the land itself. As our relationship to land is severed, these traditions erode. As our traditions erode, these built-in cultural forms of healing become less available to our maintenance as living beings.

Still, the spiritual anchors and supplements everything within our culture of healing and living, through both folkloric and religious forms. Our name for spiritual mysticisms is rouhaniyat روحانيات, coming from the word "rouh روح," meaning soul. Whether within the context of our Abrahamic practices or the animisms of our locales, these facets of practice are often rooted in the remnants of more ancient lineages of healing and kinship to place, and bound more explicitly with the earth as a primary source and vessel of the Divine's grace and revelation. While the way we seek, and who we pray to varies and transforms across eras and context, our existence is steadily sustained by the spiritual devotion of matriarchs who whisper our names to the heavens for a lifetime, and the ever-evolving forms of generational practice carried down in our homes. A broom, a basket, or a meal, the hands and voices of our elders infuse the mundane with the holy in every step that builds our cultures of life.

Ancestor Healers

On the urban streets of Beirut and scattered all across the villages of Lebanon, images of politicians and political symbols are matched only by those of our local saints. The most famous amongst them make a holy trinity of their own: St. Rafqa, Mar Charbel, and Hardini. There are no faces and figures more recognizable than theirs and the Blessed Mother Mariam's, who so often accompanies. Public altars to them are built in stone terrace walls, endless sidewalk shrines tended by neighborhood grandmothers, and wheat-pasted images on the side of buildings and shopkeepers' walls. Their silhouettes adorn bodies and homes alike—amulets, jewelry, tattoos, and figurines present every-where. These saints are not borrowed from Rome or legends in books but made from the villages and lineages still living on our lands. Their testaments are built by our own stories of miracle and redemption. Our saints are our healers, our Medicine People, our holy intermediators. They are real people, who lived deeply human lives not so long ago. Who suffered and healed amongst us, with families who neighbor us still—ancestors who lived so well that their death continues to usher life through our veneration.

In days of old, each city and town of Cana'an had a patron deity whose honor they maintained for the protection and well-being of their community and the earth. In the Christian villages across our region, this tradition has been traded for patron saints. Each village has churches named to specific saints and performs festivals honoring their celebration on their feast days. In my family, my mother chose a specific saint as guardian for each of her children, praying to each one respec-tively when she felt our lives veering off path or in need of additional support. Cultivating a relationship of guardianship that strengthens over a lifetime and generations is one of the potent keys inside the heal-ing kinships manifested. My family is not unique in this matter, nor in the numerous stories of miracles experienced in our own lives due to these holy spirits. While Christians in Cana'an are particularly associ-ated with this practice, it has maintained a significant presence amongst

Sufi communities. Kurdish, Egyptian, and Anatolian Sufi friends have taken me to numerous neighborhood shrines of similar devotion, full with people as devout in their requests to their local saints and prophets, and with similar celebrations to honor them in the villages they belong to. Some remnants of this tradition remain visible within the Sufi communities of cities like Trablos طرابلس (Tripoli) in Lebanon and Damascus. In Palestine, the shrines of al Majdoub المجدوب and Nabi Gaith مقام النبي غيث remain standing, though their visitation has decreased significantly in recent generations as Sufism gets pushed to the margins.[1]

In the mystical expressions of Islam and Christianity as well as amongst Druze, saints and prophets are honored and solicited for help of infinite kinds—particularly for healing, each with their own specialties and affinities. Many of them endured illnesses and challenges while they were alive that became associated with their healing capacities. These instances echo the archetype of "the wounded healer," human and not without tribulation, but no less capable of profound transformation, love, and service to life born from intimacy with their own wounds and masterful wisdom of the spiritual. Amongst the most famous shrines of Egypt include the Prophet Muhammad's granddaughter, Sayyida Zeinab, whose tomb is often packed with visitors because she is the saint of grief and loss, who witnessed the massacre of her own family when she was alive.* "Sayyida سيدة," a common prefix for these (female) saints, is the word for "master" in Arabic. In Islam, they are recognized as masterful "friends of God." Across the region, tombs and temples are visited by people of every sect to petition for healing, fertility, and miracles to address the most unsurmountable conditions of their lives. This is where many people resort when conventional medicine fails, or regular forms of prayer and intervention are not yielding results. It is just as much a part of our daily stewardship of protection and generational care. Acts of reciprocity and sacrifice are made to these spirits to fortify the petitions made. Sometimes this involves alms, fasting, or promises to be fulfilled as

---

* Gratitude to my friend Rena Sassi for sharing this with me.

the wish comes to fruition. For example, if the petition is for conception or healing an ill child, the child may be (re)named in the saint's honor. Other examples are promises of a behavioral change, form of ongoing service, or routine of prayer; feeding or offering money to the local community; or sometimes even religious conversion or the construction of a place of worship. Sometimes people pilgrimage by foot to the shrines of these tombs, even barefoot, when their request or devotion is dire enough. Circling the sacred places a number of times is also common.[2]

One of the primary rituals of healing embodied in these sites is through the energy of physical contact with the tombs themselves. Everywhere, people can be seen touching the feet of statues on the grounds, kneeling at the foot of the tombs, or collecting leaves or spring waters from the area to embody the blessings upon return home. Sometimes persons who have received miracles from the saints come and allow others to touch their hands or bodies in a similar transmission of barakeh, or blessings. People even sleep at their sanctuaries to immerse in the orbit of its blessings, with delegated quarters for hosting in some of the larger monasteries. It is a common tradition amongst Christians to wear amulets from these tombs. They can be gold pendants engraved with their faces, or lockets with a small piece of cloth blessed or worn by these saints inside it. These items maintain connection between the energy of the person and the saint in a sustained somatic way, believed to reinforce the prayers and blessings. Wearing robes in the colors associated with the saints is another invocation of healing and homage.[3]

Petitioners who visit these sites typically take candles, cotton soaked with oil, holy water, and frankincense blessed by the priests home with them for continued healing. In the sacrifices offered, people may leave personal items that are meaningful to them as part of an energetic exchange, but also to fortify this physical relationship of contact by leaving a part of their own energy behind. It is as often that crutches or medical aids no longer needed are left as testament to the healing miracles once complete. The tomb of Mar Charbel, a healer and saint who lived during the political turmoil of the Ottoman Empire, features many such items and an array of handmade metal votives he carved while he cultivated prayers for those who petitioned him. Some take the shape of a hand, a heart, or another limb of the body that needed healing. In Lebanon, the monastics who still live in these sites are known to cultivate land and tend the traditional crafts of our region as part of their devotional practice. Creation connects us to Creator. A life of natural simplicity and foundational self-sufficiency is understood as part of their vocation and service towards the realization of God, and ultimately in responsibility towards the Divine's creations on earth.

There is a quality of peace near these particular tombs and monasteries in Lebanon, often located on the top of a mountain. Some of them even occur in areas that were sacred temples to earlier gods, with ritual dates or customs that overlap from ancient eras, carrying over the generational cultivation of sacredness in a continuous thread of time and ancestral connection.[4] But throughout the whole of Cana'an, such worship also happens quietly in the discretion of nature. Natural landmarks are sanctified in the name of these holy spirits where devotional relationships are cultivated to leverage their blessings for the people. My friends in Jordan have taken me to visit old-growth trees in remote neighborhoods where local saints and saints-to-be are revered by their neighboring communities. An ancient tree, a natural cave or grotto, or a holy spring of water may be imbued with offerings of reverence or prayers left in the form of strings tied on branches or other such symbols.[5] These pieces of cloth or string become a physical representation of the prayer, of presence, and they establish contact between the person and the saint or prophet who is honored there, and later can be collected and shared as a vessel of their sacred energy for healing forward.[6] Old-growth terebinth and oak trees are particularly common sites of such worship, grand beings embodying their own life-giving properties to reinforce the work of miracles and medicine. There are a number of grottos and caves with this association in Lebanon, and some especially spectacular ones amongst the Druze, such as the one for the Prophet Ayyoub (Job) in Niha, covered with candles.

The elements play a significant role in the legacy of our saints, who rely on the medicine present inside the land to both self-realize and perform their healing. Their medicine is our version of vibrational or energetic healing, through alignment with the power of life/the earth. Their mere presence is enough to transmit this blessing but could also be aided by the elements and nature. When they die, people find miracle through consuming soil from their graves, cloth, water, and oil passed over their holy bodies or infused with the energy of their tombs that still emanate life. It is the candles lit with fire in their name, and the frankincense blessed at their shrines, that carry our prayers through smoke. The water collected from their springs for ablution.

In the fulfillment of their ascetic calling, saints typically devote ceremonial periods of silence, fasting on simplified plant-based diets with no sugar or fruit, and isolation within the refuge of valleys, mountains, and deserts in our region. One such valley is so famous for this in Lebanon that it is called Qadisha Valley, meaning "holy" in Aramaic, or Wadi il Qannoubine, "valley of the saints." Sufis and Christians alike have found revelation here. The valley is particularly sacred to the Maronites, whose ancestors took refuge in this valley when facing persecution from the Mamluks and other empires. It features some of the most ancient Christian monastic sites in the world, including Ethiopian, Greek, and Syriac-Maronite churches, and the gravesite of eight Maronite mummies from the tenth century AD whose robes and remnants document important insight into the cultural expressions and continuity of this ethnic group over time.[7] This valley is bound with the Eastern denominations' stories of resistance to latinization and religious conversion—some of the earliest efforts against European colonization in our region.

I remember reading about Mar Charbel's stories of communication with the snakes on the grounds of their monastery. Some of the stewards were pruning the grape vines when a huge hissing snake came towards them, ready to strike. They tried to kill it but could not capture it. Mar Charbel came out and told them to put down their tools and back down. He approached the snake with a simple gesture of his hands speaking directly to the creature to "go away from here." In a testament to some deeper attunement and respect of the sacred between them, the snake instantly slithered away, no harms committed. One of his most notable miracles involved his ability to usher away locust swarms devastating the grain fields of Annaya, where he lived in 1885. These locusts were ravaging the whole region, resulting in a famine met with harsh political rations and blockades of food by the Ottomans in power. The combination of these factors resulted in the death of almost five million Lebanese, intentionally targeting the Christian communities.[8] Mar Charbel prayed on water for the locusts to leave, and began sprinkling the water on the fields. Every single one he visited was salvaged, allowing Annaya to maintain cultivation of the life-sustaining grains which fed the entire surrounding community. The peasants in the area witnessed what was occurring and began to visit the monastery to acquire his holy water for their own farms. Each of them experienced equally miraculous results, and came to help the monastics with their harvest in a gesture of gratitude after the fact.

Many of his other stories involve mysteries of light. His first miracle was when the oil lamp in his room was traded with water by the trickster young boys who helped maintain the monastery, but somehow the fire did not extinguish for the entire night. When he died, people from various villages surrounding the mountain tomb saw mysterious lights hovering above his grave, attested even by nonbelievers in the surrounding area. Even months after his death, his body did not decompose in the way most bodies do, but rather his bones remained hard, hair and nails continued to grow, and his body produced a strange oil-like substance that soaked his robes and poured from his tombs uncontrollably for years.[9] The liquid was used for many healing miracles. These stories compel me. They rest somewhere between the cosmic and earthly, attesting to powers that heal through relationship with the universal vibrations inside life's constant becoming. Ultimately, these mysticisms harness deep earth technologies cultivated in Indigenous intimacy since the beginning of time, activating memory of the power inside our most ancient relationship to place and life itself, and returning us towards its source as ultimate redemption, possibility, and autonomy.

The saints' ancient legacy is one so tenacious and true that it transcends religious form and era. It pierces the dogmatic patina as a requirement of reverence. Their stories and the popular practice surrounding them accentuate the animistic mysticisms within Abrahamic practice, as a direct continuation of what and who preceded it. Due to this fact, folkloric rites surrounding them are sometimes shunned by the more dominant and imperialist religious leadership of certain denominations. There is something fundamentally powerful (and threatening) in their practical and magical centrality to "the people"; it re-anchors spirituality into sustained forms of self-directed relationship building through tried-and-true rituals of ancestral reverence and elemental intervention, rather than institutional affiliations that necessitate formal mediation with the Divine. Our communities are fervently anchored and self-determined in these ways because they have worked for them. They elicit a fundamental truth that often gets lost in the colonized version of more modern religious conventions: that the universal force of life itself is what contains and ushers divine consciousness and healing, and that it is most immediately accessible via mutual kinship with the miracle of our earth. It is the land that re-members us and calibrates us towards the Source of Creation, and its sanctity is directly connected to our own humanity and its stewardship. The earth is the key homeward, soulward, Godward, within life's most irreconcilable wounds and mysteries.

14

Country of
the Living:
Arz Libnan

Trees may justly be called special reservoirs of energy. The result of photosynthesis in the green portions of plants is the formation of carbohydrates, rich in energy, and the release of oxygen. Plants trap the energy of the sun and cosmos, transform it, and thereby provide for life on the planet. Modern biologists have confirmed the ancient idea: the cedar has a soul. This amazing tree has the same biological rhythms as people. The cedar displays its activity not at precisely defined times, as do other trees, but depending on external circumstances. For example, on overcast days in the summer, it "wakes up" at 10:00 a.m., while on bright days it awakens with the dawn; there is a pause in its activity from 3:00 to 4:00 p.m. In the evening, the cedar is "active" until 11:00 p.m., and then "falls asleep" for the night. In the winter, its life cycles are not suspended, as with other trees, it remains awake, but only "sleeps" much longer.

—VOZROZHDENIE [REVIVAL] FOUNDATION[1]

Cedars of Lebanon | الأرز | Cedrus libani

Atop the highest mountain in our region is tucked an ancient cedar grove, shrouded with mysticisms and stories from across our ancestors' legacies. The whole of our land and people live in the understory of this forest and its life-giving secrets, the oldest amongst them still standing in modern-day Lebanon. These trees, which live to be thousands of years old, grow into canopies of flat-topped plateaus with deep evergreen needles, up to forty meters high with trunks almost three meters wide. Their divine boughs carry both masculine and feminine parts on the same tree. Every September, their "flowers" cover the ground with divine yellow pollen, significant blooms happening every four years or so. Their cones are bright green eggs that rest firmly pointing upward on the top of their canopy outstretched, aromatic sap oozing from the inside of them down their skin onto the floor of the soft mulch ground. Inside them, they carry dozens of seeds with fragrant embryonic oil encasing them, waiting for cold and moisture to gently soften them enough to open and germinate in the earth in the essence of this luxurious holy embalming fluid. This is the water in which they are born, once considered a sacred anointment of khair, blessings, on the head of our Canaanite ancestors, according to local lore.

The way these trees grow is as ethereal as it is earthly. They are almost circular in their shape, with branches that stretch into a generous orbit of shade, and unlike other trees of this age and enormity, the roots do not reach deep into the core of the earth. Rather, they spread wide, creeping horizontally across meters of space, just as their branches. Their root systems mingle with every other plant growing in their midst, touching the earth for meters of diameter around them. Underneath this forest and surrounding it are dozens of freshwater springs, blessing canals of cold water and ice-melt that nourish this mountain and beyond. How is it that roots hovering so near to the surface of the earth could uphold trees made of such dense tons of hardwood? Their form is a metaphor for their mystical quality, a mirror of "as above, so below."

Mountains are holy places to traditional peoples all over the globe, and we are no exception. Their pyramid-like height endows closeness to the sky worlds and our reception to the mysteries of divine and cosmic realms. These cedars grow at an elevation too high for most other trees to flourish, surrounded by an ecosystem of endemic plantcestors with medicine unique to this point on the earth. In a region scarce of high mountains and dense forests in general, this one has been particularly important to the ancient peoples across the whole of the Fertile Crescent. On one hand, this forest is considered an "abode of the Gods" themselves, home of Sumerian Ea (Enki), whose primordial waters make life underneath their roots. This forest is the "Country of the Living" to the ancestors of Mesopotamia—a place of creation where life is infinite, and abundance emerges.[2] The cedar trees are sites of oracle and divine revelation, associated with immortality and considered a threshold between the mundane and spiritual worlds where gods dwell in their "garden," once even more densely lush. The Khemetic temples of Egypt used this sacred wood to build the doorways of its shrines and the tombs of its leaders within this knowing, and its oil to embalm their mummies and papyrus.[3] The Phoenicians built their divinely instructed ships from cedar trunks, star maps within their wood body whispering wayfinding genius into our ancestors' night sky navigation of the world's oceans. The temple of King Solomon was built from its timber likewise, the Bible full of references to this holy tree's strong, blessed, and purifying nature. In Islam, a majestic tree is found at the Gate of Heaven, where the Prophet Muhammad is taught how to pray by Allah during a miraculous nighttime journey ushered by the angels, amidst a time of great personal hardship and grief in his life. Some suspect this too was our cedar.[*] This same cedar that enveloped Osiris's tomb on the shores of Byblos is believed by local mystics as the place where Jesus's spirit ascended, and a gateway for all the "blessed" spirits coming and going unto our earth. Even modern mystics like Gibran Khalil Gibran and Mar Charbel have been made inside their proximity, raised inside the cedar mountain villages and called by the divine under their canopies.

---

[*] Thank you to my friend Emanne Desouky for sharing this story with me.

On the other hand, the rare access these forests offer to hard timber in a region sparse with large trees has made this ecosystem a practical commodity to the various empires who have increasingly exploited and felled them into near extinction. The resin inside these trees resists mold, insects, and bacteria and lends a type of natural sealant, making this wood resistant to water and quick decomposition. Once upon a time, they covered so much of our lands they were seen as inexhaustible, extending across the whole span of modern Lebanon and beyond. While their use amongst our early ancients was certainly notable, they were generally still felled with a degree of discretion due to their sacred association; before the Greco-Roman empire took control of Cana'an in the first century AD, the cedars were typically taken with permission from the king, who granted their timber only after receiving blessings from the gods through divination.[4] This somewhat mitigated the extent of their harvest. But between changing belief systems and more industrial technology that eventually made logging and transporting timber easier, the demand for these trees became more aggressive and reckless over time. By the end of the Greco-Roman era, plant life was seen as a lower form of life, and these trees, once used mostly to craft things of a sacred value, became completely utilitarian.[5] The Ottomans used them for things like furniture and fuel, and eventually alongside the British, also destroyed them to build railways that could enhance their empire-building efforts.[6] It seems worth mentioning that these railroads in our own lands have been obsolete since, literally with no longevity or local benefit beyond the 1970s, thanks to war and the imperial remapping of our region.

The cumulative effect of the cedars' overuse in the course of the past few thousand years has fundamentally changed the ecological reality of our entire land. In more recent years, in addition to overgrazing and overdevelopment for commercial interests such as ski resorts,[7] climate change has both impacted these trees and been affected by their degradation; these trees are experiencing infestation of damaging insects and slowly being forced to migrate towards higher elevations to survive.[8] Despite this, some of the ancient stands from these historic eras still remain standing by some miracle, with even rarer stewards who still heed their mysticisms and devote their lives to the continuation of these divine trees within an understanding that their existence is completely bound with our own. It has been one of my deepest re-membrances to immerse in the relationships of this forest and its living tenders as an ongoing ritual of my life. Their blessing is undeniably palpable, and their guardians as precious with treasured wisdoms and the healing legacies inside our land.

Medicinal Legacies

From my village in coastal Lebanon, I pilgrimage north, through the Chekka tunnel, past the cement factory, up the nearby mountain, past Koura, across the Holy Qadisha Valley, and through numerous villages quaintly lined with locally made baskets and homegrown figs sold on streetsides, to finally reach Bsharri. I stop at the bakery for a perfect man'ousheh—notably more delicious in the mountains, before the car climbs just a bit further up to arrive at the old-growth reserve known as Arz il Rab—"the Cedars of God." It takes about an hour and a half total. I arrive to the warmest greetings of a beloved friend and mentor, Hakim,** and his family, who have been tending this sacred forest for generations. They welcome me with a cup of coffee in the traditional Lebanese way, pulling up a broken plastic table and chair to talk a bit on the patio before I submerge in the forest. Hakim and his brother Karam are natural philosophers, well studied in the oral histories, eco-cultural,

---

** Out of respect for this Elder's privacy, I am using fake names to refer to him and his brother. I chose the name "Hakim," which means "wisdom," and also "doctor," and is the title we use to refer to traditional medicine practitioners of Arab medicine. Traditionally, to be a healer in our region is associated not just with technical skills to treat, but a quality of spiritual wisdom and knowledge of life—qualities aptly present in this beloved Elder and his lineage. "Karam" means "generous" or "hospitable," and expresses the essence of this family and Cana'an's mountain villages.

and medicinal legacies of this mountain. Each visit with them inspires new layers and stories, and always deepened love. They have devoted their lives to replanting thousands of trees in an effort to repopulate the endangered stands, in continuation of the work of their own father and grandfather. Despite governmental appearances, they do so with great resistance or faulty interventions from state authorities. It is clear there are many sacrifices inside their humble life, but they rarely speak about them, instead emphasizing the ways it is deeply meaningful for them to live (and give) as they do. Hakim's nephew and niece are still young but have already learned how to tend in this same legacy.

The cedar forest makes up a unique and precious bioregion, thick with endemic plants and medicinal species that locals are slowly losing generational intimacy with, many of which have also disappeared as a result of the ongoing degradation and climate collapse.[9] It is estimated that only 5 percent of what once entailed the range of these sacred trees still exists on the earth.[10] Their oldest stands are in Lebanon but their largest is in Turkey, and a smaller forest still thriving but threatened in Syria. Hakim is a knowledgeable steward and herbalist trained by time and experience in the forest, and folk wisdom passed down by his mother who was a midwife and healer. Every time I walk with him through these old growths, he teaches me of the small plants in their understory, quizzing me on my retention of knowledge and comparing folk uses in collaborative exchange. Hakim and Karam also tend baladi food gardens with impressive bounty. This is notable considering the short growing seasons and harsh conditions of the high mountains, a testament to the generational intelligence of their family's kinship with place. He tells me that the plantcestors of these forests are poten-tized with extra medicine, the clean air and cedar resins multiplying everything with antifungal, antimicrobial, and vitamin content.[11] It's so strong I can actually taste it when I eat wild roses gathered from underneath their midst. He gives me honey made from the cedar pollen, and advises me to take one spoon every morning at least fifteen minutes before eating anything; it will protect my immunity, balance my digestive flora, and bless my spirit and body with healing, he insists.

The cedar wood, resins, and young shoots are highly antioxidant, anti-inflammatory, antifungal, and antimicrobial.[12] They have been studied for effective treatment against tumors and cancers,[13] and have been used traditionally in a number of ways for healing skin conditions, respiratory disorders, and infections of many kinds. They are expectorant and have anti-aging effects on the skin and brain.[14] In folk medicine of Lebanon, the resins are incorporated into salves, and ash is made from the dead branches to treat deep infections or growths under the skin. Their smoke is used to aid constricted breathing such as asthma.[15] Given their endangerment, this medicine is not typically a first resort. What is used of it is from ground harvest or the remains from annual tending and pruning. It is still regarded as a sacred medicine to locals. Most of all, these trees are soul healers, providing deep recalibration to the nervous system, spirit, and being through their presence alone, and blessing the air of the entire mountain with healing.

It is worth noting that while the spiritual healing properties of Lebanese cedar are similar to those of American cedar honored amongst various Indigenous tribal groups within their respective bioregions, these trees are actually from different species altogether. American cedars are part of the Cupressaceae family (like juniper trees), whereas cedars are part of the Pinaceae family, reflected in their familiar needle-like foliage. Still, the cedars and redwoods of the American West Coast have endowed me with similar feelings of home and healing in my diasporic homes. There are a few species of juniper, known as lezzeb لَزّاب in Arabic, that are similarly significant to our cultural and ecological legacies. In Lebanon, these species are able to grow in even higher elevations than the cedars. Because their propagation requires their seeds to be digested through the guts of a certain bird, they face an added threat to extinction, and highlight the interconnected nature of our livelihood as species.[16]

Old-growth trees are mothers in the plant world, harboring infinite life beyond their own and containing a special role in life affirmation as well as the consciousness of humans who seek to re-member. They embody whole universes of generous nurturance, their bodies making up the habitat and sustenance of humans, birds, fungi, insects, and hundreds of other living organisms. Numerous plants flourish in their understory and receive water from their massive root systems, while their existence also helps manage the climate factors that ensure water and oxygen for humans and mammals. These trees are keystones in the formation of their ecological families across the earth, which include our species. Be they oaks, sequoias, cedars, dates, or baobabs, their presence, in more ways than one, determines our own.

Stewards of the Sacred

Hakim and I first bonded over our mutual love for plants, and a shared practice of "charging" under the oldest of these holy cedar trees. He would find and join me in my quiet ritual of sitting for minutes or hours with my back against their trunk, legs on the ground, listening and absorbing the energy present. After some time, he would begin to take me, or let me lead him, to different parts of the forest where the energies could provide greater healing. Along the way, he picks things from the ground and feeds me from the land. I ask him questions about tiny flowers. He observes my way of walking and connecting, reflecting on changes noticed year after year. Our deepest exchanges have happened within this ritual of forest submersion. Under these trees, our conversations have a different quality. Ceremonial even, a sort of infinite liminal feeling where time and space expand and disappear at once. Our words and their vibrations yield extra power, entering at the level of the spirit. Consciousness expands differently, feels wider and softer—more available. Sometimes I don't even remember the exact words exchanged once we emerge, but a quality of cellular understanding carries me forward, and I feel utterly transformed. Truth be told, I feel this even alone in these woods, my whole being recalibrating in renewal after some time spent.

Hakim says that these cedar trees have the highest electromagnetic field in the world, their aura and aromas performing psycho-spiritual healing to all who encounter them. He iterates that the larger the tree, the wider and stronger its orbit of healing reaches. He tells me of the numerous therapists, healers, and mystics from around the world who have come to visit with this intention, sharing their own anecdotes of wisdom and study along the way. Amongst the most consistently sought, he says Arabs from the Gulf regions have revisited frequently asking him for cones and resins from the forest to use for incense. Its spiritual properties are cherished even more highly than the frankincense and myrrh sacred in their own territories, and highly sought by us for use in our religious ceremonies. In fall, the hot sun beams on these trees and the aroma of these resins and pollens fill whoever is lucky enough to be there. The place transforms me. A couple days on this land renews me with clarity, bodily strength, and emotional balance. The forest itself is surrounded by mountains that become a deep shade of golden pink at sunset, illuminating everything with hues of warmth as the portal between day and night closes. The old growths are positioned perfectly in the womb of these glowing hills, cradled inside their sacred lap, collecting all their glorious energy. The feeling is purely wondersome, transformative. There is also a cumulative effect that occurs in my repetition, each visit deepening with feeling and memory, like all relationships do. Hakim acknowledges this as a result of ancestral kinship to place from generations that precede me, affirming the power of these forests to literally re-member me, and alluding to that quality of mutual recognition or bonding that fortifies with steadiness and time.

Born and raised by this mountain, Hakim profoundly embodies the sensibility of these cedars—full of Indigenous understandings emerging from within his direct relationship to this holy storied place for lineage upon lineage. It moves me how thoroughly he understands the integrity of the holistic ecosystem he is a part of. He has not studied formally, never lived or visited outside Lebanon, barely even leaves his village to go to the cities. He has not been trained in the spiritual disciplines of monasteries or other institutions, nor does he quite heed the religious conventions of those around him. His knowledge emerges almost completely from within his own relationship to his village. From within this exact place, Hakim's transmissions of both ecological and mystical understanding are profoundly astute, and often resemble the most advanced "discoveries" of scientists and leaders in these fields. I ask him sometimes how he learned this or how he knows, wondering if a teaching has been passed down by his own elders or learned some other way. His answer is usually along the lines of "I learned it through watching this forest" or through trial and error of his own "scientific" process. He tells me about how he would study the patterns of the bugs and organisms inside it since he was a child. He shows me how he eats from the seasons of the land, what diets and processes of immersion support him towards clarity and spiritual reception. He is a child of this land, a purest student of its most minute details of soul and soil entailed. His reflections illuminate the universal threads of truth that weave through earth-based knowledge systems which within their numerous specificities, ultimately emerge from the same source: the earth. While there are various aspects of such wisdom present in fragments all across Cana'an's villages and mysticisms, the quality of depth, meaning, and cohesion Hakim conveys has become very rare and increasingly convoluted within the pressure cooker of modernization and imperialism. His existence reminds me viscerally that there is no deeper source, no truer and more direct avenue to re-membrance, revelation, and healing than direct relationship with the land of place. That regardless of every fragment lost, taken, or buried, every species erased and ancestor forgotten, the earth beneath and inside us is still complete in its knowing and readily awaits our communion.

Hakim's existence also reinforces the critical position of our sacred sites and ancestral stories of becoming. While earth itself is our source—a full microcosm of life's wisdom and healing wherever we are—this particular forest Hakim has grown in is not just any place. These trees are part of our spiritual power and cosmological existence. That these stories alone have maintained a presence in our lives after thousands of years and many iterations of cultural transformation and erasure since seems as destined as these trees somehow, still standing despite all attempts to annihilate and extract. Hakim emphasizes to me that these trees exist as long as we do. Rather, that our own existence is dependent upon theirs. That once they cease to be, we fall quickly behind. Our souls are necessarily bound together. Beyond national symbols, corporate, and political co-optations of these legendary trees as a nationalistic symbol, there is a deeper story inside their power that ripples despite and through us. This forest is the "garden of the gods" that made us. Its quality of immortality and divinity is reflected directly by the biodiversity of life that is harbored in its midst. When we ourselves immerse in it, life's consciousness and mysteries imbue us, re-members us homeward.

Cosmologies of Reverence and Desecration

Karam told me that before this place was called Arz il Rab, it was called Arz Il (or El), "Il" being the ancient title for gods as well as the name for the chief god amongst the Canaanites and Sumerians and their Abrahamic descendants.[17] He shared a story about an ancient king who became angry when he learned that some people living in a mountain forest of cedars atop Lebanon began to call the place in God's name. In a typical display of patriarchal power holding, what place could be grander than he, after all? He grabbed his beard with one hand, and his hair with the other, pulling the strands from his face and head with anger, and vowed to go confront them himself. He traveled up the mountain to find them. Once he got there, he was stunned, in awe at the glory he did witness. A dense evergreen forest, the bough of each tree more than a foot thick, the floor covered with inches upon inches of fragrant resins. It was unlike anything he had ever seen or felt before. His spirit was transformed by merely being in its midst, the incense entering his lungs and soul and rewiring him completely. He left converted, agreeing that this place was not only to be named for the gods, but that the trees were to be protected and treated with correspondent reverence. Hakim said that once upon a time, a circle of stones would be placed around a thing to mark it as sacred. At first, it was one huge tree in the center that they surrounded in such a way. But the circles kept growing and growing until eventually, the whole grove was surrounded with a stone wall. This phenomenon would continue across the ages and empires. Even many who began with a will to exploit these trees would, by some circumstances of nature, be brought to their knees with mercy for their glory and undeniable power. Sadly, like most of the creation sites and stories across our land, this forest has recorded as much violence and desecration as it has holiness.

Their story of the king's visitation reminisces the Epic of Gilgamesh, one of the most famous and ancient written stories, and one of the most complete of the Mesopotamian clay tablets transcribed from almost 4,000 years ago:

> Gilgamesh was the King of Uruk. He was ⅔ man and ⅓ god, with dominion over many things, but he was not granted immortality like the gods. He needed to conquer something grander to be remembered for eternity. He convinced his resistant friend Enkidu, once a child of these forests himself, to join him towards the Country of the Living. Here, he would kill the holy monster Humbaba, divinely delegated guardian of the cedar forest.

> They went to Shamash god of the Sun, the Council of the Elders, and Gilgamesh's mother to ask permission and blessings to make their journey. Though they each deterred him with disapproval, his insistence and fragility around his mortality evoked enough pity from the gods to grant his wish. . . .

> It took them 3 nights to arrive at the foothills, and 3 more days to cross seven mountains before they reached the gate of the forest. They made offerings at every significant transit along the way. They received dreams of guidance and affirmation each time, until they finally arrived at the gate of the forest. There, they stood, admiring the beauty and peace of this beautiful Cedar place, home of the gods and throne of the goddess Ishtar.

> They were in utter awe of its thickness and lushness, so entangled with trees that there was barely a pathway in. A strong cacophony of birds and monkeys chattering. Sacred sap that fell like

waterfalls along the trees, more precious than gold and with a fragrance that intoxicated them with peace. Giglamesh dug a well to bathe in and make another offering, as they were instructed. They poured grains to the earth at sunset. Their dreams spoke of victory. The next day, they awoke for the final battle.

Gilgamesh felt weakness come over him, as Enkidu once assured him he would. But they had come so far and it was now Enkidu's turn to encourage his friend and remind him of his strength. Gilgamesh took his axe and fell one Cedar, immediately calling the attention of Humbaba who was enraged at the sound of it. He went immediately to interrogate who had come to commit such a crime. He thought Enkidu returning home would be a blessing, but instead he brought with him a threatening intruder. Betrayal overcame him. An intense battle ensued and they succeeded in killing Humbaba . . .

For miles, the Cedars shuddered and shivered at the sight of this loss. The mountains began to change their shape, their fierce guardian no longer present to protect. The symphony of birds and animals paused in silence, ran for refuge as these men entered this holy forest, and began to fell the Cedars one by one to take back with them to their city.

Enkidu looked back on what they were doing, even more regretful and ashamed now that the task was done. He turned to his brother Gilgamesh and proclaimed to him, "my friend, we have reduced the forest to a wasteland. How shall we answer to Enlil now? What was this wrath of yours that you went trampling the forest!?" . . .

When they were done with their harvest, Gilgamesh took the head of the guardian Humbaba, kissed the ground and presented it there to Enlil, the God of all Gods and all of Creation.

Enraged at them for acts which they had no righteousness to violate under his law, he scolded them harshly and in anger, warning them of the destiny they had just carved for themselves, and the retribution that would soon be made as a result of their life-desecrating choices. It was not only victory that would follow them home, but reparations. And so it would unravel in the stories to come.[18]

As our regional cosmologies so often do, this story warns of the endangerment and exploitation these sacred trees have faced for thousands of years now, and the dark side of "civilization," patriarchy, and empire on the desecration of the holy earth. Furthermore, it illuminates the rawest emotions in the human condition, and our responsibility or destruction of life within their negotiation. The epic describes in detail the density of life and diversity of species once protected in this forest, which seemed more like a jungle then.[19] The earth *is* the home of the gods, its vitality explicitly nurturing our own, and its destruction ultimately diminishing our peace forward. The gods convene to devise a plan for appropriate consequences after the numerous violations Gilgamesh has committed, which began with the murder of Humbaba and the logging of the forest and continued with his insulting the primary goddess of fertility, Ishtar, and killing her Bull of Heaven. They argue about their own responsibility and regretful support of Gilgamesh in his initial pursuits, and finally determine that one of these men must die to restore the disruptions within this violation. Enkidu falls ill and dies a death of no glory—the kind that will not be remembered. His loss sends Gilgamesh into a deep spiral of grief and regret, and an even greater terror of his own mortality. He embarks on a journey across mountains and oceans, killing numerous lions, bears, hyena, and other animals along the way, and spurning every helper on his path. To his surprise, when he finally meets Utanapishtim, a human turned immortal by Ea, he sees familiarity in his being and is disarmed for a moment as the man reminds Gilgamesh of his own privileges. The moment is short lived. Gilgamesh returns to a self-centered, aggressively fearful, and frustrated disposition within his ongoing realization that there is no escaping death for him. Utanapishtim's wife helps Gilgamesh prepare for the eventual return to his city, where he begins his journey of reparations, both to the gods and to the wilds.

This story is rich with relevance and hints about the digressions of our modern world, and the "cultures of severance" perpetuated within the separation of humans from the earth and the divine within. Gilgamesh embodies the shift from connective reverence and life-affirming values to securing personal power driven by fear, insecurity, and underlying inferiority. He begins as the archetype of male fragility and dominance at once. Ultimately though, his trauma and fear cannot be bypassed. His spiral of grief and violence eventually put him "in his lane," offering a different possibility of development and "civilization" that's aided within the reverence of the gods (the earth) rather than the narcissistic impulse to supersede them. Enkidu, on the other hand, began as a child of the divine forest and was forcefully "civilized" in earlier chapters of this epic, eventually leading him on a path that was contrary to his own essence and resulted in a painful death characterized by regret and dishonor. He symbolizes the colonial wounding of severance from the earth's nurturance and our nature as a part of it. The eventual immortality of Gilgamesh does get fulfilled by this famous epic, which for the most part, ironically, puts his most human imperfections and disgraces on vast display, hopefully in the ultimate service of a deeper teaching and warning for descendants to avoid these same mistakes. The details within these stories carry their own remedies and secrets through tribulations of our very real lives on earth, including detailed depictions of familiar human emotions and the behavioral tendencies within their neglect, as well as the arch of their possible healing and atonement.

One message highlighted by the Garden of the Gods is that the natural world abides its own laws and balance, and violation of its life-affirming nature results in eventual consequence to keep said balances in check. Whether we are conscious and diligent towards our innate interdependence with the earth and cosmos, it is a biological fact of our existence. So much so that to harm the natural world is to harm ourselves, because we are the natural world. Development and empire do not alter this reality. The symphony of life on earth requires each part to fulfill its purpose for the next part to remain on course, and the system as a whole will repurpose what needs to be reconfigured in order to ensure this cascade of co-creative relations persists—it adapts in order for life to continue. These sacred trees are close to us on an essential soul level, a kinship so deep that when violated, it responds with sharp immediacy.

Every time I visit Hakim, I hear a new story demonstrating the way Enkidu's retribution has continued in the lives of those who commit harm against these trees or disrespect the natural order of its sacred grounds in any way. Many of these stories are things Hakim has personally witnessed or experienced in his own family, and some are more historical anecdotes passed down. He told me once of a dream his mother had during his childhood. They had some sheep they had kept close to their home, and they needed a barrier to block them into a small pen they created in the rocks to ensure they would not escape. So his father or brother went into the forest and grabbed a piece of wood to serve this purpose. His mother wasn't even aware this had happened, but when they fell asleep, she had a dream about it instructing her to ensure the wood was returned. They immediately did so, reminded that even for them as stewards, to take anything from those grounds should not be taken for granted. That respect requires intention, permission, and purpose that is conscious and mutual so we may not veer into the nonchalance and extraction that ushers many of the horrors inside these ancestral stories.

Hakim told me another such story about how the Ottomans eventually came to respect this forest, despite themselves:

There was an Ottoman ruler whose daughter was delegated as the leader of his army force in the area. One day, he asked her to take her troops to the Cedar forest and cut down their trees to bring to him. She and her troops went up to do what was ordered and she commanded them to begin cutting down trees. But something came over them, a force beyond explanation stopping their arms mid-swing with axes. They, like Gilgamesh, became weak as soon as they entered the old-growth garden, and the commander stood in awe as they took pause to reassess their plan of action. It wasn't long before her father came marching in on a horse, yelling and scolding her and the troops for not committing the order, determined to enter and do the deed himself. His horse quickly kicked him off its back and the ruler lay unconscious on the ground. His daughter, convinced by the eerie mystery of this forest, got down towards her father and petitioned the trees in his favor. "To the power that lives inside this forest, I ask you, please spare my father his life and I promise that I will work everything in my power to protect and guard you with respect thereafter." The Spirits of the Forest heard her and granted her that blessing, and from that time on, the Ottomans delegated the old-growth cedars of Arz il Rab to be a protected holy area, off limits for timber.

This effort was soon followed by the British Queen Victoria, who funded the construction of the wall around the old-growth reserve in 1867, which has since helped prevent goats from overgrazing on the young trees. Both these empires had a hefty hand in logging the forest for their own utility, these stories echoing the premonitions within Gilgamesh's story, which eventually end in some form of amends, however insufficient they ultimately are at addressing the systems of damage being perpetuated against our earth and ecosystems; their regeneration ultimately depends on the sovereignty of Indigenous stewards around the world who have been dispossessed from their lands and cultural knowledge by the hands of these very same empires. And yet there is irony in Gilgamesh's determination to be immortal, a wish that is fulfilled somehow through this pertinent story being told thousands of years later. Foolish as he looks within it, his prayer somehow enchanted it into rare survival; this epic is amongst the few and most intact records of our cosmological legacy, numerous sacred artifacts like it still being actively looted and destroyed across our region to this day.[20] This holy forest has been as enduring in its reverential insistence, named to (the) God(s) even as their nature of worship has shifted and transformed over eras. This portal of cosmic heaven on earth remains standing despite all odds and efforts, with lessons to heed so that we may continue onward in re-membrance, inshallah ان شاء الله (God willing).

The Earth Re-Members

I asked Hakim and Karam what they themselves would like to transmit from the memory of this forest, this holy mountain inside their blood.

They emphasized most of all the importance of returning to the land, starting slowly and simply. Karam said to begin with a mere visit, then learn to grow your own food, or at the least, eat the food that grows locally where you are from. Food, they both insisted, is an accessible and intimate avenue that will open most who have been severed back to the memory and mysteries inside the natural world and its kinship and healing. They spoke specifically and extensively about the importance of returning to visit ancestral lands. When I explained to them that many living in diaspora either do not have the ability to do this, or struggle to integrate once they do, they insisted that it was much deeper yet. Karam emphasized three points of importance in regards to this:

1. Il rouh ma bit moot الروح ما بتموت. The soul never dies. There is a fundamental essence that cannot be lost inside of us, nor through time or space. Its truths are steadfast, always accessible and operating inside of us and inside of life, no matter how long or how far we have been severed. This truth is in some sense, inevitable, despite the ways we ourselves repress or ignore it. Or at the very least, always accessible if we choose to nurture and return to it. We reactivate it when we cultivate these kinships to the living world.

2. Asar il ajdad أثر الأجداد. The ripples of our ancestors—their inherited effect on us. Their energy and stories retain gravity and a pulse in our lives. No matter how long you have been separated from the land or ways of your ancestors, their legacy continues inside of you and the earth you come from. To relate to the land, foods, plants, ways of your ancestors is to awaken and rekindle them. You cannot be separated from your ancestors and their legacies, even if you have forgotten or been away. We are made of them, their imprint continuing to inform and guide who we are, even unconsciously. Karam emphasized the ways the ancestors' ripples are registered inside the soil and land itself, echoing the Plantcestral Re-Membrance philosophies my own practice centers upon, and reminding me of the power inside relating to the land where we come from, to reactivate ancestral legacies of memory and wisdom that do not die. But also, the secrets in relating to any land at all, which will ultimately lead us to this same source of truth inside us.

3. Fikr فكر. Thought. Consciousness is pivotal, and is what allows us to move from the dissociative amnesia of loss and severance, towards reconnection with these fundamental truths and the healing they provide. To engage the land in the ways suggested here is part of what opens and builds this consciousness, not by inserting something that wasn't there, but by reflecting and activating the dormant wisdoms that are already inside of you. To engage and work with your own mind and being towards understanding, expansion, and integrous choices is also a part of this process. As earlier sections of this text have reiterated, the flowers and trees of our earth are one avenue to support this aspect of cultivation, vibrationally expanding perceptions and deeper knowledge—but we must use all of our human faculties to re-member, including our mental ones.

These teachings highlight the relationship between us, our minds and spirits, the lands we come from, and our lineages as fundamental parts of us that have the power to yield life-affirming wisdom, connective re-membrance, and transformative healing. Hakim has left me with something yet more practical and profound in its directness and simplicity; a teaching he has emphasized repeatedly, and shared quite concisely with a group of friends from the region I once brought to sit with him is "hafzu a'ala jugrafiyitcon حافضوا على جغرافيتكن *Focus on your geography—the place where you are.*" Or in the impression left by my grandmothers: *tend the life in front of you.* Hakim says that the way to re-membrance and the recalibration of our consciousness is to drink the water where you live, eat the food grown there, immerse in the elements of place. This is the most foundational road homeward towards the prevailing truths and integrity of our worlds. He emphasized that "your geography" is about where you are from, where you are born. And when I asked him what that means then for diaspora-born like myself, he suggested that where I was born physically is significant in this picture, and where my spirit was born is always a woven part of that. Similarly to what Karam emphasized—that the ancestors ripple through me/us, our bodies a remnant of their original blood-land no matter where we are, but they are built forward by where we dwell today. My spirit retains a connection to Cana'an and the diasporic homes that ushered me to life, mutually, and to relate to the place of my universe, I must immerse in the elements of each of these homes that make me.

The consciousness of these Indigenous tenders emphasizes that to connect to land where we are is a sacred act and a practical one at once. These are life-affirming truths that reattune our source, our souls. Belonging is realized through stewardship and embodiment with land, no matter where we may find ourselves. This is the fundamental relationship that returns us to who we are and have ever been.

15

The Ritual of Belonging

THERE IS THIS distinct quality of cohesion I observed in my parents growing up—this way they do not seem to doubt or crumble under the pressure of external worlds. Regardless of what tribulations or hostility faces them, something essential inside of them remains intact, steady. It does not push them off their own soul's axis. It is as though they are spiritually tethered to their own inherent dignity. It took me years to grasp what was beneath this state of trusting security that felt so fragmented and fragile within my siblings and me raised in diaspora, and so many of the peers and students of my generation who I have witnessed over the years. I did not detect its source until I internalized the stories alive in my father's village, immersing myself in them bodily over and over. Until I loved my grandmother as an adult, truly witnessing and joining the ways her body made home in foreign earth.

When I am in Lebanon, the summer is for the sea, and the sea is a place of family, thick with memory. My father's coastal village is one of the few remaining clean public beaches in all of Lebanon, and it functions as the communal living room of local folk of every age who gather there ritually, day after day. His cousins and extended kinships await me at 4 p.m. to immerse together. We settle on the rock under my cousin's house to swim to the cold spring at the te'a rock, and then return to bask on the sun-warmed boulders till we dip again. All chattering, all jokes along the way. Each reef and route is familiar, familial, a testament to relationships curated over generations by the people of this place that I happen to be a part of. Each rock we rest on is named endearingly, like the te'a, meaning window, where, as children, my father and his cousins would rinse in the cool fresh spring water before returning home for the day. Or the maghsal, meaning sink, where they bathed the sheep and learned to swim in the shallow sheltered pool formed by the massive boulders. My father's stories of his childhood are anything but lonely. Even amidst pain and the natural reckonings of growing up, the human shortcomings we each carry. Even after generations of colonizer after colonizer in exactly these places, each turn eroding a bit of something Indigenous inside of us. The children of my father's village would gather daily in spite of everything time had taken, continuing their own ritualized routes and rhythms, with all the aunties dwelling shoreside watching and bathing them like her own.

Every part of my dad's village marks some kinship, some mishap, or memory made thru relationship with the elements already existing there and the care embedded by the people who naturally pulsated in unison with the place itself. He and his siblings spent the school year mostly in Beirut, but my father's formation is an intimate, living imprint of this village. These places inhabit him bodily. As I witness him there, feel aspects of him each time I bathe inside the sea that raised him, I finally understand that tethering thread. It is the spirit of this land that is my father. It defines and fortifies him, enshrouds and emanates from even thousands of miles and decades away. The relationships of care it constructed through his upbringing linger inside of him, making him who he is and me who I am by extension, however fractured. This foundation of love rooted firmly and specifically in place protects him, realizes him, embeds that unwavering sense of belonging and responsibility in the earth of his own spirit and body, everywhere it lands.

There have been so many iterations of colonization and erasure in Lebanon that it awes me how this rootedness in place managed to remain intact up to my father's generation. That despite languages and customs lost and taken, the land can always maintain a deeper story, weave a wholesome type of care inside its inhabitants, endow its own memory and power to a kinship that withstands despite all efforts and odds—and transcends surface notions of belonging to nation, with identity anchored in the creative power of place itself. I ask my father if he thinks this still exists in Lebanon, in his village now. He notes the ways more recent iterations of military occupation have since planted seeds of mistrust and disrupted safety in the social structure that is long to repair. Be it war or departure, to rupture a people's relationship to their place is to sever something fundamental and holy. Despite this, I myself feel unexplainable healing in those waters thick with memory, and learn deep lessons of "belonging" from those who remain still on their shores. Not because it is seamless or given, but because it is something lived in my flesh, (re)built in ongoing kinship.

Immersing in the elements of my lineage homes has re-membered me profoundly. Generational memories of place help reactivate the earth inside a person, the soul of those unwavering truths our modern world so aptly severs. But what connecting to them has illuminated more than anything is that the relationships built in bodily communion are what sow a sense of belonging and home. It is Hakim's call to "focus on your geography," Teta's acts of "tending the life in front of her," it is the earth inside my baba's body that nourishes life everywhere he goes. Belonging is about relating to place, everywhere that may be. This applies doubly in diaspora.

Diasporic Dysphoria

Having a generational relationship to place is so powerful because its familiarity is built over decades, reverberating cellularly in expansive and integral ways. The intimacy of this continuity yields understanding and revelation from within the land, and profound co-creative kinship between its stewards and creatures across species. For those who feel rootless and are able to, visiting ancestral lands is highly advisable. "Belonging" is complex and requires mutual relationships that can take time to rebuild, even if only recently separated. You may not feel at "home" there right away or at all, even if you have lived in a nearby city all your life. Yet there remains the land itself, and its reverberations carry their own consciousness with an incredible power to re-member, even if you don't detect it consciously. To find a body of water, a desert, a mountain or spring, a grove of trees or meadow of flowers, a cross-breeze of gentle wind and simply immerse in it, is a truly ceremonial reunion—an offering to the ancient imprint of memories inside of you, and a somatic bridge of healing towards what lives beyond it through your mere existence. To allow your being to commune with these elements of place and do what it will with you—even if only once in your life—can be transformative and propel a whole array of revelations and reconnections into motion.

I am viscerally aware of how much this alone is a privilege, especially amongst the diasporas of Cana'an, many of whom live in exile, unable to enter their lineage lands due to the militarized borders of settler-colonial states and political dictators alike. There are many even upon return who have no villages left to return to, demolished by empires recent and past, or are not free to commune with land and water for whatever plethora of reasons. Even immersing in the ancestral sea I touch almost daily in Lebanon is a mere aspiration for my friends living in Occupied Palestine who belong to these exact same waters—not because it is geographically far, but because their mobility is restricted by the Zionist state oppressing them and restricting access to their own generational land. I do not take for granted how such severance looms across the expanse of our region. Even for me whose mobility and access is greater than most, the instabilities of Lebanon and its surrounding borders have reminded me more than once in just my lifetime that return is never promised, and often not simple. Generations of exile and land loss lurk somewhere in each of our family lines, and often fluctuate within our very own lifetimes. My hope is that one day it will just as suddenly turn in our favor, restoring our lands to their borderless integrity, and its belonging to our lineages who have tended and loved upon it for thousands of years continuously. For those unable to return to lineage lands but longing for this connection to their ancestral homes, cultivating a relationship with a plantcestor of your lineage is another powerful way to bring the land intimately close to you. Belonging is a human need, and some form of connection with land and lineage is an avenue available to everyone, no matter where we live on this earth.

There is a stark pattern of dysphoria amongst the displaced communities scattered across the cities of the Global North. I repeatedly witness students, peers, and acquaintances become frozen in consuming levels of unacknowledged grief, which oftentimes manifest into chronic pain, debilitating illness, and unshakeable mental health conditions; we are the earth, and we carry the systemic transgressions against our lineages and the land in our flesh. Generational wounds untended, traumas never addressed, losses not yet mourned, all flush our system in a cascade of spiraling emotions with no place to express but our bodies, when the proper containers and witness to honor it are not present.

One of my wisest teachers spoke often about this intersection of emotional, physical, and ancestral wounding. Doña Lucia Perez Santiz is a Maya-Tzeltal curandera from Chiapas, Mexico, and she insists that 95 percent of the physical wounding we experience is rooted in the unreconciled emotional. I could theorize about the ways that the comforts of diaspora outside our region signal just enough physical distance from war and its memories to allow the aches of generations prior to surface in the body—particularly for those generations who did not migrate themselves. Cultural and physical factors of displacement and dissociation, with inadequate social structures to support emotional integration surely don't help. The culture of the Global North is too often painfully individualistic and deficient in love to properly hold this. But Doña Lucia would say that regardless of physical distance, what occurs within our ancestral place and people at the time we are born will ripple through us for resolution, and that it is only through studying these ancestral inheritances from our past several generations that we can begin to liberate ourselves from them, and harness the gifts within. To know our ancestors is to know ourselves. Just as Hakim would say to immerse in their land is to realize their memory, Doña Lucia calls on us to become conscious of the stories within our own bodies and beings. All these elements are what make up the ecosystems of who we are and our state of wellness. Our mental health is a conversation with our collective story and homelands across time and space, and it directly affects our sense of belonging in this world. Alas, it often strikes me how much this emotional expression differs amongst those living in the homelands where these wounds are open and the conditions of life are frequently more severe. This is due at least in part to the spiritual and collectivist character, cultural continuity of place, and traditional customs built in to ritualize life and loss.

The truth is, practical (im)possibilities of "return" aside, re-membrance is a realm charred with grief. To live within these ruptures is excruciating. To thaw from them is a reckoning full of tenderness and relentless confrontation with loss—thick with rage and despair for how lost and estranged from relationship itself we have become in the process. We yearn profoundly for returns—physical and otherwise—we will likely never quite know, and miss many glimpses of it because our desperation makes us insatiable or full of doubt. We grieve, swimming in feelings of spiritual orphanage and abandonment that seem to deepen with each generation displaced. Even in return to the land, to our homes, to ourselves, many of us are haunted by isolated and tenuous pathways, forgotten languages and clumsiness in the face of even the most simple skills we no longer know how to perform. There is often as much shame in forgetting, as there is pain and hope in remembering and return.

There is so much irreparable. Even the most merciful moments of reconnection are born ultimately alongside the species, traditions, and lands already gone. In this era, even the animals lose their relatives more quickly. The plants disappear before our eyes. The trees and rivers live on the brink. Even the shorelines shrink in front of us. Boulders of memory crumble in their water to make way for another resort. Plastic fills the bellies of its majestic creatures. Oil from war ships suffocates the floor of its primordial grounds. Relatives seeking refuge sink to the bottom of its sea on dinky ships. Wildfires swallow whole ecologies of life in front of our very face. War resounds in its continuation. Dictators determine our inability homeward as they destroy it. And so many of us have barely touched this land before it disappeared.

In all the holiness and desecration alike, there is inevitable aching. The diasporic longing to "belong" from this displaced land of the in-between propels a search that evokes the rawness of it all more distinctly. The call of return to the earth and our lineages places us inside the source of life and the visceral site of its losses all at once, and everything feels true enough to propel us, but still too far to touch. Our loss is what compels us to re-member. It signals the void of something so essential, it never completely leaves us; our yearning towards it is its own testament of continuation. All things born and re-membered considered, this way is loaded with emotion and breaking open as we stumble through the mysteries of it all.

For the multiple generations removed, this diasporic grief is often paired with a nostalgic longing towards a homeland or cultural lifeways one has never known bodily, or mixed feelings about one they have been alienated from. Reconnecting "homeward," literally and otherwise, can be complex for multiple reasons: gender, language, cultural barriers, sexuality, religion, family abuse or estrangement, and so on.

Reconnecting to land can be as tender when we have been severed for some time. For some of us, our ancestral relationships with land-tending have been exploited or looked down upon due to class or racialized violence, and there is healing of another level to be had. For those in North America, Australia, and elsewhere, this sense of displacement from motherland is often echoed by the chilling reality of living as uninvited guests on other Indigenous people's unceded land, alongside the prevailing sense of nonacceptance into white American hegemonies and the pressure to adapt to them or disappear completely.

I have seen these layers translate into a pervasive sense of shame and deep disconnection, a non-belonging and lack of permission to "be," anywhere. This deep need to connect to land, identity, and home lives without a sense of how and where to find one's self in it. Folks are neither fully connected or "allowed" where they are, nor where they come from, oftentimes displaced from inside their own bodies and beings as a result. This is often multiplied for those living in recent exile, whose integration into a new home can feel like betrayal—a somatic admittance that the determination to return to one's rightful home has been surrendered for the comfort of somewhere new. The dysphoric condition of nonconnection this creates makes living in the most basic sense unbearably difficult. This trauma of the colonial wound ripples in every aspect of inner and communal life.

We also live in a colonized time when the impulse to remember sometimes turns into a need to claim some distant Indigenous ancestor, cultural identity, mysticism, or role of healing that gives one a sense of authority that somehow validates their permission to belong—particularly for those acculturated in the Global North. Without a rooted relationship and mutual recognition from within these communities and homelands we claim, these reclamations become dangerously hollow. Seeking from a state of loss and dysphoria, it can be easy to be led astray. Alienation results in searching everywhere but where we are. This makes sense, since where we are often doesn't feel safe. Traumatic wounds sever us, and fracture our fundamental sense of belonging and security in our own body and being. We seek connection homeward because a deeper part of us knows this relationship is what will redeem us from these wounded states. But belonging homeward has less to do with nominal identity and fixation on the past than it does with sincere relationships nurtured in the ecology of the here and now. Our ancestors reveal and live through us. Our authenticity and well-being is what facilitates their continuation, and hones our connection to them, ultimately. The in-between is its own sacred place, the gestational grounds of the everything and the nothing which is ours to embrace and nurture.

Re-membrance is a constant becoming, not likely an arrival. For the colonized, return is ongoing and perpetual, not eventual.

In so many ways, we live in a time of unyielding rupture, the utter darkness of decomposing and becoming to re-member at once. Amidst it all, the earth persists. A future is still sown from the ancient inside our bones who don't forget as readily. The dualities are uncomfortable and miraculous. Our yearning forges a new road out of sheer need, and there are plenty of dead ends and fertile mysteries within it. Babies are still born. Ancient grains of wheat come back to life. Whales adapt to survive. Dreams remind us who we are. We are brought to our knees in a field of poppies that fill us with childlike wonder for a mere moment. The ocean liberates us into a catharsis of tears returned. We create something beautiful, find love in something simple, hang on to rare moments of connection so savored they linger longer. The miniscule joys become a lifeline that do not replace sovereignty, but reattune us to the possibilities inside creation and liberation when it begins to feel impossible. Re-membrance offers some hope of reconnection and reconciliation forward through these disconcerting terrains.

Our roots are fundamental to understanding who we are and what we bring to the table. They provide an anchor and a profound reservoir of resilience and meaning. But how can one feel cohesive and connected to any place, community, or sense of self to access this, if they are dissociated from where they are? If they are severed from the basic safety and "home" of their own bodies?

Humans learn and self-realize through reflection. There is no "self" without the other, no healing without relationship. The people and places we relate to every day inform how we understand, express, and become. They are the elements that usher our life today, nurturing the cellular foundations laid in our ancestral bodies. Through stewardship of the ecology we inhabit here and now and immersing in the familiar elements that imbue life, our bodies begin to mend the ruptures of traumatic wounding with the aid of the plantcestors and earth. Neglecting land anywhere in the world that we exist not only perpetuates colonial patterns of severance and extraction, but reinforces the wedge of dysphoria, spiritual displacement, and non-belonging to life and lineage that hurts so many diasporic and modern people. Where belonging to culture, identity, and social communities is its own complex battle for many in the modern world, it also can never replace an integrated kinship with the earth—the source that unites and makes us. Cultivating relationship to place where we are is not just possible but a necessary part of balance, liberation, and restoration to the Indigenous truth of our earth worldwide. It returns us homeward and restores universal integrity to the ecosystems of life our species inhabits.

Belonging Is a Practice

Village life itself has taught me: there is nothing automatic about "home." Whether Indigenous, traditional, or diasporic—ancestral, displaced, or continuous across time, belonging is a practice. A cultivated relationship that deepens with presence and repetition, illuminates with the culmination of eras and efforts.

Village life is a ritual that sustains and regulates through its continuity. It's a routine of lifeways that anchor even when everything else collapses—so steady and rhythmic it becomes familiar and familial. Every day, when I come down the stairs towards the rocks where I swim, a precious young boy offers me flowers. I offer them in turn to the sea. I know exactly who I will see once I arrive there, or who I won't, based on the time of day. Which folk I will find on which rocks. Which will fish onshore and which will submerge. The trails they will choose inside the water, and the way they will dive in. Like clockwork, I know which tetas will be sitting on their balcony watching me, greeting me. Inspecting the company I am with.

Every day, my dad's cousin parks his tractor along the coastal highway after a full day's work and climbs to the rock between the te'a and my cousin's house. I have never seen him swim, just catch fish after fish for hours until the sun is close to setting. First he fishes to the right side of the rocks, and then to the left. When I see him driving in his tractor through the village, he smiles and waves at me, his fisher's hat on his head and his kind face ready to welcome me, sincerely. Here, he is so deep in his devotion that he rarely notices my greetings from inside the water. My dad says he has been practicing this way since they were children.

Imagine. Through occupations and multiple wars, through economic crisis, food shortages, and pandemic, through deaths and births and all life's valleys, this a'amo عم(uncle) and his ritual with the sea have endured. Each night, he eats and feeds his family from this communion. The fish of its water build the nourishment of his very bones.

When I leave the sea, I drive along the mina ميناء road to get back home. The people who live in the house with the huge plumeria tree wave at me from their balcony. They don't know who I am, except by virtue of my routine past their house. "Howle," they tell me. Stop in for a visit. Every once in a while they scold me for never actually doing so. A few doors down, the men from the fish restaurant gather in front of the garage. They nod their head at me in acknowledgment as they carry on. Just down the way, an elder with white hair and big glasses sits with his wife, cane in hand. He stares at me every day, but never smiles back. The road and its inhabitants are as predictable as the companions on shore, as steady with arrival.

There are a million cycles of repetition like this in the village ecosystem. As I ripen inside of them, they educate and elucidate layers of understanding I wasn't actively seeking. My body acclimates in its own repetition of return, and I find myself veering towards the patterns of locals with an unexpected regularity. It's an atypical one, really. Each year a deeper rhythm of unison happens unwittingly. My days used to be each one on a different rock, at a different time of day, a constant fluctuation inspired by moods or a wish for solitude. But this land has slowly absorbed me into its chorus over time. I become more like a bird inside a flock, whose movements are directed by the seasons of land. Our wings don't touch, but we move in some form of attunement.

By 4 p.m., the village is hot, absorbing multiple hours of southern sun. Submerging in the sea relieves me and regulates the temperature of my body for the entirety of the evening to come. Who doesn't swim finds a balcony with a crossbreeze to enjoy. We are all looking for reprieve. We cross paths in our search for it, intersecting in the ritual of these elements, ultimately. Sun clocks and water turn into routines. Routines turn into recognition. What was solitary becomes cycles in unison. Familiarity is sown by steadiness. My own belonging becomes about this presence, repeated. Not who I am or if I agree—not my thoughts, my accent, my way of dress—not even who my father or uncle is. Simply, that I come and go over and over again weaves me into some network of witness. Some unspoken agreement of mutual guardianship. Some recognition that I am becoming a part of this place with them.

"Home" becomes in the elements of this land frequented over and over again. It is the place itself that eventually belongs. My body has learned to crave the hue of water on still September days, the shape of rocks whose path I've eventually remembered. The smiling face of children with hands full of flowers. The fragrance of tayyoun resin in the heat of August. The amnesiac grandmother's exact same question every day. The feeling of the cedar forest that becomes deeper each time I repeat. Even the mosquitos don't itch as much as they used to. This elemental immersion builds a homeward pattern of recall, a cellular calibration. The ritual in the land itself is what synchronizes me with the people who also live inside of it.

There is so much difficulty in the broader realities of our cities and lifetimes. We each live worlds apart. Yet now, when the children are in need, their mother knows she can confide in our joint care. When A'amo isn't on the rocks for a few days in a row, I know to inquire if he is well. Belonging becomes anchored in the grace of these faces who ritual with me, more often than an enveloping sense of seamlessness in my own identity or sameness. A care, some dignity is woven beyond this, as dictated by the land and its cycles of togetherness heeded. These rituals of place endow every needed grace somehow. They sustain life,

288

re-member souls, fortify strength in the simplicity of their withstanding truths.

When place anchors habit, relationships of belonging and culture naturally form over time. When belonging is built around social identities without anchorage in the ecosystem, it leaves a fundamental gap in the formation of "home." Our places make us. Not just the ones we come from, but the ones we live in every day. This is often the piece that gets lost in diasporic community formation and modern concepts of the self, fostering eternal rootlessness that multiplies with its aches.

Tending the Life in Front of Us

Migration is a natural phenomenon: birds, seeds, whales, butterflies— even desert sands and winds—travel from one part of the earth to the opposite in cycles that life necessitates and mutually supports. Humans are part of these land routes and waterways, following them for sustenance and evolution along with the rest of creation. For thousands of years before colonialism, migrational relationships of exchange between human societies have taken place in generally mutual regard. We move, we evolve, we change and grow over time, we connect so that we may continue. What are not natural are nation-states, borders, empire, settler occupation, genocide, and chattel slavery. These political systems of exploitation and oppression have drastically changed how modern migration looks today and why it occurs. A primary quality of difference between settler-colonial cultures and historic migrations boils down to extraction vs. relationship and consent. Where the very foundation of modern migrational relationships has been violated and manipulated to create the nation-states we currently live in, we need not normalize nor adopt cultural habits of severance and exploitation in our everyday relationships as diasporic people, even living within these incredible complexities.

There is a common ethos within traditional cultures and amongst Cana'an's ancestors that when you visit another person's home or territory, you live in accordance with their laws, and that you never come empty handed. Reciprocity and generosity are embedded values of practice that must be extended in relationship to land and its original stewards in the diasporic context likewise. This is not merely a matter of formality; this ethic contains deeper wisdom towards the integrity of life and its ability to mutually flourish for the longevity of our earth. These values of respect and reciprocity are part of how relationship has been cultivated in sustaining ways across time, and they are something we have learned from the land itself. Just as we knew, loved, and became with the food, plants, and weather of our ancestral lands, we graciously learn about our new homes through time invested, and wisdom gleaned via adherence to the protocols developed generationally by those who have known them since the beginning of time.

In a context where consent from the original people was not a part of our homemaking—in some cases not even a part of our own—living with active regard and care for the place we dwell is a minimum pathway towards repair and integrity. Such care cannot happen if we are in denial about the lands we are a part of every day, our existence within the land, and our very own bodies. Wherever we find ourselves in the world, to ignore the elements of place is dissonant, offensive, and damaging to earth and its people, and a denial of our own fundamental well-being and ancestral connection in the process. It is colonial wounding that puts us in this state of non-relating and grief for where we are; at times I have even witnessed this show up as resentment of the lands one lives on. Ultimately it is our responsibility to humbly tend the ecologies we make home, in whatever capacity we can. Our mutual and multispecies liberation depends on care steadily given and received, and depends perhaps most importantly on the quality of connection repaired in the process of such stewardship. Our souls need this to be well. Our communities need this to be well. Our ancestors need this to be well. We are the earth, and when we nourish it, we nourish ourselves forward and back. This responsibility is in fact, a gift of primordial healing.

Practicing relationship to place itself—the actual fullness of the ecosystems we are a part of and living from every single day—is an ultimate act of love and reciprocity to our ancestors and future, the earth, and life-affirming cultures globally. Feeding into the land helps heal ruptures of colonial damage where we live, and repairs its wounding of separation inside of us. To reconnect with the elements of place is a form of deep re-embodiment that begins to thaw dysphoria and trauma on the personal, ecological, and generational levels. Mending those lingering places of loss rebuilds our kinship and responsibility to life, and begins to restore pathways to belonging and place through recentering Indigenous continuation and the source that makes us all. While it is often our grief and colonial wounding that cause us to feel separated from our diasporic homes, connecting to them often makes way for the reconciliation we actually long for. The land is part of our community, and when we commune with it, we become harmonized with everyone and everything that thrives alongside us. Over time then, home becomes an integrated experience—your new place blending with the gifts you have brought in order to relate in presence and harmony for mutual continuation.

One of the most impactful and accessible ways I have found to begin this reconciliation is by deepening intimacy and stewardship with the native plantcestors of my diasporic home. Meaning, the ones that grow Indigenously to that particular place on earth. Tending plantcestors and ecologies of place returns the land to its own balance, regenerating the habitat and supporting its Native cultures, while reverberating with radical healing and repair in every direction. It is an act of care to the Indigenous livelihoods where we are, as much as it is to our own selves and lineages. Even within the vast dispossession of Indigenous people from their traditional lands across this planet, their communities are responsible for the most biodiverse ecosystems still thriving on our earth.[1] Lands managed by Indigenous communities emit at least 73 percent less carbon.[2] Though Indigenous people inhabit only 15 percent of the land on this planet, their territories make up 40 percent of the protected ecosystems of the entire globe.[3] Yet they are in a constant battle to maintain the integrity of these homes that our whole planet relies on for survival. Within the erosion of localized habitats and the life-affirming lifeways and cultures of generational wisdom they yield, the integrity of our broader earth suffers in every dimension.

In an era of climate collapse, there is also a direct role for native grasses, plants, and trees in sequestering carbon dioxide from the environment, mitigating impending damage and securing the whole interwoven cascade of multispecies life we are a part of.[4] There are plants that hold the soil of the earth together, plants that clean water and regenerate soil, fungi that transmute contamination in the earth— organisms of infinite kinds that work with the plants to restore entire ecosystems of life. There is a lot we do not have immediate control over in the scope of these devastating systems of domination that destroy for profit, though our efforts to resist them are invaluable and necessary. While we engage in the long-term political struggles to interrupt imperialism and capitalism ravaging our earth, we also have the capacity to contribute to these habitats and the Indigenous communities maintaining them, in direct ways right now.

Growing native plants can be as simple as planting a seed in one pot on your balcony and adding a new plant every season or year, or pulling out your lawn and replanting it with local species. It can be as elaborate as actually returning a piece of land to your local tribal community to steward in the time-tested traditional methods they see fit. I have found it most impactful to familiarize myself with the plants and ecologies of place directly through the initiatives of Indigenous people in my cities who are leading this work, whether it's enrolling in educational offerings, joining a river cleanup or habitat restoration effort, or purchasing native plants or seeds from their nurseries. One of my greatest teachers of native land regeneration on this is Olivia Chumacero of Everything Is Medicine. Olivia is a brilliant artist of Raramuri descent who has taught numerous inhabitants of Tongva (Los Angeles) about the local plantcestors through inviting co-stewardship of a land along the LA River. She guided the process of its transition to a lush native medicine garden over the course of eight years, before it was destroyed by developers for a "Wi-Fi" park. One of the most powerful things Olivia shared with me is that simply removing invasive species from a space for a sustained amount of time is often enough for the plantcestors of place to return on their own. This powerful mirror from the earth speaks volumes about our nature and the possibilities of re-membrance living beings contain: we are created to adapt and fulfill our life-affirming purpose, intelligently navigating changing conditions in order to protect our ability to do so. Native seeds can rest dormant in the ground for decades until they have the space and conditions safe and suitable enough for their gestation and revival.

Sowing Home

Immersing in the elements of where we are is a critical part of integration and realization. It begins to weave us into the vibrational wisdom, kinships, and story of places we make home. When my father first took me back to my kindred village sea, I will admit that while I enjoyed it, it was unfamiliar at first. My version of a sea was the cold water of the Pacific Ocean, with waves more massive than me that tumbled me inside them. It was long stretches of sand, starfish and sand dollars, and feeling dizzy at the edge of the shore where my feet sunk into receding water and sand. My earliest memories of the earth are the feeling and color of bright green moss and the softness of California sycamore seeds being scattered between my childhood hands on my elementary school playground. However scarce these moments became as I matured, their feeling calls me back to myself every time I feel the coolness of moss, or the fuzz of a sycamore tree. "Focus on your geography" comes to mind here. Be it submersion in the ocean, or eating a California wild rose on my hike through the creek, to immerse is a critical pathway to re-membrance.

One of the embedded generosities of the earth is that as we tend it, it multiplies in its offerings back to us. Through stewardship of plants, we have the opportunity to learn about their uses as medicine and food and to participate in their life cycles as we tend to their seasonal needs. While connecting with ancestral medicines has great power and is necessary for our deeper well-being, our current bioregions are ultimately the relationships of care we rest on every day. There are no Lebanese cedar trees or tayyoun plants when I'm in California; there are yarrow and oaks. Maramiye does not grow on the Pacific coast, but each time I bring native Pozo Blue sage in from garden trims, my mom says, "It smells like my village," and a new kind of connection is formed. Local plantcestors become familiar over time, evoking a sense of companionship and care where we are. This realm of kinship with land is one of deep affection, mutual care, and prolific beauty, beyond only practicality.

As Hakim suggested, eating, drinking, and growing food from the local bioregions is part of how these places become a deeper part of us, and how we calibrate to the integrity of land, lineage, and our part in it. Just as deepening with the plantcestors of my villages has transformed my life, native plants of my diaspora home have initiated a whole series of meaningful kinships and re-membrances, facilitating connections to my own lineage in the process. The earth re-members us, no matter where in the world we are. The plantcestors themselves teach this aptly, finding ways to survive and adapt in new homes and oftentimes even becoming part of the cultural medicines of the Indigenous who live there. Traditional people relate to the living abundance of place, even while it changes.

Generational memory is built with time. Ancestral cuisines reverberate with foundational ancient parts of us because of our long relationships, while foods from the Indigenous terrains of our diasporic homes help us integrate and realize new bridges of kinship with where we live, who we are today, and with respectful possibilities of belonging between these worlds. Their sustenance, through our cultivation, usher new intimacies and consciousness inside of us. Both these layers have potent implications in our spiritual and physical well-being and cannot simply replace each other. Foods of address and origins can help educate our internal landscapes to attune more harmoniously with the ecosystems we are part of today, as we participate in their reproduction and the continuation of the whole network of life and culture they uplift. Our diasporic aunties and grandmothers often embody this naturally when they arrive somewhere new. They are used to scouting the landscapes where they live to learn what is familiar and what isn't, and traditional recipes become supplemented by local ingredients out of necessity, if nothing else. Sometimes our own ancestral plants have become invasive in our diasporic homes. An example is black mustard (*Brassica nigra*), a noxious edible weed that runs rampant in North America in damaging ways. I have found "foraging" wild invasives from their root for food or medicine is a constructive way to aid the local habitat, while attuning to the environment I am a part of, in order to meet communal needs. On the other hand, the native edibles growing in my garden give me a chance to work with them as I also cultivate their care, while not further taxing their stands in the wild. Growing a local sumac tree or grape vine for use in our ancestral recipes, or interweaving buckwheat instead of regular wheat in a dessert, gives me a new chance to integrate and connect as I merge and deepen within my worlds and learn to find home where I am. This is part of the fertile co-creation that diaspora itself yields, evolving into its own futures and new expressions of culture.

There was a qualitative shift in my relationship to diaspora and my own being when I began explicitly connecting at the axis of both the land and people of the places where I lived—whether it was in diaspora, or my generational villages. It helped me feel more at "home" not only in a physical sense but in a spiritual and ancestral one too. In this intersection, the land where I am, and the land in my blood merge seamlessly for a rare union of true re-membrance. When I am crouching down to feel the tiniest flower on Mt. Doyembele (Diablo) with a giggling friend, dancing towards the waves of the Pacific Ocean near an urban pier, or singing in a traditional arbor with Native aunties, belonging is bodily. My ancestors join the ancestors of place through my somatic union with the land and its cultures, and "belonging" is all the places I have been and gone to at once. For a moment, I am returned to this source where we all emerge mutually. It is less desolate, more lush to exist in this connection. My spirit and nervous system recalibrate there, allowing me rare moments of arrival and clarity. And my soul reorients to the cellular part of me that constantly knows and forgets and knows again, that there is nothing and no one superfluous or alone on this earth.

☙

Seeds contain a complete roadmap of fulfillment, deep cellular memory, lineages of story, and generational resilience built from their origins, and ultimately activated by the minerals of soil, sun, and seasons where they are planted. Even the shape of seeds are made for journeys on the wind, fur, or in the belly of a bird traveling wayward towards new homes, yet full with the knowledge of its origins. Seeds are built to sow futures of longevity by virtue of connection to where they land; this communion with place is the kinship that nourishes continuation.

The terrain of in-betweens is one of expansive becoming, in which all the worlds we come from and the ones we live in are constantly in conversation. For the spiritually displaced and distraught with non-belonging, the stewardship of connection and care towards the land wherever we live can deeply revolutionize our way of feeling, being, and moving towards belonging in the world. A return to our planetary mother is a return of transformative and regenerative proportions that allows us to give to the life that is giving to us every moment.

The earth is an archive of memory and love—an infinite key and a mirror, our primordial healer. Its elements are an oracle of futures being made in our cells, memory that still stirs with creation beneath our feet, inside our marrow, between our breath and the trees, the life-giving water and the moon that sways us in unison. Amidst everything forgotten and ruptured, our most foundational relationship homeward persists from within our bones and the soil we stand on. The earth is our invitation to belong, readily awaiting our return from everywhere we are.

The land offers moments of reprieve. There is redemption, if nothing else, in the nurturance towards life. There is salvation in connection, however fleeting "belonging" might in fact be. Perhaps the life-tending way of my grandmothers is no more than graceful surrender, submission to the beauty within survival that often aches. Like my mother always says, "Money is not for the grave." We give to what needs us, today. Our love offers meaning to a moment, dignity to a life, simply because it exists.

There is healing in the stewardship of making life out of everything you touch. In the rhythmic cycles of the garden, the stitches, the kneading of dough, the body softens towards what memory rests inside of it. Inner secrets unfurl alongside the flowers of the earth that also bloom in the spirit of life's tending. A way is paved that is deeper in insight than it may appear. My thinking mind has often led me into deeper confusion or lost resonance with time, where these ancestral legacies of seemingly basic care have anchored me over and over into deeper truths. In the craftsmanship of our handmade efforts, be they bread, a basket, or something beautiful to wear, the rhythms of our bodies synch up with the earth's, and our essence is what expands ultimately. There is home and repair in the bodily way of tending for the sake of life and love, as my elders always have. And their service was not mere chore imposed, but a way much deeper. Teta Renee would sing, orate poems while she sewed. Recite phrases of prayer and affirmation. Open her curtains just wide enough to see her rose peeking through from the garden. She would talk to her greens as she plucked and prepared them to eat, the earth of her new home carrying her forward with as much love mutually as the ones she left. Jiddo Salloum would improvise verses as he visited his fig trees. He would come home with two banged-up tomatoes in a batch of seven because "the storekeeper needs to feed his family, too." Tetitna Hind would immerse in our world for moments or hours, deep with presence to love and understand our lives in sincere curiosity and wisdom, and the second we left the room, she would lift a rosary in our name to pray our path forward. These ways were imbued with soul, with kinship and spirit that mend us despite all lost.

This devotion is where re-membrance emerges—not in the esoteric inventory of forgotten pasts or anxious calculations for what happens next, but in our responsibility towards life's sanctity in the here and now. This cultivation of care is a practice of hope that tethers, a pragmatism of ancestral love that births new roads. These lifeways of stewardship retrieve what colonial rupture has dispersed and taken. They are a secret of the earth that recalibrates us towards the source of truths that constantly make and remake us. They are the foundations of our sovereignty and our way back towards it. These relationships are our redemption.

Meaningful
Language Glossary

EARTH and LAND | Throughout this book, I often refer to "land" and "earth." Humans are part of land/earth, not separate from it. Please note that when I speak of "land" or "earth," I am often using these words to encompass all the elements of place, the whole ecology of relationships and also the earth's place as part of a cosmic universe. "Land" for me may encompass the waterways, the animals and organisms, and the humans of a place. "Earth" includes the oceans and seas, the whole planet, and its place as a cosmic entity that relates to and reflects what is in the stars beyond. I am, in many cases, using these words in these expansive capacities.

✽

INDIGENOUS and TRADITIONAL | "Indigenous" refers to the people, plants, and species that have originated in a particular place, and the cultures and lifeways which have emerged from their specific relationship to it. Beyond blood, indigeneity is about extended generational relationships to place, culture, and a mutual recognition/belonging within it. In the contemporary reality of a highly colonized world, there are some added layers and nuances inside what this word means within different contexts, making it important to clarify my own use of it throughout this text.

One of these layers is the political reality of this era, in which peoples who have maintained indigeneity are disproportionately subjected to violence, displacement, occupation, ethnic cleansing, and the desecration of their ancestral lands and lifeways, constantly in a battle for basic self-determination and sovereignty over their own lives and the care of their territories and traditions. They are often faced with such threats not only from external forces, but also the ruling classes and dominant cultures of the states their territories exist within. I use "Indigenous" to refer not only to the identities of people with bloodlines that originate in a particular place, but those who also maintain a level of continuity in their ancestral relationship to it: stewardship and proximity to its earth-based customs, pre-colonial languages and cultures, original paradigms of understanding, relationships to land and water, concepts of self and oral knowledge, ancestral practices and rituals, place-based cosmologies and identities, and mutual recognition within community kinships/generational social structures. I understand that these are not often neatly cut lines in the contemporary context, as culture naturally evolves and adapts, geographic displacement is rampant, and colonialism has simultaneously touched nearly everyone on today's earth, influencing aspects of this in some degree or another even within continuous Indigenous cultures.

This can be particularly complex to grapple with in a region like the one represented in this book, which has been colonized repeatedly by different forces for over thousands of years, each one altering, erasing, or influencing localized relationships to place/culture in varying degrees of aggression and totality. I use the language of "traditional people," village folk, fallahi or baladi, to honor those ways and lineages who are native to the places discussed and have maintained a level of specific and localized culture and land stewardship that has evolved within broadly colonized or assimilated identities. Yet I reserve the language of "Indigenous" to those parts of our ancestries and contemporary communities who actively and consciously steward pre-colonial place-based cultures, lifeways, and identities, or are in active political struggles for sovereignty and the protection of their ancestral land bases, original cultures, and distinct ways of tending them.

PLANTCESTORS | In this text, I share and explain my usage and meaning of the word "plantcestors," a word that I coined in 2014 to express the axis of my Plantcestral Re-Membrance methodology, but whose underlying wisdom is embedded in traditional earth-based paradigms and systems of practice that precede me by far. The concept of "plants are our ancestors" is Indigenous knowledge, understood and honored in cultural expressions of various traditional communities across this earth, from the prehistoric caves of Armenia to the sweat lodge of the Lakota. Throughout this book, I extend some of my own understandings regarding this concept, as well as some related wisdoms offered by cherished elders in Cana'an. While the language of "plantcestors" is my own, many traditionalists from Indigenous and traditional lineages, especially those extending from the Americas, the African continent and its diasporas, and the broader Crossroads region (aka Southwest Asia/the Middle East), have conveyed aspects of its underlying wisdom to me over the years in ways both subtle and direct that have contributed immensely to my own consciousness. The first time someone spoke to me explicitly about the plants as ancestral entities, I was in a dream circle in California in 2010, hosted by my dear friend Atava Garcia-Sweicecki, founder and teacher of Ancestral Apothecary located in Huichin Ohlone Territories in (Oakland) California. She often brought plants to accompany and support our dream space, and one day she shared this understanding with me as we were conversing after class. I did not start my formal training with plants until soon after that, inspired by a series of dreams I have heeded since. It impacted me to think of the plants in the language of ancestry so early in my path as an herbalist, and influenced the way I unfolded and deepened in my own work with them in the years to follow.

I have held and shared the word "plantcestors" to anchor and express my own relationship and practice as a sort of prayer. Specifically, reconnecting to plants of lineage was part of a spiritual transmission in my life to aid efforts of collective re-membrance and healing from colonial and generational rupture that have motivated me since I was a young adult. I embrace this language and the specific way of working that came alongside it as a direct gift from my own ancestors, and my personal contribution within and towards an ongoing lineage of cultural healing work. I do so with explicit honor, permission, and acknowledgment of the accumulated traditional wisdom that precedes and makes me, and with a hope to recenter the consciousness within that promises life forward as rooted in our original ways, and is still tended by steadfast Indigenous and traditional peoples across this earth. It is my hope that this language and my personal way of practice and continuation honors them and reveres the lineages and lands they/ we come from, and especially that it supports a more reciprocal and reverential way of relating to the plantcestors and earth itself—one that is anchored in relationship and regeneration, instead of the extraction and consumption that have become disturbingly normalized. One that acts as a healing bridge across generations and dimensions, towards the liberation and rematriation of our world, all leading us ultimately to our own re-membrance "homeward."

Herbal Actions Glossary

Borrowed with permission from Shabina Lafleur-Gangji, co-founder of Seeds, Soil & Spirit School

Abortifacient induces abortion, miscarriage, or premature removal of a fetus

Adaptogen works through the endocrine system to modulate the physical, mental, and emotional effects of stress and increase resistance to physiological imbalances and disease by strengthening the immune system

Analgesic relieves pain

Anesthetic induces loss of sensation or consciousness due to the depression of nerve function

Antibacterial destroys or stops the growth of bacteria

Anticatarrhal reduces inflamed mucous membranes of head and throat

Antidiarrhetic prevents or treats diarrhea

Antiemetic stops vomiting

Antifungal destroys or inhibits the growth of fungus

Antihemorrhagic controls hemorrhaging or bleeding

Anti-inflammatory controls inflammation, a reaction to injury or infection

Antimicrobial destroys microbes

Antipruritic prevents or relieves itching

Antipyretic reduces fever (febrifuge)

Antirheumatic eases pain of rheumatism, inflammation of joints and muscles

Antiseptic produces asepsis, removes pus, blood, etc.

Antispasmodic calms nervous and muscular spasms or convulsions

Antitussive controls or prevents cough

Antiviral opposes the action of a virus

Anxiolytic reduces anxiety

Aphrodisiac increases the capacity for sexual arousal

Aromatic an herb containing volatile oils, fragrant odor, and slightly stimulating properties

Astringent constricts and binds by coagulation of proteins

Bronchodilator relaxes spasms or constriction of the bronchi or upper part of the lungs, thereby improving respiration

Cardiotonic increases strength and tone (normal tension or response to stimuli) of the heart

Carminative causes the release of stomach or intestinal gas

Cholagogue increases flow of bile from gallbladder

Demulcent soothes and protects inflamed and irritated mucous membranes both topically and internally

Diaphoretic increases perspiration (synonym: sudorific)

Digestive promotes or aids the digestion process

Diuretic increases urine flow

Emetic produces vomiting and evacuation of stomach contents

Emmenagogue regulates and induces menstruation

Emollient softens and soothes the skin

Estrogenic causes the production of estrogen

Expectorant facilitates removal of mucus and other materials

Febrifuge reduces or relieves fever

Galactagogue promotes the flow of milk

Hemostatic controls or stops the flow of blood

Hepatic having to do with the liver

Hypertensive raises blood pressure

Hypnotic strong-acting nervous system relaxant (nervines) that supports healthy sleep

Hypotensive lowers blood pressure

Laxative loosens bowel contents

Lithotriptic a substance that causes kidney or bladder stones to dissolve

Mucilaginous polysaccharide-rich compounds that coat and soothe inflamed mucous membranes

Narcotic induces drowsiness, sleep, or stupor, and lessons pain

Nervine affects the nervous system

Nutritive a herb containing nutrients required to nourish and build the body

Purgative causes the evacuation of intestinal contents; laxative

Refrigerant relieves thirst with its cooling properties

Relaxant tends to relax and relieve tension, especially muscular tension

Rubefacient reddens skin, dilates the blood vessels, and increases blood supply locally

Sedative exerts a soothing, tranquilizing effect on the body

Sialagogue increases the production and flow of saliva

Stimulant increases body or organ function temporarily

Tonic strengthens an organ or system or the whole body

Vermifuge expels worms from the intestines

Vulnerary aids in healing wounds

Notes

Introduction

1 "UNHCR Lebanon at a Glance," UNHCR, 2021, https://www.unhcr
.org/lb/at-a-glance.

2 "Program for Economic and Urban Resilience in Lebanon," Urban Projects Finance Initiative, n.d., https://upfi-med.eib.org/en/projects/multi
-city-urban-development-programme-in-lebanon/.

3 "Painful Reality and Uncertain Prospects Poverty in Lebanon Multidimensional Poverty," United Nations Economic and Social Commission for Western Asia, 2021, https://www.unescwa.org/sites/default/files
/news/docs/21-00634-_multidimential_poverty_in_lebanon_-policy
brief-_en.pdf.

4 UN ESCWA, "Painful Reality."

5 Amer Shibani, "From Cities to Villages: Reverse Migration on the Rise in Lebanon," Beirut Today, September 22, 2021, https://beirut-today
.com/2021/09/22/from-cities-to-villages-reverse-migration-on-the
-rise-in-lebanon/.

Chapter 1: Re-Membering the Crossroads

1 Senem Aslan, *Nation-Building in Turkey and Morocco: Governing Kurdish and Berber Dissent* (Cambridge: Cambridge University Press, 2015); Niveen Kassem and Mark Jackson, "Cultural Trauma and Its Impact on the Iraqi Assyrian Experience of Identity," *Social Identities* 26, no. 3 (May 3, 2020): 388–402, https://doi.org/10.1080/13504630.2020.1762557; Maja Janmyr, "Nubians in Contemporary Egypt: Mobilizing Return to Ancestral Lands," *Middle East Critique* 25, no. 2 (February 29, 2016): 127–46, https://doi.org/10.1080/19436149.2016.1148859.

2 Kelly Duquette, "Environmental Colonialism," Postcolonial Studies at
   Emory, January 2020, https://scholarblogs.emory.edu/postcolonialstudies
   /2020/01/21/environmental-colonialism/.

3 Mazin B. Qumsiyeh and Mohammed A. Abusarhan, "An Environmental
   Nakba: The Palestinian Environment under Israeli Colonization," *Science
   under Occupation* 23, no. 1 (2020), https://magazine.scienceforthepeople
   .org/vol23-1/an-environmental-nakba-the-palestinian-environment-under
   -israeli-colonization/; Adib Dada and Maya Maroni, "Nature-Empowered
   Liberation: A Pathway to Lebanese Political Reform," Slow Factory, October 29, 2022, https://slowfactory.earth/readings/tbd-the-other-dada.

4 Nader Noureldeen Mohamed, "Negative Impacts of Egyptian High
   Aswan Dam: Lessons for Ethiopia and Sudan," *International Journal of
   Development Research* 9, no. 8 (August 2019), https://www.journalijdr
   .com/sites/default/files/issue-pdf/16178.pdf.

5 Ashok Swain, "Challenges for Water Sharing in the Nile Basin: Changing
   Geo-Politics and Changing Climate," *Hydrological Sciences Journal* 56, no.
   4 (June 2011): 687–702, https://doi.org/10.1080/02626667.2011.577037;
   Marina Ottaway, "Egypt and Ethiopia: The Curse of the Nile," Wilson
   Center, July 7, 2020, https://www.wilsoncenter.org/article/egypt
   -and-ethiopia-curse-nile.

6 Jonathan Drury, "Byblos and Its Relationship with Egypt," *Retrospect Journal*, April 18, 2021, https://retrospectjournal.com/2021/04/18/byblos
   -and-its-relationship-with-egypt/.

7 John Scott, "The Phoenicians and the Formation of the Western World,"
   Comparative Civilizations Review 78, no. 78 (2018): 4, https://scholars
   archive.byu.edu/cgi/viewcontent.cgi?article=2047&context=ccr; Ivan
   Van Sertima, *They Came before Columbus: The African Presence in Ancient
   America* (New York: Random House, 2003).

8 Scott, "Phoenicians and the Formation."

9 Kristin Romey, "Living Descendants of Biblical Canaanites Identified
   via DNA," *National Geographic*, July 27, 2017, https://www.national
   geographic.com/history/article/canaanite-bible-ancient-dna-lebanon
   -genetics-archaeology.

10 Christopher Ehret, S. O. Y. Keita, and Paul Newman, "The Origins of
   Afroasiatic," *Science* 306, no. 5702 (December 3, 2004): 1680.3–1680,
   https://doi.org/10.1126/science.306.5702.1680c; Don Jaide, "The Semites
   of Africa," Rasta Livewire, March 13, 2006, https://www.africaresource
   .com/rasta/sesostris-the-great-the-egyptian-hercules/the-semitic
   -speakers-of-africa/.

11 Edward W. Said, *Orientalism* (Brantford, ON: W. Ross Macdonald School,
   Resource Services Library, 1978).

12 Wongi Park, "The Blessing of Whiteness in the Curse of Ham: Reading Gen 9:18–29 in the Antebellum South," *Religions* 12, no. 11 (October 25, 2021): 928, https://doi.org/10.3390/rel12110928; Haroon Bashir, "Black Excellence and the Curse of Ham: Debating Race and Slavery in the Islamic Tradition," *ReOrient* 5, no. 1 (2019): 92, https://doi.org/10.13169 /reorient.5.1.0092; Robert Warrior, "Canaanites, Cowboys, and Indians: Deliverance, Conquest, and Liberation Theology Today," *Christianity and Crisis* 49, no. 12 (1989), https://www.academia.edu/17688887/Canaanites _Cowboys_and_Indians_Deliverance_Conquest_and_Liberation_Theology _Today; Robin Law, "The 'Hamitic Hypothesis' in Indigenous West African Historical Thought," *History in Africa* 36 (2009): 292–98, https://doi .org/10.1353/hia.2010.0004.

13 Franck Salameh, "Adonis, the Syrian Crisis, and the Question of Pluralism in the Levant," *Bustan: The Middle East Book Review* 3, no. 1 (March 1, 2012): 36–61, https://doi.org/10.1163/187853012x633526.

14 Yolande Knell, "Gaza Farmer Finds 4,500-Year-Old Statue of Canaanite Goddess," BBC News, April 26, 2022, https://www.bbc.com/news /world-middle-east-61228553; Marc Haber et al., "Continuity and Admixture in the Last Five Millennia of Levantine History from Ancient Canaanite and Present-Day Lebanese Genome Sequences," *American Journal of Human Genetics* 101, no. 2 (August 2017): 274–82, https://doi .org/10.1016/j.ajhg.2017.06.013.

15 Yohannes Mekonnen, *Ethiopia: The Land, Its People, History and Culture* (Yohannes Mekonnen, 2013), Google Books; Graham Hancock, *Sign and the Seal: The Quest for the Lost Ark of the Covenant* (New York: Simon and Schuster, 1993), Google Books.

16 William Davison, Solomon Yimer, and Kibreab Beraki, "Violent Qemant Dispute Fueling Explosive Amhara-Tigray Divide," Ethiopia Insight, December 16, 2018, https://www.ethiopia-insight.com/2018/12/16 /violent-qemant-dispute-fueling-explosive-amhara-tigray-divide/; Sanyika Bryant, "Bilad il Asmar: Where Does Africa End?," interview by Layla K Feghali, SWANA Ancestral HUB, February 15, 2017, https:// www.riverroseremembrance.com/ancestralhub-posts/2017/02/15 /where-does-africa-end-bilad-il-asmar-an-opening-conversation-with -sanyika-bryant.

17 Philip K. Hitti, *Lebanon in History* (New York: Macmillan, 1957), Internet Archive, https://archive.org/details/dli.ernet.53848/.

18 J. Benjamin, "Of Nubians and Nabateans: Implications of Research on Neglected Dimensions of Ancient World History," *Journal of Asian and African Studies* 36, no. 4 (January 1, 2001): 361–82, https://doi.org /10.1177/002190960103600403.

19 Ali Mazrui, "Afrabia: Africa and the Arabs in the New World Order,"
    Ufahamu: A Journal of African Studies 20, no. 3 (1992), https://doi.org
    /10.5070/f7203016755.
20 Bryant, "Where Does Africa End?"
21 Chouki El Hamel, *Black Morocco: A History of Slavery, Race, and Islam* (Cam-
    bridge: Cambridge University Press, 2014); Jok Madut Jok, *War and Slavery
    in Sudan* (Philadelphia: University of Pennsylvania Press, 2003); Bina Fer-
    nandez, "Racialised Institutional Humiliation through the Kafala," *Journal
    of Ethnic and Migration Studies* 47, no. 19 (February 3, 2021): 1–18, https://
    doi.org/10.1080/1369183x.2021.1876555; Tessa Talebi, "National Identity
    in the Afro-Arab Periphery: Ethnicity, Indigeneity and (Anti)Racism in
    Morocco," Project on Middle East Political Science, June 16, 2020, https://
    pomeps.org/national-identity-in-the-afro-arab-periphery-ethnicity
    -indigeneity-and-antiracism-in-morocco; Menna Agha, "Nubia Still Exists:
    On the Utility of the Nostalgic Space," *Humanities* 8, no. 1 (January 31,
    2019): 24, https://doi.org/10.3390/h8010024.
22 "Oromia Region," OromianEconomist, 2014, https://oromianeconomist
    .com/tag/oromia-region/; Cheikh Anta Diop, *Nations Nègres et Culture:
    De l'Antiquité Nègre Égyptienne Aux Problèmes Culturels de l'Afrique Noire
    D'aujourd'hui* (Paris: Présence Africaine, 2018); Martin Bernal, *Black
    Athena* (Ithaca, NY: Cornell Alumni Federation, 1992).
23 Joanna Allan and Raquel Ojeda-García. "Natural Resource Exploitation in
    Western Sahara: New Research Directions," *Journal of North African Studies*
    27, no. 6 (April 21, 2021), https://doi.org/10.1080/13629387.2021.1917120;
    Ashok Swain, "Challenges for Water Sharing in the Nile Basin: Changing
    Geo-Politics and Changing Climate," *Hydrological Sciences Journal* 56, no. 4
    (June 2011): 687–702, https://doi.org/10.1080/02626667.2011.577037.
24 Edith R. Sanders, "The Hamitic Hypothesis; Its Origin and Functions
    in Time Perspective," *Journal of African History* 10, no. 4 (1969): 521–32;
    Robin Law, "The 'Hamitic Hypothesis' in Indigenous West African His-
    torical Thought," *History in Africa* 36 (2009): 293–314, https://doi.org
    /10.1353/hia.2010.0004; Bernal, *Black Athena*.
25 Franck Salameh, "Adonis, the Syrian Crisis, and the Question of Plural-
    ism in the Levant," *Bustan: The Middle East Book Review* 3, no. 1 (March 1,
    2012): 36–61, https://doi.org/10.1163/187853012x633526; Decolonize Pal-
    estine, "Myth: Palestinians Are Arabs That Arrived in the 7th Century,"
    March 14, 2021, https://decolonizepalestine.com/myth/palestinians
    -are-arabs-that-arrived-in-the-7th-century/; Saad D. Abulhab, "The
    Case for Early Arabia and Arabic Language: A Reply to the New
    Arabia Theory by Ahmad Al-Jallad," City University of New York

(CUNY), 2020, https://academicworks.cuny.edu/cgi/viewcontent. cgi?article=1018&context=oaa_pubs.

26 Abulhab, "Case for Early Arabia"; Cristoph Correll, "Ma'lula. 2. The Language," in *The Encyclopaedia of Islam*, vol. 6, 103–104, Malhun-Mand, Prepared by a Number of Leading Orientalists, ed. C. E. Bosworth et al. (Holland: Brill, 1987); Michael Erdman, "From Language to Patois and Back Again: Syriac Influences on Arabic in Mont Liban during the 16th to 19th Centuries," 2017, https://www.academia.edu/34245489/From _Language_to_Patois_and_Back_Again_Syriac_Influences_on_Arabic _in_Mont_Liban_During_the_16TH_to_19TH_Centuries; Elie Wardini, "Some Aspects of Aramaic as Attested in Lebanese Place Names," *Orientalia Suecana 61 Suppl.*, 2012, https://www.diva-portal.org/smash/get /diva2:635253/FULLTEXT02.pdf.

27 Rodrigo Cámara-Leret and Jordi Bascompte, "Language Extinction Triggers the Loss of Unique Medicinal Knowledge," *Proceedings of the National Academy of Sciences* 118, no. 24 (June 8, 2021): e2103683118, https://doi .org/10.1073/pnas.2103683118; Janet Blake, "Safeguarding Endangered and Indigenous Languages—How Human Rights Can Contribute to Preserving Biodiversity," *Environmental Sciences* 10, no. 1 (2013), https:// envs.sbu.ac.ir/index.php/Economicsandmodeling/search/journal /journal/article_94887_86a3760661098741617454872 3b268ea.pdf; Albert Marshall, Karen F. Beazley, Jessica Hum, shalan joudry, Anastasia Papadopoulos, Sherry Pictou, Janet Rabesca, Lisa Young, and Melanie Zurba, "'Awakening the Sleeping Giant': Re-Indigenization Principles for Transforming Biodiversity Conservation in Canada and Beyond," *FACETS* 6 (January 1, 2021): 839–69, https://doi.org/10.1139/facets-2020-0083.

28 Ibrahim A. Ghalioum, "Search for Identity in Post-War Lebanon: Arab vs Phoenician" (master's project, University of Alaska Fairbanks, May 2019), https://scholarworks.alaska.edu/handle/11122/10943.

29 Edith R. Sanders, "The Hamitic Hypothesis; Its Origin and Functions in Time Perspective," *Journal of African History* 10, no. 4 (1969): 521–32.

30 Norman Myers et al., "Biodiversity Hotspots for Conservation Priorities," *Nature* 403, no. 6772 (February 2000): 853–58, https://doi .org/10.1038/35002501.

31 Zeina Hassane, "Biodiversity Status of Lebanon," Ministry of Environment, Lebanon, n.d. https://www.cbd.int/doc/c/d460/8092 /86b588a498ec733c737897a6/chmws-2018-01-item-04-lb-en.pdf.

32 Marta Coll et al., "The Biodiversity of the Mediterranean Sea: Estimates, Patterns, and Threats," *PLoS ONE* 5, no. 8 (August 2, 2010): e11842, https://doi.org/10.1371/journal.pone.0011842.

33 Birdlife International, "Ecosystem Profile Mediterranean Basin Biodiversity Hotspot," 2017, https://www.cepf.net/sites/default/files/mediterranean-basin-2017-ecosystem-profile-english_0.pdf.

34 Omar Said and Stephen Fulder, "Steps towards Revival of Graeco-Arabic Medicine in the Middle East: A New Project—American Botanical Council," *Herbalgram*, no. 83 (2009): 36–45, https://www.herbalgram.org/resources/herbalgram/issues/83/table-of-contents/article3431/; Scott, "Phoenicians and the Formation"; Cheikh Anta Diop and Mercer Cook, *African Origin of Civilization: Myth or Reality* (San Antonio: Chicago Review Press, 1989).

35 E. F. Frey, "The Earliest Medical Texts," *Clio Medica* (Amsterdam) 20, no. 1-4 (1985): 79–90, https://pubmed.ncbi.nlm.nih.gov/2463895/; Reginald Campbell Thompson, *Assyrian Medical Texts from the Originals in the British Museum* (Oxford University Press, 1923).

36 Ismail Serageldin, "Ancient Alexandria and the Dawn of Medical Science," *Global Cardiology Science and Practice* 2013, no. 4 (September 2013): 47, https://doi.org/10.5339/gcsp.2013.47; Aeron Haworth, "Egyptians, Not Greeks, Were True Fathers of Medicine," University of Manchester, May 9, 2007, https://www.manchester.ac.uk/discover/news/egyptians-not-greeks-were-true-fathers-of-medicine/; Kayley Boddy, "Imhotep and Asclepius: How Egyptian Medical Culture Influenced the Greeks," *Hayley Classical Journal* 1, no. 2 (2022), https://issuu.com/haleyclassicaljournal/docs/the_haley__issue_ii_final/s/10730817.

37 Rachel Hajar, "The Air of History Part III," *Heart Views* 14, no. 1 (2013): 43, https://doi.org/10.4103/1995-705x.107125.

Chapter 2: Plantcestral Re-Membrance

1 Linsay Rosenfeld, "The Body in Remembrance: Dhikr in Moroccan Sufism," University of North Carolina at Chapel Hill, 2013, https://globalstudies.unc.edu/wp-content/uploads/sites/224/2013/11/Rosenfeld-Lindsay-BODY-IN-REMEMBRANCE.pdf.

2 Audre Lorde, *Sister Outsider: Essays and Speeches* (Berkeley, CA: Crossing Press, 1984), 53–59.

Chapter 3: Tending "Weeds"

1 Faith Lagay, "The Legacy of Humoral Medicine," *AMA Journal of Ethics* 4, no. 7 (July 1, 2002), https://doi.org/10.1001/virtualmentor.2002.4.7.mhst1-0207; Ismail Serageldin, "Ancient Alexandria and the Dawn of Medical Science," *Global Cardiology Science and Practice* 2013, no. 4 (September 2013): 47, https://doi.org/10.5339/gcsp.2013.47.

2 Riccardo Orlandi et al., "'I Miss My Liver,' Nonmedical Sources in the History of Hepatocentrism," *Hepatology Communications* 2, no. 8 (August 2018): 986–93, https://doi.org/10.1002/hep4.1224.

3 Jing-Juan Li et al., "The Genus Rumex (Polygonaceae): An Ethnobotanical, Phytochemical and Pharmacological Review," *Natural Products and Bioprospecting* 12, no. 1 (June 16, 2022), https://doi.org/10.1007/s13659-022-00346-z.

4 Andrea Vasas, Orsolya Orbán-Gyapai, and Judit Hohmann, "The Genus Rumex: Review of Traditional Uses, Phytochemistry and Pharmacology," *Journal of Ethnopharmacology* 175 (December 2015): 198–228, https://doi.org/10.1016/j.jep.2015.09.001.

5 João Cleverson Gasparetto, Cleverson Antônio Ferreira Martins, Sirlei Sayomi Hayashi, Michel Fleith Otuky, and Roberto Pontarolo, "Ethnobotanical and Scientific Aspects of *Malva sylvestris* L.: A Millennial Herbal Medicine," *Journal of Pharmacy and Pharmacology* 64, no. 2 (2011): 172–89, https://doi.org/10.1111/j.2042-7158.2011.01383.x.

6 Sabri Fatima Zohra, Belarbi Meriem, and Sabri Samira, "Some Extracts of Mallow Plant and Its Role in Health," *APCBEE Procedia* 5 (2013): 546–50, https://doi.org/10.1016/j.apcbee.2013.05.091.

7 Seyyed Mojtaba Mousavi et al., "A Review on Health Benefits of *Malva sylvestris* L. Nutritional Compounds for Metabolites, Antioxidants, and Anti-Inflammatory, Anticancer, and Antimicrobial Applications," *Evidence-Based Complementary and Alternative Medicine* 2021 (August 14, 2021): 5548404, https://doi.org/10.1155/2021/5548404.

8 Safaa Baydoun et al., "Ethnopharmacological Survey of Medicinal Plants Used in Traditional Medicine by the Communities of Mount Hermon, Lebanon," *Journal of Ethnopharmacology* 173 (September 2015): 139–56, https://doi.org/10.1016/j.jep.2015.06.052.

9 Tabaraki Reza, Yosefi Zeynab, and Asadi Ali. "Chemical Composition and Antioxidant Properties of *Malva sylvestris* L.," 2012; Gasparetto et al., "Scientific Aspects of *Malva sylvestris* L."

10 Fonyuy E. Wirngo, Max N. Lambert, and Per B. Jeppesen, "The Physiological Effects of Dandelion (*Taraxacum officinale*) in Type 2 Diabetes," *Review of Diabetic Studies* 13, no. 2-3 (2016): 113–31, https://pubmed.ncbi.nlm.nih.gov/28012278/.

11 H. Jane Philips, "Lebanese Folk Cures" (PhD diss., Columbia University, 1958).

12 Baydoun et al., "Ethnopharmacological Survey of Medicinal Plants."

13 Philips, "Lebanese Folk Cures."

14 Ajay Kumar et al., "A Review on Bioactive Phytochemicals, Ethnomedic-
inal and Pharmacological Importance of Purslane (*Portulaca oleracea* L.),"
May 10, 2021, preprint, https://doi.org/10.21203/rs.3.rs-501982/v1.

15 Amal Alachkar et al., "Traditional Medicine in Syria: Folk Medicine in
Aleppo Governorate," *Natural Product Communications* 6, no. 1 (January
2011): 1934578X1100600, https://doi.org/10.1177/1934578x1100600119.

16 Ammar Khammash, "Blue Globe," Khammash Architects, July 2003,
https://www.khammash.com/research/blue-globe.

17 Baydoun et al., "Ethnopharmacological Survey of Medicinal Plants."

18 "Internal Information in the Yusef A-Shawamreh Killing Reveals: Com-
manders Ordered Live Fire Ambush of Teens, Though They Posed No
Danger. The Result: A 14-Year-Old Killed, No One Held Accountable,"
B'tselem: The Israeli Information Center for Human Rights in the Occupied Territories (blog), June 16, 2015, https://www.btselem.org
/accountability/20141106_shawamreh_investigation_impunity.

19 Hassan Azaizeh et al., "The State of the Art of Traditional Arab Herbal
Medicine in the Eastern Region of the Mediterranean: A Review," *Evidence-
Based Complementary and Alternative Medicine* 3, no. 2 (2006): 229–35,
https://doi.org/10.1093/ecam/nel034.

20 Nissim Krispil, "*Inula viscosa* Traditional Medicine," Avisco Ltd., 1987,
http://www.inulav.com/Inula_viscosa_Traditional_Medicine.html.

21 Rami Zurayk and Salma Talhouk, *Plants and People: Ethnobotanical Knowledge from Lebanon* (American University of Beirut, 2009).

Chapter 4: Man'oushet Za'atar: Street Food Staples

1 Reem Abu Alwafa, Samer Mudalal, and Gianluigi Mauriello, "*Origanum
syriacum* L. (Za'atar), from Raw to Go: A Review," *Plants* (Basel, Switzer-
land) 10, no. 5 (May 1, 2021), https://doi.org/10.3390/plants10051001.

2 Alachkar et al., "Traditional Medicine in Syria."

3 Mohammad Qneibi et al., "The Neuroprotective Role of *Origanum syriacum* L. and *Lavandula dentata* L. Essential Oils through Their Effects on
AMPA Receptors," *BioMed Research International* 2019 (March 11, 2019):
5640173, https://doi.org/10.1155/2019/5640173.

4 Abd Al-Majeed Al-Ghzawi, Shahera Zaitoun, Nawaf Freihat, and Ahmad
Alqudah, "Effect of Pollination on Seed Set of *Origanum syriacum* under
Semiarid Mediterranean Conditions," *Acta Agriculturae Scandinavica, Section B—Soil & Plant Science* 59, no. 3 (2009): 273–78, https://doi
.org/10.1080/09064710802093862.

5 United Nations Development Program and LAR, *Conservation Guidelines for Medicinal and Aromatic Plants in Lebanon* (Lebanese Agricultural
Research Institute, 2013).

6 UNDP and LAR, Conservation Guidelines.

7 Jumana Manna, "Where Nature Ends and Settlements Begin," *E-Flux Journal*, no. 113 (November 2020), https://www.e-flux.com/journal/113/360006/where-nature-ends-and-settlements-begin/.

Chapter 5: Floral Foods

1 Richard Bach, *The Twelve Healers and Other Remedies* (CW Daniel, 1941).

2 Andrzej Górak and Eva Sorensen, *Distillation, Fundamentals and Principles* (Amsterdam: Elsevier Academic, 2014).

3 Mahbubeh Tabatabaeichehr and Hamed Mortazavi, "The Effectiveness of Aromatherapy in the Management of Labor Pain and Anxiety: A Systematic Review," *Ethiopian Journal of Health Sciences* 30, no. 3 (May 1, 2020), https://doi.org/10.4314/ejhs.v30i3.16.

4 Ipek Suntar et al., "An Overview on *Citrus aurantium* L.: Its Functions as Food Ingredient and Therapeutic Agent," *Oxidative Medicine and Cellular Longevity* 2018 (May 2, 2018): 7864269, https://doi.org/10.1155/2018/7864269.

5 Soner Kazaz, Hasan Baydar, and Sabri Erbas, "Variations in Chemical Compositions of *Rosa damascena* Mill. and *Rosa canina* L. Fruits," *Czech Journal of Food Science* 27, no. 3 (2009), https://www.agriculturejournals.cz/publicFiles/5_2009-CJFS.pdf.

6 K. Hüsnü Can Başer, "Rose Mentioned in the Works of Scientists of the Medieval East and Implications in Modern Science," *Natural Product Communications* 12, no. 8 (August 2017): 1934578X1701200, https://doi.org/10.1177/1934578x1701200843.

7 Naheed Mahmood et al., "The Anti-HIV Activity and Mechanisms of Action of Pure Compounds Isolated From *Rosa damascena*," *Biochemical and Biophysical Research Communications* 229, no. 1 (December 1996): 73–79, https://doi.org/10.1006/bbrc.1996.1759.

8 Muhammad Akram et al., "Chemical Constituents, Experimental and Clinical Pharmacology of *Rosa damascena*: A Literature Review," *Journal of Pharmacy and Pharmacology* 72, no. 2 (November 11, 2019): 161–74, https://doi.org/10.1111/jphp.13185.

9 Alachkar et al., "Traditional Medicine in Syria"; Philips, "Lebanese Folk Cures"; Azaizeh et al., "State of the Art of Traditional Arab Herbal Medicine."

10 Juliette De Baïracli-Levy, *Common Herbs for Natural Health* (Woodstock, NY: Ash Tree, 1997).

11 Philips, "Lebanese Folk Cures."

12 Ali A. Samaha et al., "Antihypertensive Indigenous Lebanese Plants: Ethnopharmacology and a Clinical Trial," *Biomolecules* 9, no. 7 (July 2019): 292, https://doi.org/10.3390/biom9070292.

13 Chadi Khatib, Abdulhakim Nattouf, and Mohamad Isam Hasan Agha, "Ethnobotanical Survey of Medicinal Herbs in the Western Region in Syria (Latakia and Tartus)," March 31, 2021, preprint, https://doi.org/10.21203/rs.3.rs-355008/v1.

14 S. N. Kramer, *History Begins at Sumer* (University of Pennsylvania Press, 1988).

15 Hannah Bauman and Monica Silva, "Food as Medicine: Caper (*Capparis spinosa*, Capparaceae)," *HerbalEgram* no. 5 (May 2008), https://www.herbalgram.org/resources/herbalegram/volumes/volume-14/number-5-may/food-as-medicine-caper-capparis-spinosa-capparaceae/food-as-medicine-caper/.

16 Hassan Annaz et al., "Caper (*Capparis spinosa* L.): An Updated Review on Its Phytochemistry, Nutritional Value, Traditional Uses, and Therapeutic Potential," *Frontiers in Pharmacology* 13 (July 22, 2022): 878749, https://doi.org/10.3389/fphar.2022.878749.

17 Bauman and Silva, "Food as Medicine: Caper."

18 "*Capparis spinosa* L. (Capparaceae) Caper, Caperbush (Medicine)," What When How, n.d., https://what-when-how.com/medicine/capparis-spinosa-l-capparaceae-caper-caperbush-medicine/.

19 Hanan Bou Najm, Lebanese, lives in and originates from Aley. Oral teaching through personal communication. August 21, 2022.

20 Mohamed Azzazy and Azza Ezzat, "The Sycamore in Ancient Egypt: Textual, Iconographic, and Archaeopalynological Thoughts," in *Liber Amicorum–Speculum Siderum: Nūt Astrophoros: Papers Presented to Alicia Maravelia*, ed. Nadine Guilhou, Egyptology 17 (Archaeopress, 2017), e-book.

21 Moshe A. Flaishman and U. Aksoy, *Advances in FIG Research and Sustainable Production*, CAB International, 2022.

22 Ephraim Lansky et al, "Ficus Spp. (Fig): Ethnobotany and Potential as Anticancer and Anti-Inflammatory Agents," *Journal of Ethnopharmacology* 119, no. 2 (2008): 195–213, https://doi.org/10.1016/j.jep.2008.06.025.

23 Hanna Bauman and Jayme Bisbano, "Food as Medicine: Fig (*Ficus carica*, Moraceae)," *HerbalEgram* 14, no 8. (August 2016), https://www.herbalgram.org/resources/herbalegram/volumes/volume-14/number-8-august/food-as-medicine-fig/food-as-medicine-fig/.

24 A. R. Gohari, S. Saeidnia, and M. K. Mahmoodabadi, "An Overview on Saffron, Phytochemicals, and Medicinal Properties," *Pharmacognosy Review* 7, no. 13 (2013): 61–66, https://www.ncbi.nlm.nih.gov/pmc/articles/PMC3731881/.

25 Philips, "Lebanese Folk Cures."

26 Maud Grieve, *A Modern Herbal*, vol. 2 (Dover, 1971).

27 Benton Bramwell, "*Arum palaestinum* as a Food-Medicine," *Natural Medicine Journal* 11, no. 2, (February 2019), https://www.naturalmedicine journal.com/journal/2019-02/arum-palaestinum-food-medicine.

Chapter 6: Fruit of the Tree

1 Ann Christensen, "Sumac (Wu Bei Zi / Yan Fu Zi)," White Rabbit Institute of Healing, n.d., https://www.whiterabbitinstituteofhealing.com /herbs/sumac/.

2 Hasan Korkmaz, "Could Sumac Be Effective on COVID-19 Treatment?," *Journal of Medicinal Food* 24, no. 6 (August 18, 2020), https://doi.org /10.1089/jmf.2020.0104.

3 de Baïracli-Levy, Common Herbs for Natural Health.

4 Mark Plotkin, "The Ethnobotany of Wine as Medicine in the Ancient Mediterranean World," *HerbalEgram*, no. 129 (2021): pp. 56–71, https:// www.herbalgram.org/resources/herbalgram/issues/129/table-of -contents/hg129-feat-ethnobotany-wine/.

5 Plotkin, "Ethnobotany of Wine as Medicine."

6 de Baïracli-Levy, *Common Herbs for Natural Health*.

7 S. A. Baydoun et al., "Ethnobotanical and Economic Importance of Wild Plant Species of Jabal Moussa Bioreserve, Lebanon," *Journal of Ecosystem and Ecology* 7 (February 2017): 245, https://doi.org/10.4172/2157-7625 .1000245.

8 Azaizeh et al., "State of the Art of Traditional Arab Herbal Medicine."

9 Elsa Sattout and Hala Zahreddine, *Native Trees of Lebanon and Neighboring Countries: A Guidebook for Professionals and Amateurs* (Notre Dame University Press, 2013).

10 Philips, "Lebanese Folk Cures."

11 Sattout and Zahreddine, *Native Trees of Lebanon.*

12 Philips, "Lebanese Folk Cures"; Alachkar et al., "Traditional Medicine in Syria"; Baydoun et al., "Ethnopharmacological Survey of Medicinal Plants."

13 Zurayk and Talhouk, *Plants and People.*

14 Sabine Beckmann, "Resin and Ritual Purification: Terebinth in Eastern Mediterranean Bronze Age Cult," in *Athanasia: The Earthly, the Celestial and the Underworld in the Mediterranean from the Late Bronze and the Early Iron Age*, ed. N. Stampolidis, A. Kanta, and A. Giannikouri, 27–40 (Iraklion, 2012).

15 Mahbubeh Bozorgi et al., "Five Pistacia Species (*P. vera, P. atlantica, P. terebinthus, P. khinjuk,* and *P. lentiscus*): A Review of Their Traditional Uses, Phytochemistry, and Pharmacology," *Scientific World Journal* 2013: 219815, https://doi.org/10.1155/2013/219815.

16 Zurayk and Talhouk, *Plants and People.*

17 Beckmann, "Resin and Ritual Purification."

18 Berrin Ozçelïk, Ufuk Koca, Durmuş Kaya, and Nazim Sekeroglu, "Evaluation of the in Vitro Bioactivities of Mahaleb Cherry (*Prunus mahaleb* L.)," *Romanian Biotechnological Letters* 17 (2012): 7863–72.

19 Philips, "Lebanese Folk Cures."

Chapter 7: Zeitoon, Tree of Life

1 Dionysiaca Nonnus, trans. William Henry Denham Rouse (1863–1950), Loeb Classical Library, Cambridge, MA, Harvard University Press, 1940, https://topostext.org/work/529#40.391.

2 Omar M. Sabry, "Review: Beneficial Health Effects of Olive Leaves Extracts," *Journal of Natural Sciences Research* 4, no. 19 (2014), https://iiste .org/Journals/index.php/JNSR/article/view/15864/16658.

3 Alachkar et al., "Traditional Medicine in Syria."

4 Anna Boss et al., "Evidence to Support the Anti-Cancer Effect of Olive Leaf Extract and Future Directions," *Nutrients* 8, no. 8 (August 19, 2016): 513, https://doi.org/10.3390/nu8080513.

Chapter 8: Birth Is a Sacred Threshold

1 Hiba Abbani, "Medical Patriarchy: The Case of Legal Midwives in Lebanon," *Kohl* 5, no. 2 (Summer 2019), https://kohljournal.press/legal -midwives-lebanon.

2 Abbani, "Medical Patriarchy."

3 Abbani, "Medical Patriarchy."

4 Aref Abu-Rabia, *Indigenous Medicine among the Bedouin in the Middle East* (2015; repr., Berghahn Books, 2020).

5 Abu-Rabia, *Indigenous Medicine among the Bedouin.*

6 Abu-Rabia.

7 Abu-Rabia.

8 "White Broom," Mahmiyat, n.d., https://www.mahmiyat.ps/en/flora -and-fauna/400.html.

9 Rosina-Fawzia B. Al-Rawi, *Grandmother's Secrets: The Ancient Rituals and Healing Power of Belly Dancing*, trans. Monique Arav (Interlink: 2012).

Chapter 9: Postpartum Protocols for the Nafseh

1 Layla B. Rachid, *Revive Reclaim Restore: Traditional Moroccan Wisdom to Heal the New Mother in the First Forty Days* (Self-Published, 2020), www .laylab.co.uk.

2 Amal Akour, Violet Kasabri, Fatma U. Afifi, and Nailya Bulatova, "The Use of Medicinal Herbs in Gynecological and Pregnancy-Related

Disorders by Jordanian Women: A Review of Folkloric Practice vs. Evidence-Based Pharmacology," *Pharmaceutical Biology* 54, no. 9 (2016): 1901–18, https://doi.org/10.3109/13880209.2015.1113994.

3 Philips, "Lebanese Folk Cures."

4 Asie Shojaii and Mehri Abdollahi Fard, "Review of Pharmacological Properties and Chemical Constituents of *Pimpinella anisum*," *ISRN Pharmaceutics* 2012: 510795, https://doi.org/10.5402/2012/510795.

5 Mohaddese Mahboubi and Mona Mahboubi, "*Pimpinella anisum* and Female Disorders: A Review," *Phytomedicine Plus* 1, no. 3 (August 1, 2021): 100063, https://doi.org/10.1016/j.phyplu.2021.100063.

6 Imane Es-safi et al., "Assessment of Antidepressant-Like, Anxiolytic Effects and Impact on Memory of *Pimpinella anisum* L. Total Extract on Swiss Albino Mice," *Plants* 10, no. 8 (July 30, 2021): 1573, https://doi.org/10.3390/plants10081573.

7 Philips, "Lebanese Folk Cures."

8 Daniel Zohary and Maria Hopf, *Domestication of Plants in the Old World* (Oxford: Oxford University Press, 2000).

9 Bahare Salehi et al., "Nigella Plants: Traditional Uses, Bioactive Phytoconstituents, Preclinical and Clinical Studies," *Frontiers in Pharmacology* 12 (April 26, 2021), https://doi.org/10.3389/fphar.2021.625386.

10 Mousa Al Reza Hadjzadeh et al., "The Effects of Hydroalcoholic Extract of *Nigella sativa* Seeds on Serum Estradiol and Prolactin Levels and Obstetric Criteria due to Hypothyroidism in Rat," *Advanced Biomedical Research* 6, no. 1 (2017): 166, https://doi.org/10.4103/2277-9175.221860; Md. Abdul Hannan et al., "Black Cumin (*Nigella sativa* L.): A Comprehensive Review on Phytochemistry, Health Benefits, Molecular Pharmacology, and Safety," *Nutrients* 13, no. 6 (May 24, 2021): 1784, https://doi.org/10.3390/nu13061784.

11 Amin F. Majdalawieh and Muneera W. Fayyad, "Recent Advances on the Anti-Cancer Properties of *Nigella sativa*, a Widely Used Food Additive," *Journal of Ayurveda and Integrative Medicine* 7, no. 3 (July 1, 2016): 173–80, https://doi.org/10.1016/j.jaim.2016.07.004.

12 Joseph A. Bailey II, "Dignity's Ancient African Origin," Voice, January 3, 2017, https://theievoice.com/dignitys-ancient-african-origin/.

13 Aref Abu-Rabia, "Ethnobotany among Bedouin Tribes in the Middle East," in *Medicinal and Aromatic Plants of the Middle-East*, ed. Z. Yaniv and N. Dudai, Medicinal and Aromatic Plants of the World, vol. 2 (Dordrecht: Springer, 2014), https://doi.org/10.1007/978-94-017-9276-9_3.

14 S. A. Siddiqui et al., "Anti-Depressant Properties of Crocin Molecules in Saffron," *Molecules* 27, no. 7 (2022): 2076, https://doi.org/10.3390/molecules27072076.

15 Baydoun et al., "Ethnopharmacological Survey of Medicinal Plants."

16 Philips, "Lebanese Folk Cures."

17 Fazeleh Moshfegh et al., "*Crocus sativus* (Saffron) Petals Extract and Its Active Ingredient, Anthocyanin Improves Ovarian Dysfunction, Regulation of Inflammatory Genes and Antioxidant Factors in Testosterone-Induced PCOS Mice," *Journal of Ethnopharmacology* 282 (January 2022): 114594, https://doi.org/10.1016/j.jep.2021.114594; Yan Liu, Xuying Qin, and Xiaofen Lu, "Crocin Improves Endometriosis by Inhibiting Cell Proliferation and the Release of Inflammatory Factors," *Biomedicine & Pharmacotherapy* 106 (October 2018): 1678–85, https://doi.org/10.1016/j.biopha.2018.07.108.

18 Philips, "Lebanese Folk Cures."

19 de Baïracli-Levy, Common Herbs for Natural Health.

20 Philips, "Lebanese Folk Cures."

21 Philips, "Lebanese Folk Cures."

22 Abu-Rabia, Indigenous Medicine among the Bedouin.

23 Marcela A. Garcia Probert, "Twigs in the Tawfik Canaan Collection of Palestinian Amulets," in *Amulets and Talismans of the Middle East and North Africa in Context*, ed. Marcela A. Garcia Probert and Petra M. Sijpesteijn, 253–74 (Brill, 2022), https://brill.com/display/book/edcoll/9789004471481/BP000011.xml.

24 Grace M. Crowfoot and Louise Baldensperger, *From Cedar to Hyssop: A Study in the Folklore of Plants in Palestine* (London: Sheldon Press, 1932).

25 Saad Dagher, Palestinian, lives in Bani Zaid, Palestine. Oral teaching, personal communication, September 17, 2022.

26 Abu-Rabia, *Indigenous Medicine among the Bedouin*; Crowfoot and Baldensperger, *From Cedar to Hyssop*.

27 de Baïracli-Levy, *Common Herbs for Natural Health*.

28 Abu-Rabia, *Indigenous Medicine among the Bedouin*.

29 Elizabeth Price, Palestinian Heritage Center, and Sunbula, *Embroidering a Life: Palestinian Women and Embroidery* (Bethlehem, Palestine: Palestinian Heritage Center, 1999); Diana Krumholz McDonald, "The Serpent as Healer: Theriac and Ancient near Eastern Pottery," *Source: Notes in the History of Art* 13, no. 4 (July 1994): 21–27, https://doi.org/10.1086/sou.13.4.23205619.

30 Philips, "Lebanese Folk Cures."

31 Abu-Rabia, "Ethnobotany among Bedouin Tribes."

32 Philips, "Lebanese Folk Cures."

33 Philips, "Lebanese Folk Cures."

34 Khaleeq Raheman, Arshiya Sultana, and Rahman Shafeequr, "*Gossypium herbaceum* Linn: An Ethnopharmacological Review," *Journal of*

Pharmaceutical and Scientific Innovation 1, no. 5 (2012), https://www
.researchgate.net/publication/285331150_Gossypium_Herbaceum_Linn
_An_Ethnopharmacological_review.

35 Claudia Jeanne Ford, "Weed Women, All Night Vigils, and the Secret Life
of Plants: Negotiated Epistemologies of Ethnogynecological Plant Knowledge in American History," (PhD diss., Antioch University, 2015), http://
aura.antioch.edu/etds/221.

36 Cara Terreri, "Black History Month: The Importance of Black Midwives,
Then, Now and Tomorrow," Lamaze International, February 22, 2019,
https://www.lamaze.org/Connecting-the-Dots/black-history-month
-the-importance-of-black-midwives-then-now-and-tomorrow-1.

37 Ford, "Weed Women, All Night Vigils."

38 Karen L. Culpepper, "Cotton Root Bark as Herbal Resistance," *Journal of
the American Herbalists Guild* 15, no. 2 (2017), https://www.american
herbalistsguild.com/sites/americanherbalistsguild.com/files/sample
-articles-pdfs/jahg_autumn_2017_cotton_root_culpepper.pdf.

39 Beshara Doumani, *Rediscovering Palestine: Merchants and Peasants in Jabal
Nablus, 1700–1900* (Berkeley: University Of California Press, 2000), chapters 2 and 3.

40 Doumani, *Rediscovering Palestine*; Aaron G. Jakes and Ahmad Shokr,
"Finding Value in Empire of Cotton," *Critical Historical Studies* 4, no. 1
(March 2017): 107–36, https://doi.org/10.1086/691060.

41 John P. Dunn, "King Cotton, the Khedive, and the American Civil War,"
South Writ Large, 2015, https://southwritlarge.com/articles/king-cotton
-the-khedive-and-the-american-civil-war/.

42 Dunn, "King Cotton, the Khedive."

43 Jakes and Shokr, "Finding Value in Empire of Cotton."

44 Jack Lashendock, "Uninvited Protector: An Assessment of Egyptian Autonomy during British Occupation," Institute for a Greater Europe, September
25, 2021, https://institutegreatereurope.com/uninvited-protector-an
-assessment-of-egyptian-autonomy-during-british-occupationdraft/.

45 Sherine Abdel-Razek, "The Economic Roots of Egypt's 1919 Revolution,"
Ahram Online, March 8, 2019, https://english.ahram.org.eg/NewsContent
P/1/327837/Egypt/The-economic-roots-of-Egypts--Revolution.aspx.

46 Rachid, *Revive Reclaim Restore*.

47 Rachid, *Revive Reclaim Restore*.

48 Tawfīq Kanʿān, "The Decipherment of Arabic Talismans," *Berytus Archae-
ological Studies* 4 (1937): 69–110; 5 (1938): 141–51.

49 Amots Dafni et al., "Ritual Plants of Muslim Graveyards in Northern
Israel," Journal of Ethnobiology and Ethnomedicine 2, no. 1 (September
10, 2006), https://doi.org/10.1186/1746-4269-2-38.

Chapter 10: Raqs Baladi:
A Spiritual and Somatic System of Health

1 Al-Rawi, *Grandmother's Secrets.*
2 Al-Rawi, *Grandmother's Secrets.*
3 Maha Al Musa, *Dance of the Womb: The Essential Guide to Belly Dance for Pregnancy & Birth* (Self-Published, 2008), www.mahaalmusa.com.
4 Brunem Washam, "Polyvagal Herbalism," *Journal of the American Herbalists Guild* 19, no. 1 (2021): 29–36; Brigitte Leeners et al., "Pregnancy Complications in Women with Childhood Sexual Abuse Experiences," *Journal of Psychosomatic Research* 69, no. 5 (November 2010): 503–10, https://doi .org/10.1016/j.jpsychores.2010.04.017.

Chapter 11: Wayfinding

1 Giorgio Milos, "Coffee's Mysterious Origins," *Atlantic*, August 6, 2010, https://www.theatlantic.com/health/archive/2010/08/coffees -mysterious-origins/61054/.
2 Siamak Bidel and Jaakko Tuomilehto, "The Emerging Health Benefits of Coffee with an Emphasis on Type 2 Diabetes and Cardiovascular Disease," *European Endocrinology* 9, no. 2 (2010): 99, https://doi.org/10.17925 /ee.2013.09.02.99.
3 Sana Abbasi, "A Study of the Evil Eye Phenomenon and How It Is Translated into Modern Fashion, Textiles, and Accessories," *Indian Journal of Scientific Research* 13, no. 1 (2017): 137–43, https://www.ijsr.in/upload /108373904925.pdf.
4 Zacharias Kotzé, "The Evil Eye of Sumerian Deities," *Asian and African Studies* 26, no. 1 (2017), https://www.sav.sk/journals/uploads/0530144305 _Kotze_FINAL.pdf.
5 Christiane Gruber, "The Arts of Protection and Healing in Islam: Water Infused with Blessing," Ajam Media Collective, April 30, 2021, https:// ajammc.com/2021/04/30/water-infused-with-blessing/.
6 Kanʿān, "Decipherment of Arabic Talismans."
7 Samuel Thrope, "What Should Be Done with the Magic Bowls of Jewish Babylonia?" Aeon, May 24, 2016, https://aeon.co/essays/what-should -be-done-with-the-magic-bowls-of-jewish-babylonia.
8 Abbasi, "Evil Eye Phenomenon."
9 Karim ReFaey et al., "The Eye of Horus: The Connection between Art, Medicine, and Mythology in Ancient Egypt," *Cureus* 11, no. 5 (May 23, 2019): e4731, https://doi.org/10.7759/cureus.4731.
10 A. Wallis, *The Literature of the Ancient Egyptians* (Good Press, 2020), 71.

11 Issa Tapsoba et al., "Finding out Egyptian Gods' Secret Using Analytical Chemistry: Biomedical Properties of Egyptian Black Makeup Revealed by Amperometry at Single Cells," *Analytical Chemistry* 82, no. 2 (January 15, 2010): 457–60, https://doi.org/10.1021/ac902348g.

12 Tapsoba, "Egyptian Gods' Secret."

13 Kan'ān, "Decipherment of Arabic Talismans."

14 Wafa Ghnaim, Palestinian from Safad, lives in Oregon. Oral teaching from online tatreez workshop with SWANA Ancestral HUB, January 6, 2021.

15 Price, Palestinian Heritage Center, and Sunbula, *Embroidering a Life.*

16 Tala Khanmalek, "Esfand: Warding off the White Gaze," Ancestral HUB, July 2, 2015, https://www.riverroseremembrance.com/ancestralhub -posts/esfand.

17 "Neolithic Site of Çatalhöyük," UNESCO World Heritage Centre, 2012, https://whc.unesco.org/en/list/1405/.

18 Mina Cheraghi Niroumand, Mohammad Hosein Farzaei, and Gholam-reza Amin, "Medicinal Properties of *Peganum harmala* L. In Traditional Iranian Medicine and Modern Phytotherapy: A Review," *Journal of Traditional Chinese Medicine* 35, no. 1 (February 2015): 104–9, https://doi .org/10.1016/s0254-6272(15)30016-9.

19 Maryam Vahabzadeh, Ali Banagozar Mohammadi, and Mohammad Delirrad, "Abortion Induced by *Peganum harmala* Ingestion in a Pregnant Woman: A Case Report and Literature Review," *International Journal of Medical Toxicology and Forensic Medicine* 9, no. 3 (2019): 165–70, https:// doi.org/10.32598/ijmtfm.v9i3.25910.

20 Noam Sienna, "Henna in the Ancient World," Henna by Sienna, n.d., http://www.hennabysienna.com/henna-in-the-ancient-world.html.

21 Catherine Cartwright-Jones, "Ancient Sunrise Henna for Hair Chapter 2, the History of Henna Hair Dye Part 1: The Evolution and Migration of Henna into Cultural Practices," 2018, http://www.hennapage.com /henna/tdlarchive/AS_henna_for_hair/chapters/chap2/Mycenaean _henna.pdf.

22 Noam Sienna, "Eshkol HaKofer: The Hennaed Dove: Henna in Palestinian Culture," Eshkol HaKofer, October 14, 2016, http://eshkolhakofer. blogspot.com/2016/10/the-hennaed-dove-henna-in-palestinian.html.

23 Patricia Kelly Spurles, "Henna for Brides and Gazelles: Ritual, Women's Work and Tourism in Morocco," 2004, https://www.academia.edu /233356/Henna_for_Brides_and_Gazelles_Ritual_Womens_Work _and_Tourism_in_Morocco.

24 Kurt Seligmann, *Magic, Supernaturalism and Religion* (New York: Pantheon, 1975).

25 Laura M. Zucconi, "Medicine and Religion in Ancient Egypt," *Religion Compass* 1, no. 1 (2007).

26 J. Donald Hughes, "Dream Interpretation in Ancient Civilizations," *Dreaming* 10, no. 1 (2000): 7–18, https://doi.org/10.1023/a:1009447606158.

27 Hughes, "Dream Interpretation in Ancient Civilizations."

28 Alexis Pauline Gumbs, "Freedom Dreams and the Nightmare of Policing," INDY Week, June 24, 2020, https://indyweek.com/news/voices/freedom-dreams-nightmare-policing/.

29 Assata Shakur, *Assata: An Autobiography* (London: Zed Books, 2014).

Chapter 12: Holy Archetypes of the Mother and Their Plantcestral Legacies

1 "The Mysterious Origins of the Language of the Maronites," SyriacPress, January 5, 2021, https://syriacpress.com/blog/2021/01/05/the-mysterious-origins-of-the-language-of-the-maronites/; Mousa Ismail et al., "The Influence of Canaanite and Aramaic Languages on the Recent Palestinian Dialects," *International Journal of Academic Research in Business and Social Sciences* 9, no. 2 (February 18, 2019), https://doi.org/10.6007/ijarbss/v9-i2/5523.

2 Correll, "Ma'lula. 2. The Language."

3 Erdman, "Syriac Influences on Arabic"; Wardini, "Aramaic as Attested in Lebanese Place Names."

4 Nassim Nicholas Taleb, "No, Lebanese Is Not a 'Dialect Of' Arabic," Medium, East Med Project: History, Philology, and Genetics, January 2, 2018, https://medium.com/east-med-project-history-philology-and-genetics/no-lebanese-is-not-a-dialect-of-arabic-e95320c164c; Erdman, "Syriac Influences on Arabic"; Ismail et al., "Influence of Canaanite and Aramaic Languages."

5 "Our Lady of Ilige," National Apostolate of Maronites, n.d., https://www.namnews.org/index.php?page=ELIGE#sthash.rd5ZfbsW.dpuf.

6 Reverend Joseph Mahfouz, *"Os Santos Lebaneses Maronitas" / the Lebanese Maronite Saints,* trans. Fr. Leo P. Rothrauff (General Secretariat of Catholic Schools in Lebanon, 2009).

7 Cherifa Selmani, Djamila Chabane, and Nadia Bouguedoura, "Ethnobotanical Survey of *Phoenix dactylifera* L. Pollen Used for the Treatment of Infertility Problems in Algerian Oases," *African Journal of Traditional, Complementary and Alternative Medicine* 14, no. 3 (March 2017): 175-186, https://www.ncbi.nlm.nih.gov/pmc/articles/PMC5412223/; A. Mazlan, "Uses and Benefits of Date Palm That Will Surprise You," RemedyGrove, March 6, 2013, https://remedygrove.com/traditional/The-Various-Uses-of-Date-Palm-Tree.

8 O. Al-Kuran, L. Al-Mehaisen, H. Bawadi, S. Beitawi, and Z. Amarin, "The Effect of Late Pregnancy Consumption of Date Fruit on Labour and Delivery," *Journal of Obstetrics and Gynaecology* 31, no. 1 (2011): 29–31, https://www.ncbi.nlm.nih.gov/pubmed/21280989/.

9 N, Khadem & A., Sharafy & Latifnejad Roudsari, Robab & N., Hammod & Ebrahimzadeh, Samira, "Comparing the Efficacy of Dates and Oxytocin in the Management of Postpartum Hemorrhage," *Shiraz E Medical Journal* 8, no. 2 (2007): 64–71, https://brieflands.com/articles/semj-93686 .html.

10 J. A. Black, G. Cunningham, E. Fluckiger-Hawker, E. Robson, and G. Zólyomi, "The Electronic Text Corpus of Sumerian Literature," 1998–2001, https://etcsl.orinst.ox.ac.uk/edition2/etcslmanual.php.

11 J. Grahn, "Ecology of the Erotic in a Myth of Inanna," *International Journal of Transpersonal Studies* 29, no. 2 (2010): 58–67, http://dx.doi.org/10 .24972/ijts.2010.29.2.58.

12 Lorenzo Nigro and Federica Spagnoli, "Pomegranate (*Punica granatum* L.) from Motyaand Its Deepest Oriental Roots," *Vicino Oriente* 22 (2018): 49–90, http://www.journal-vo.it/Publicazioni/VO%20XXII/VO_XXII _PDF_Autori/VO_XXII_049-090_Nigro-Spagnoli.pdf.

13 A. R. Ruis, "Pomegranate and the Mediation of Balance in Early Medicine," *Gastronomica* 15, no. 1 (2015): 22–33, https://doi.org/10.1525 /gfc.2015.15.1.22.

14 Nigro and Spagnoli, "Pomegranate (*Punica granatum* L.)."

15 Ruis, "Pomegranate and the Mediation."

16 Ruis, "Pomegranate and the Mediation."

17 Ruis, "Pomegranate and the Mediation."

18 Philips, "Lebanese Folk Cures."

19 Avicenna, *Herbs*, Avicenna Aromatic Waters Booklet (Ceredigion, UK: Self Published, 2016).

20 A. Dafni, Z. Yaniv, and D. Palevitch, "Ethnobotanical Survey of Medicinal Plants in Northern Israel," *Journal of Ethnopharmacology* 10, no. 3 (1984): 295–310.

21 Zurayk and Talhouk, *Plants and People*.

22 Dafni et al., "Ritual Plants of Muslim Graveyards."

23 UNDProgram and LAR, *Conservation Guidelines*.

24 Milka Mileva et al., "Rose Flowers—a Delicate Perfume or a Natural Healer?," *Biomolecules* 11, no. 1 (January 19, 2021): 127, https://doi.org /10.3390/biom11010127.

25 Akram et al., "Clinical Pharmacology of *Rosa damascena*."

26 Seyedeh Atefeh Koohpayeh et al., "Effects of *Rosa damascena* (Damask Rose) on Menstruation-Related Pain, Headache, Fatigue, Anxiety, and

Bloating: A Systematic Review and Meta-Analysis of Randomized Controlled Trials," *Journal of Education and Health Promotion* 10 (2021): 272, https://pubmed.ncbi.nlm.nih.gov/34485569/; Qamar Riazi et al., "Effect of *Rosa damascena* on the Severity of Depression and Anxiety in Postmenopausal Women: A Randomized, Double-Blind, Placebo-Controlled Clinical Trial," *Evidence Based Care* 11, no. 1 (April 1, 2021): 35–43, https://doi.org/10.22038/ebcj.2021.57608.2506.

27 Akram et al., "Clinical Pharmacology of *Rosa damascena*"; Tabatabaeichehr and Mortazavi, "Aromatherapy in the Management of Labor Pain and Anxiety."

28 Karim Dolati, Hassan Rakhshandeh, and Mohammad Naser Shafei, "Antidepressant-like Effect of Aqueous Extract from *Rosa damascena* in Mice," *Avicenna Journal of Phytomedicine* 1, no. 2 (September 1, 2011): 91–97, https://doi.org/10.22038/ajp.2011.127.

29 Abu-Rabia, "Ethnobotany among Bedouin Tribes."

30 Abu-Rabia, *Indigenous Medicine among the Bedouin*.

31 IUCN Centre for Mediterranean Cooperation, *A Guide to Medicinal Plants in North Africa* (Malaga, Spain, 2005), https://portals.iucn.org/library/sites/library/files/documents/2005-093.pdf.

32 Krystina Friedlander, "The Flower of Maryam," Baraka Birth, June 18, 2018, https://www.barakabirth.com/blog/2013/11/08/the-flower-of-maryam.

33 metras_global, Instagram, https://www.instagram.com/metras_global/.

34 Azaizeh et al., "State of the Art of Traditional Arab Herbal Medicine."

35 Nejibeddine Assamarkandi, *Pharmacopeia: On the Classification of Causes, 1222 A.D.*, trans. Dr. Georges Tohme (Librairie du Liban Publishers, 1994).

36 Philips, "Lebanese Folk Cures."

37 A. Vogel, "*Cyclamen europaeum* L.," Plant Encyclopaedia, https://www.avogel.com/plant-encyclopaedia/cyclamen_europaeum.php.

Chapter 13: Rouhaniyat: Mystical Traditions and Elemental Healing Lineages

1 "Friends of God: The Origins and Evolution of Sufism in Rural Palestine," Sufi Trails in Palestine, n.d., http://www.sufitrails.ps/etemplate.php?id=35.

2 Nour Farra-Haddad, "Shared Rituals through Ziyārāt in Lebanon: A Typology of Christian and Muslim Practices," in *Performing Religion: Actors, Contexts, and Texts*, ed. Ines Weinrich, 37–51 (Orient-Institut Beirut, Ergon-Verlag GmbH, 2017), https://www.themathesontrust.org/papers/comparativereligion/Farra-Shared_Rituals_through_ziyarat.pdf.

3 Farra-Haddad, "Shared Rituals through Ziyārāt."

4 Farra-Haddad, "Shared Rituals through Ziyārāt."

5 Tawfiq Kanaan, *Mohammedan Saints and Sanctuaries in Palestine* (The Journal of Palestine Oriental Society, 1980).

6 Garcia Probert, "Twigs in the Tawfik Canaan Collection."

7 Rachelle Haddad, "Out of the Valley of Qadisha Modern Syro-Maronite Identity and Its Impact on Relations with the Arab Islamic World" (master's thesis, University of Saint Paul-Ottawa, 2020), https://ruor.uottawa .ca/handle/10393/40497.

8 Paul Daher, *Saint Charbel* (Annaya, Byblos, Lebanon: St. Maron's Monastery, St. Charbel's Tomb, 2012).

9 Daher, *Saint Charbel.*

Chapter 14: Country of the Living: Arz Libnan

1 Vozrozhdenie [Revival] Foundation, "The Cedar: Grandeur in Each Crown," The Ringing Cedars of Russia, 2013, https://www.ringing cedarsofrussia.org/iu/Apr-29-2013/cedar-resin-healing-properties.html.

2 N. K. Sanders, "The Epic of Gilgamesh," Assyrian International News Agency, n.d., http://www.aina.org/books/eog/eog.pdf.

3 Amy L. Balogh, "Mapping the Path to Ecological Reparation: An Ecopsychological Reading of the *Epic of Gilgamesh* and Its Implications for the Study of Religion," *Journal of the American Academy of Religion* 90, no. 1 (February 22, 2022): 86–120, https://doi.org/10.1093/jaarel/lfac020.

4 Balogh, "Mapping the Path."

5 Balogh, "Mapping the Path."

6 S. Khuri, M. R. Shmoury, R. Baalbaki, M. Maunder, and S. N. Talhouk, "Conservation of the *Cedrus libani* Populations in Lebanon: History, Current Status and Experimental Application of Somatic Embryogenesis," *Biodiversity and Conservation* 9, no. 9 (2000): 1261–73, https://doi .org/10.1023/a:1008936104581.

7 Khuri et al., "Conservation of the *Cedrus libani.*"

8 Lara Hajar et al., "*Cedrus libani* (A. Rich) Distribution in Lebanon: Past, Present and Future," *Comptes Rendus Biologies* 333, no. 8 (August 2010): 622–30, https://doi.org/10.1016/j.crvi.2010.05.003.

9 Marcello Rossi, "Can Lebanon's Cedars Outlive Climate Change and a Pesky Insect?," Al Jazeera, April 20, 2019, https://www.aljazeera.com /news/2019/4/20/can-lebanons-cedars-outlive-climate-change-and -a-pesky-insect.

10 Khuri et al., "Conservation of the *Cedrus libani.*"

11 Vozrozhdenie [Revival] Foundation, "The Cedar."

12 Antoine M. Saab et al., "Phytochemical and Pharmacological Properties of Essential Oils from Cedrus Species," *Natural Product Research* 32, no. 12 (July 3, 2017): 1415–27, https://doi.org/10.1080/14786419.2017.1346648.

13 Andree Elias et al., "In Vitro and in Vivo Evaluation of the Anticancer and Anti-Inflammatory Activities of 2-Himachelen-7-Ol Isolated from *Cedrus libani*," *Scientific Reports* 9, no. 1 (September 6, 2019), https://doi.org/10.1038/s41598-019-49374-9.

14 Olivier Bezes, "Lebanon Cedar," Mahmiyat, n.d., https://www.mahmiyat.ps/en/flora-and-fauna/522.html.

15 Philips, "Lebanese Folk Cures."

16 Dana Hourany, "Juniper Trees: A Means to Preserve Lebanon's Environment," Fanack, September 22, 2022, https://fanack.com/lebanon/geography-of-lebanon/juniper-trees-a-means-to-preserve-lebanons-environment/.

17 Ira Spar, "The Gods and Goddesses of Canaan," Department of Ancient Near Eastern Art, Metropolitan Museum of Art, April 2009, https://www.metmuseum.org/toah/hd/cana/hd_cana.htm; Hitti, *Lebanon in History*.

18 Chenoy Ceil, "Epic of Gilgamesh," SSRN Electronic Journal, 2012, https://doi.org/10.2139/ssrn.2030863.

19 F. N. H. Al-Rawi and A. R. George, "Back to the Cedar Forest: The Beginning and End of Tablet v of the Standard Babylonian Epic of Gilgameš," *Journal of Cuneiform Studies* 66, no. 1 (2014): 69, https://doi.org/10.5615/jcunestud.66.2014.0069.

20 Andrew Curry, "Here Are the Ancient Sites ISIS Has Damaged and Destroyed," *National Geographic*, September 1, 2015, https://www.nationalgeographic.com/history/article/150901-isis-destruction-looting-ancient-sites-iraq-syria-archaeology.

Chapter 15: The Ritual of Belonging

1 Marshall et al., "Re-Indigenization Principles for Transforming Biodiversity Conservation."

2 Jake M. Robinson et al., "Traditional Ecological Knowledge in Restoration Ecology: A Call to Listen Deeply, to Engage with, and Respect Indigenous Voices," *Restoration Ecology* 29, no. 4 (May 2021), https://doi.org/10.1111/rec.13381.

3 Nadia S. Santini and Yosune Miquelajauregui, "The Restoration of Degraded Lands by Local Communities and Indigenous Peoples," *Frontiers in Conservation Science* 3 (April 25, 2022), https://doi.org/10.3389/fcosc.2022.873659.

4 Pawlok Dass et al., "Grasslands May Be More Reliable Carbon Sinks than Forests in California," *Environmental Research Letters* 13, no. 7 (July 1, 2018): 074027, https://doi.org/10.1088/1748-9326/aacb39.

Index

About the Author

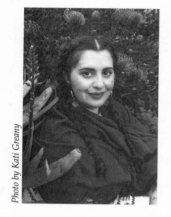

Photo by Kati Greany

Layla K. Feghali lives between her ancestral village on the northern coast of Lebanon and California, where she was born and raised. Her work is about restoring relationships to earth-based ancestral wisdom as an avenue toward eco-cultural stewardship, liberation, and healing collective trauma within diasporic and colonized communities.

Layla is a cultural worker and folk herbalist, inspired greatly by the life-tending imprint of her grandparents. Her practice is anchored by relationships with plants of place and lineage—or the "plantcestors"—as keepers of profound cultural memory, story, and healing that have the capacity to awaken deep reservoirs of embodied and taken knowledge in the soil of our own blood and bones. Her cultural work re-engages community relationships with medicinal plants, ancestral stories, and various folk traditions as a pathway to re-membrance. Layla offers Plantcestral Re-Membrance Circles, a line of herbal medicine, and other culturally rooted educational resources through her practice, River Rose Re-Membrance. She also hosts the Ancestral HUB (formerly SWANA Ancestral HUB), an online space for the cross-pollination of ancestral knowledge across diasporic and home communities from the Crossroads.

Layla has cultivated both formal certifications and colloquial training in various herbal, therapeutic, cultural, and traditional practices for over a decade. Alongside relationships with the plants and village elders of her own lineage lands, her work has been informed in proximity to Ifa and the African diasporas, Curanderismo, and Indigenous elders and communities from across Turtle Island (North America), who have contributed to her understandings in profound generosity throughout her diasporic upbringing. Layla also supports birth-tending processes and is a certified teacher of EmbodyBirth/BellydanceBirth. Her current work builds on a background in movement building, and an MSW, in which she specialized in cultural interventions for addressing trauma and grief.

About North Atlantic Books

North Atlantic Books (NAB) is an independent, nonprofit publisher committed to a bold exploration of the relationships between mind, body, spirit, and nature. Founded in 1974, NAB aims to nurture a holistic view of the arts, sciences, humanities, and healing. To make a donation or to learn more about our books, authors, events, and newsletter, please visit www.northatlanticbooks.com.